T0313874

A Dissociation Model
of BORDERLINE
PERSONALITY
DISORDER

The Norton Series on Interpersonal Neurobiology
Allan N. Schore, PhD, Series Editor
Daniel J. Siegel, MD, Founding Editor

The field of mental health is in a tremendously exciting period of growth and conceptual reorganization. Independent findings from a variety of scientific endeavors are converging in an interdisciplinary view of the mind and mental well-being. An interpersonal neurobiology of human development enables us to understand that the structure and function of the mind and brain are shaped by experiences, especially those involving emotional relationships.

The Norton Series on Interpersonal Neurobiology provides cutting-edge, multidisciplinary views that further our understanding of the complex neurobiology of the human mind. By drawing on a wide range of traditionally independent fields of research—such as neurobiology, genetics, memory, attachment, complex systems, anthropology, and evolutionary psychology—these texts offer mental health professionals a review and synthesis of scientific findings often inaccessible to clinicians. The books advance our understanding of human experience by finding the unity of knowledge, or consilience, that emerges with the translation of findings from numerous domains of study into a common language and conceptual framework. The series integrates the best of modern science with the healing art of psychotherapy.

A Norton Professional Book

A Dissociation Model

of BORDERLINE PERSONALITY DISORDER

Russell Meares, MD

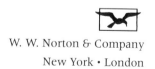

W. W. Norton & Company
New York • London

For information about permission to reproduce selections from this book, write to
Permissions, W. W. Norton & Company, Inc., 500 Fifth Avenue, New York, NY 10110

For information about special discounts for bulk purchases, please contact
W. W. Norton Special Sales at specialsales@wwnorton.com or 800-233-4830

Manufacturing by Quad Graphics, Fairfield
Book design by Charlotte Staub
Production manager: Leeann Graham

Library of Congress Cataloging-in-Publication Data

Meares, Russell.
  A dissociation model of borderline personality disorder / Russell Meares. — 1st ed.
    p. cm. — (Norton series on interpersonal neurobiology)
  "A Norton professional book."
  Includes bibliographical references and index.
  ISBN 978-0-393-70585-0 (hardcover)
  1. Borderline personality disorder. I. Title.
  RC569.5.B67M42 2012
  616.85'852—dc23   2011050072

ISBN: 978-0-393-70585-0

W. W. Norton & Company, Inc., 500 Fifth Avenue, New York, N.Y. 10110
www.wwnorton.com

W. W. Norton & Company Ltd., Castle House, 75/76 Wells Street, London W1T 3QT

1 2 3 4 5 6 7 8 9 0

CONTENTS

Expanded Contents

Acknowledgments

IMPETUS TOWARD THE EVENTUAL PRODUCTION of this book began in the early 1980s when a group of enthusiastic young people at Westmead Hospital, Sydney, mainly trainee psychiatrists and senior psychiatric nurses, set out with me and some senior colleagues to develop a program for the treatment of a condition then deemed intractable—borderline personality disorder (BPD) —which had only recently been given recognition as a formal diagnostic entity. Out of these efforts developed a much larger program. I wish to thank all those who took part in that pioneering effort.

Four people who took part in that initial endeavour were able to continue with the project. They are Joan Haliburn, George Lianos, Michael Williamson, and Janine Stevenson, who together with Philip Graham, Leo van Biene, Tessa Philips, Anthony Korner, and Jai Bains form the faculty of Master of Medicine (Psychotherapy) at Sydney University, which is devoted to training psychiatric and other mental health professionals in the treatment of BPD by means of the Conversational Model. This faculty has contributed, through seminars, conferences and so forth, to the development of an understanding of BPD derived not only from clinical data, but from neurophysiology, linguistics, and developmental data. I have been extremely fortunate in having such people join me in the quest which this book reflects. They have provided me with immense support.

The research program initially focused on outcome studies, the data for which was mainly gathered by Janine Stevenson. I thank her for her tireless efforts. An essential neurophysiological component was added to the research endeavor by the work of Evian Gordon, who developed a scientific group now called the Brain Dynamics Centre, and led by Lea Williams. This group included Dmitri Melkonian, a mathematician and neurophysiologist. His work has been invaluable in providing the data central to the development of the thesis of psychic disintegration, which is the core of this book. I am very grateful to him for the energy, commitment, and creativity he has brought to the program. Lea Williams and her colleagues have provided another essential element in the research background to this book. She has been studying the cerebral processing of emotion, with a particular focus on the effect of trauma. These findings have provided a unique understanding of the unconscious perception of traumatic experience. She and her collaborators in this venture, Richard Bryant and Kim Felmingham, have given me great support and stimulus.

Help in understanding the phenomena of dissociation and the borderline experience has also come from further afield, from Onno van der Hart in Holland and Bessel van der Kolk at Harvard. I have valued greatly the contribution they have made to the development of our work through their visits to Sydney and other venues.

Our third research theme, linguistics, has been led by David Butt. I thank him for the generosity of his contributions to the program and for the intellectual excitement he has brought to our discussions.

I have also been very lucky in my editors. Allan Schore has been an unfailing source of stimulation and encouragement. His important notion of right-brain-to-right-brain relating in mother–infant interaction marries perfectly with the disintegration theory of BPD outlined in this book, and is an essential element of it. Deborah Malmud's patience and guidance was a great support while I struggled with this work.

The person to whom I am most particularly grateful is Michelle Phillips, my secretary and assistant. Without her unflagging efforts, skills, and competence in a number of areas, and her steadiness and good humor, I do not think I could have completed this work.

Finally, I thank my wife Susanne, who has provided the necessary "surround" in which creativity can grow.

A Dissociation Model
of BORDERLINE
PERSONALITY
DISORDER

Chapter 1

INTRODUCTION
THE BORDERLINE EXPERIENCE

FOR MANY YEARS what is now called borderline personality disorder (BPD) was considered an intractable condition. Those who suffered from it were deemed "unanalyzable." In the early 1990s, however, therapies specifically designed to treat BPD began to emerge (Linehan et al., 1991; Stevenson & Meares, 1992). These were followed by a number of reports on the effect of other ways of treating BPD (Bateman & Fonagy, 1999; Clarkin et al, 2007; Giesen-Bloo et al., 2006).

At present, however, as pointed out in a recent authoritative review, "there is no evidence to suggest that one specific form of therapy is more effective than another. Further research is needed on the diagnosis, neurobiology, and treatment of borderline personality disorder" (Leichsenring et al., 2011, p. 74). The next phase in the search for effective treatment of BPD will depend upon an understanding of the central disturbance of BPD, which will provide a logical basis for treatment methods that must be directed toward the core of the condition. This book outlines a proposal concerning such a core. The origins of this proposal are found in the typical experience of those afflicted with BPD.

The heart of BPD is conveyed by our first meeting with Adele, a woman of about 30. Our conversation begins with her struggle to find words, as she tries to say what it is that troubles her most and what brings her to the clinic. She speaks of a barely expressible pain of living, of moving not merely from day to day, but from minute to minute, each step seeming impossible, as if paralyzed by an overwhelming sense of emptiness. Underlying it, and so omnipresent as to be part of normal existence, is fear, which is without shape or object. Some of it involves aloneness. Time by herself is hardly to be endured yet in the presence of others she feels an isolate and unknown. She lives as if on the edge of a void, which those who suffer this illness often call "the black hole." From time to time, she is thrown over, usually by some circumstance of daily life. A suicide attempt might follow. She has attempted suicide many times.

Adele has undergone much intermittent treatment for the past 10 years, receiving heavy medication without substantial benefit. She senses that she is "in the 'too hard' basket," and that nobody is able to help her. She is shifted back and forth between mental health facilities, from one professional to another. In this process, she feels she has never been responded to as a person, never been heard. She believes that this perceived invisibility has contributed to her sense that, as she put it, "I don't know who I am." She says, "When I look in the mirror, I don't see me." With this expression she intimates, albeit indirectly, the main theme of this book: that a disturbance of the experience of self is the core of this painful and frequently disabling condition. The central feature of the disturbance is a feeling of disconnection in several life domains. Psychic life is as if fragmented, and there is an alienation from those in the social environment. There is also an alienation from self, a sense of estrangement evident in the statement "When I look in the mirror, I don't see me."

Adele has a pleasant demeanor. She is attractive in an unobtrusive way, and has a nice smile. Those who know her find it hard to believe that there is anything seriously wrong with her, and they are unaware of her sense of alienation. For the first 15 minutes or so of my meeting with her, this demeanor prevailed. When, however, she began to tell of the abuse she had received, this "front," as she called it, broke, and she began to cry.

Was this front a defense, as she implied by the use of this word, or was it something else as well? Those with BPD frequently behave in a way that belies an underlying state of, for example, anxiety or desolation. Yet, for the most part, this front, which is discontinuous with the individual's emotional state, does not seem like a defense. Rather, it seems to represent yet another aspect of her disconnectedness. There is a "split" between what C.S. Myers, in his observations on the aftereffects of shell shock, called an "apparently normal personality" and another, "emotional personality" (Myers, 1940).

The estrangement implicit in Adele's experience on confronting the mirror is a central feature of the phenomenon of dissociation. The main thesis of this book is that the core disturbance of BPD is an experience of personal existing, or self, which resembles authoritative descriptions of dissociation. The *Diagnostic and Statistical Manual of Mental Disorders—Fourth Edition* (DSM-IV), for example, states that "the essential feature of the Dissociative Disorders is a disruption in the usually integrated functions of consciousness, memory, identity, and perception of the environment" (American Psychiatric Association, 1994, p. 477). No better term than *dissociation* is available for the subtle impairments in sense of self experienced by Adele. It is used in this book with an awareness of its unsatisfactory nature and the fact, as Paul Dell has remarked, that current conceptions of dissociation are often "vague, confusing, even controversial" (Dell, 2009, p. 225).

A main theme evolving throughout this book is that the disconnectedness of personal existence in BPD is underpinned by disconnectedness in brain function, in which areas of neural activity that usually function together fail to do so. The structure of the book resembles an extended hypothesis. An attempt has been made to give a semblance of narrative coherence as the story moves from chapter to chapter. This objective, however, can only be partially achieved when approaching the complexity of BPD. Although I am choosing a particular path through this complexity, I have tried to cover most of the areas of current research in order to provide a general guide to this emergent field of study. The main purpose of this opening chapter is to provide an outline of the structure of the book and an indication of how the story will unfold in the following chapters.

The story of BPD begins with modern medicine, in the second half of the 19th century. It appeared then under the name of "hysteria." The two conditions are not precisely equivalent syndromes since a personality is shaped by the culture in which it arose. The behaviors that excited the interest of the medical system in the 19th century are not the same as those of the present. Nevertheless, the fundamentals are the same. The pioneering efforts of Pierre Janet in elucidating some of these fundamentals through his studies provide a crucial background to the formulation of a *dissociation model of BPD*. He was the original descriptor of dissociation and remains a principal authority on the subject.

Janet proposed a "disintegration" theory of hysteria reflected in multiple shifting and inconstant symptoms (Janet, 1901, p. 505). He saw this disintegration as the manifestation of a failure of "personal synthesis." His ideas and the cultural context in which they arose are introduced in Chapter 2, where a brief history is given of the waning of Janet's influence during the mid-20th century and the concurrent demise of hysteria. It was officially abolished as a diagnostic term in 1980, when the DSM-III also formally recognized the clinical entity of borderline personality disorder.

The 1980 revisions had a major effect. A condition that had been ignored and neglected, like those who suffered from it, became an important subject of research and clinical endeavor.

These efforts revealed a condition that was serious and disabling. Some studies showed a suicide rate of nearly 10% (Kullgren, 1988; Paris et al., 1987; Stone, 1990), a rate similar to that for patients with schizophrenia or major depressive disorders. BPD can be diagnosed in 20% of psychiatric inpatients and 10% of outpatients (Widiger & Frances, 1989). Its prevalence in the general population is similar to schizophrenia: 1.3 or 1.4% (Coid et al., 2009; Lenzenweger et al., 2007; Torgersen et al., 2001). Like that illness, BPD imposes a heavy burden on the health system, as Zanarini, Frankenberg et al. (2001) point out. These patients receive an enormous amount of psychiatric treatment, including more extensive outpatient, inpatient, and pharmacological treatment and all forms of psychosocial therapies, than those with depressive disorder (Bender et al., 2001) or other personality disorders (Zanarini, Frankenberg et al., 2001).

Such data spurred a quest to find suitable means of alleviating the suffering surrounding BPD, which is experienced not only by the patients themselves but by those around them, particularly children (e.g., Hobson et al., 2009).

Adele's experience, however, of being placed in the "'too hard' basket" and of being passed backward and forward between people who seemed unable or unwilling to treat her, attests to the fact that there remains considerable doubt in the minds of most practitioners who do not specialize in personality disorder about how those with BPD should be treated. An aim of this book is to provide an understanding of the symptoms of BPD, largely based on research findings. Some emphasis is given to neurobiological data since experiential and developmental aspects of the condition are considered in more detail in previous volumes (Meares, 2000, 2005).

A first step in establishing an understanding of a condition is an awareness of what is fundamental to it, the nature of its core disturbance. This core disturbance is suggested by Adele's story. Her most salient symptoms were emptiness, fear of being alone, and an ill-developed sense of self. This triad, which can be called the "self-triad," is sometimes confused with depression (Silk, 2011), since it is associated with a painful affect that is difficult to describe precisely. In Chapter 3, a study is described that gives support to the idea that this constellation of features, which are three of the nine diagnostic criteria for BPD catalogued in the DSM-IV, is the core of BPD, whose primary characteristic is "painful incoherence" (Wilkinson-Ryan & Westen, 2000).

Incoherence refers to a lack of cohesion of self. In order to conduct a scientific study of this state, it is necessary to start with what is meant by the term *self*. Chapter 4 is devoted to this subject. Hughlings Jackson's hierarchial model of self, supported by William James's descriptions, forms the mainstay of the definition.

Jackson's writings are condensed and somewhat gnomic. They were not properly understood by his peers, who nevertheless considered him a near-genius. His neural model of self was the first of its kind. Nothing comparable had emerged until the proposals of Damasio (1996), with which it is broadly compatible. Jackson considered "self"—which is identified by, but not the same as, the capacity for an awareness of inner events—to be a special form of consciousness that appeared late in evolution and is likely to be unique to the human primate. He understood its emergence in terms of the brain, the organization of which has been laid down by evolutionary history. He believed that the new kind of consciousness, which is characterized by an enhanced voluntary control over mental life, does not depend upon the evolution of new structures or new forms of neural tissue. Rather, the elaboration of existing structures, notably the prefrontal cortex, allows a greater coordination between areas of brain activity than was previously possible. "Self" is the outcome of such enhanced coordination.

Jackson's ideas provide a way of testing the hypotheses concerning the "painful incoherence" at the heart of BPD. They suggest that underpinning this relative lack of cohesion in the experience of self is a "concomitant" (to use Jackson's word) disconnectedness among systems of brain function. Chapter 5 reports on a study that tests the hypothesis that this disconnectedness is found in the brains of those with BPD. The method involved a novel technique for the analyses of the effect of a single stimulus on the electrical patterns evoked in the brain (Melkonian, Blumenthal, & Meares, 2003; Melkonian, Gordon, & Bahramali, 2001). The event-related potential (ERP) has a major component appearing about 300 milliseconds after the presentation of the stimulus. This component, the P3, reflects major attentional processing. It is a large monophasic wave, produced by the coordination of two main generators, resulting in a single output. The two generators are reflected in two aspects of P3, called *P3a* and *P3b*. In patients with BPD these aspects are no longer coordinated, as the hypothesis predicted.

A second study comparing patients with PTSD who dissociate and those who do not gave support to the idea that the central disturbance in BPD is dissociative. The dissociative patients with PTSD showed the same forms of disturbance in P3 as those with BPD.

Although the capacity to introspect identifies the self, it does not give us a way of conceiving the fragmentation that characterizes, in varying degrees, the psychic life of those with BPD. This conception, however, is given by Jackson's more complete definition of self. He called awareness of an event, inner or outer, *object consciousness*. This object consciousness is always linked to subject consciousness, which is a continuous state, an omnipresent background, somewhat analogous to the Jamesian "stream." Object consciousness "comes out of" subject consciousness (Jackson, 1958, p. 93), which is symbolized by the pronoun *I*. This symbolization makes the Jacksonian concept of self complex, strange, and not easily grasped. Nevertheless, the notion of subject consciousness provides a means of figuratively conceiving the "broken-upness" of the experience of those with BPD. It is this "half" (p. 93) of self in which the disconnectedness is to be found.

This idea could have had no scientific value until recently because there were no means of testing it. In the last decade, however, a new area of inquiry has opened up concerning the "default mode network." This system of neurocircuitry is active during periods when object consciousness is absent, when the individual is not focused on any particular task or event. It seems to be the neural basis of the subject consciousness that Jackson implied was the matrix of mind. This neurocircuitry, together with the possibility that failures in its neurocircuitry may be the basis of BPD, is discussed in Chapter 6.

The disconnectedness implied in the term *painful incoherence* is being called, in this book, *dissociation*. It is necessary, therefore, to know what the term *dissociation* means since, to quote Paul Dell again, dissociation remains "an elusive concept . . . vague, confusing, and even controversial" (Dell, 2009, p. 225), despite much recent investigation. An extended discussion is given to the subject in Chapter 7. In essence, dissociation is seen to have two main forms, "primary" and "secondary," which correspond with the respective, and apparently contradictory, conceptions of Janet and Freud. The two theorists were right in different ways.

The basic form of dissociation, "primary dissociation," is understood in terms of a hierarchy of consciousness, a conception necessary to Janet's fundamental descriptions of a phenomenon to which he gave no overarching name but, instead, applied descriptive terms to its several aspects.

Dissociation is not merely a state of mind. It is also part of a larger system that includes a form of relatedness. A linguistic study of this important but neglected aspect of dissociation is described in Chapter 8. It focuses on an overt dissociative episode occurring during a therapeutic session with a patient with BPD, whose permission has been given for this transcript to be pub-

lished. Analyses of this text show that dissociation is characterized not only by a disconnection between elements of thought
that usually go together but also by connection between areas
of experience that are usually separated, such as past–present,
inner–outer, subject–object. This state of the simultaneous, and
paradoxical, experience of disconnection and fusion is mirrored
by a strange form of relatedness encountered in working with
those with BPD, of coexisting fusion and alienation.

The fusion and disconnection described in Chapter 8 is a state
brought on by the remembrance of traumatic past events. The
repeated triggering of such memories by the circumstances of everyday life overthrows a frail sense of self and impedes the progress of maturation. Identification of these states and fostering
their integration into the larger consciousness of self are principal therapeutic aspects of working with those with BPD.

Unlike the case described in Chapter 8, traumatic memory frequently produces an unconscious effect. The subject is unaware
that he or she is in the grip of memory. In such circumstances,
the individual plays out a role decreed by a "script" (Meares,
1998) derived from the original traumatic situation, which is
typically generic. The memory system represents an accumulation of traumata of similar kind, such as emotional abuse, going
on day after day. With the triggering of this system, whether by
external events that resemble certain kinds of its features or by
internal associations, the relational configuration is activated.
The attributes of self and other given by the script now become
present reality. Aspects of these unconscious relational configu-
rations are briefly discussed in Chapter 9.

Two of these reflections of unconscious traumatic relatedness
were evident in the story told by Adele. The first was the effect of
the "expectational field," in which the individual's script-driven
expectations of the other are often fulfilled—a consequence, it is
suggested, of the other's subliminal detection of the subject's
bodily signs (Meares, 2005, pp. 114–125). Adele's experience of

being placed in the "'too hard' basket" was very like her experience of early life. Her parents had split when she was a baby. She was an impediment in both their lives, and so was thrown back and forth between them.

Adele described spontaneously a second kind of traumatic relatedness. There were times when she became, suddenly and in a way that frightened her, aggressive, loud, and abusive—quite unlike her usual self. Although she was not actually violent during these episodes, violence was implicit in her tone. She seemed out of control. Afterward, she would worry about the effect of this tone on her children. In these episodes, the roles of the traumatic script are switched and, in a "reversal" (Meares, 1993a, pp. 87–100; 1993b, 2005, pp. 104–113), she plays the abusive father, as if inhabited by him. Patients, in describing this experience, talk of being demonized, of having something alien, an "it," active within them.

We might understand reversals, at least in a figurative way, as aspects of the disintegration of self. In this unintegrated state these aspects are as if "loose," able to swing between the poles of the traumatic script. A consequence of the unintegrated nature of traumatic memory systems is speculatively considered in Chapter 10.

In a patient with BPD, there is likely to be a number of traumatic memory systems derived from different caregivers, and from individual caregivers in different traumatic modes: for example, controlling/intrusive, abandoning/nonresponsive, fearful/fear inducing. Furthermore, the same kind of traumatic situation may have different effects on the same child at different ages. For example, when an alcoholic single mother who is prone to violence when drunk flings a child down a staircase on one occasion, her child may when very young have attacks of terror in which he seems to be frozen. Somewhat older, he is conflicted between attachment longings and fear of his mother. His behavior shows this confusion in "disorganized attachment." Somewhat older, he develops an unexpected way of behaving; he shows a precocious maturity and takes on the role of caregiver to his mother. All these various traumatic systems are as if sequestered from each other and from the consciousness of self. In Chapter 9 it is suggested that the Axis I disorders that are diagnosed during the lifetime of those with BPD are not generally comorbid in the usual sense. Rather, they are part of the same systematic disturbance, with each kind of Axis I illness having its basis in a particular traumatic memory system.

The individual suffering from BPD switches from state to state, dependent upon his or her relationship with the environment. Each of these states involves not only different forms of relatedness but also differences in emotional expression. There is evidence in these states of emotional dysregulation, exemplified by aspects of Adele's story. Affect and impulse dysregulation are sometimes seen as the core disturbance of BPD. In this book, they are conceived as secondary to disintegration of the self, which involves, as predicted by the Jacksonian model, a loss of higher-order inhibitory capacities. This loss is demonstrated by an abnormally large P3a characteristic in patients with BPD and in those who dissociate (Chapter 5). The issue of affective instability in BPD is discussed in Chapter 11. It is a subject of considerable complexity involving more than a disturbance in the inhibitory capacity alone.

The disturbance in the inhibitory systems is likely to be involved in the persisting and painful affective state described by Adele. It is as if her central nervous system is unable to modify the intensity of this experience. Actual pain is also a feature of the BPD syndrome. Although central to Briquet's (1859) classical description of hysteria, it finds no place in the DSM-IV list of BPD criteria. This kind of somatization is discussed in Chapter 12. The pain processing system overlaps with, and is part of, the medial neurocircuitry involved in emotional processing.

Pain is not the only kind of somatization experienced by those with BPD. Other forms of somatization include the so-called conversion disorders (Chapter 7) and a somewhat neglected category of phenomena that Janet called "accidents." As discussed in Chapter 13, these are representations of fragments of trauma that are as if imprinted upon the skin. They are understood as particular aspects of neural disconnectedness in BPD. In BPD, the autonomic system acts apparently independently of other systems, including of the orbitofrontal cortex, which Damasio (1996) has identified as necessary to the self system. Moreover, the parasympathetic and sympathetic components of the autonomic nervous system do not properly coordinate. The autonomic system acts as a primitive representing mechanism through control of the vascular bed of the skin.

Chapter 14 deals with another rather neglected aspect of the borderline syndrome: the paranoid ideation and occasional delusion formation that compose the ninth diagnostic criterion, together with dissociation, included in the DSM-IV (American Psychiatric Association, 1994). This chapter follows the implication of this pairing by arguing for a disintegrative, or dissociative, basis for delusion formation in BPD. The story of Lord Byron is given as an example of the paranoid stance in BPD. He understood the borderline experience, writing on one occasion to his future wife of the painful experience of the void, the characteristic experience of BPD, and the ways that are used to avoid it. He wrote of "sensation—to feel that we exist—even though in pain —it is this 'craving void' which drives us to Gaming—to Battle— to travel" (Lord Byron, letter, Sept. 6, 1813). For Adele, the 'craving void' drove her to food.

Chapter 15 returns to the study reported in Chapter 5 and enlarges on the finding regarding the pathologically large amplitude of P3a, which is suggested as a biological marker of self, and thus of BPD—or, more particularly, of dissociation. Data are presented showing that the abnormality of P3a is right-hemispheric. The fact that the right hemisphere is concerned with the shaping of sensory impressions and the discernment of patterns gives rise to the possibility that the basis of the "painful incoherence" at the core of BPD is a deficiency in the right-hemispheric function of creating coherence. This idea leads to the topic of Chapter 16: the proposal that a central aspect of the treatment of BPD should foster the emergence of right-hemispheric function. A particular kind of conversation is required that is reminiscent of the right-brain to right-brain engagement between mother and child postulated by Allan Schore (2001, 2002, 2003). I am calling this kind of conversation "analogical relatedness." The treatment implications of a dissociation model of BPD, however, are not touched upon in any detail, since they are the subject of a parallel volume (Meares et al., 2012 in press).

Chapter 2

FROM HYSTERIA TO BORDERLINE
A Brief History

THE MAIN MENTAL ILLNESSES were all described and named before the First World War. Borderline personality disorder emerged half a century later, as if it were a new disease. It had, however, a long history, under a different name, stretching back to the origins of Western medicine. BPD's predecessor was the syndrome of "hysteria." The story of this illness, at least during the modern period when mental illness became the subject of scientific inquiry, is highly relevant to the main thesis of this book and to an understanding of the syndrome currently called *borderline*.

HYSTERIA AND CULTURE

In her history of hysteria Ilza Veith remarks that "whenever it appears it takes on the colours of the ambient culture and mores" (1965, p. 1). Conceptions of the disorder mirrored periods of relative cultural enlightenment and also times of darkness, superstition, religious dogmatism, and cruelty. The apparent disappearance of hysteria during the first part of the 20th century can be seen as a reflection of the zeitgeist of the West during much of that century. In its brief history, the shifting attitudes toward BPD, as was the case for hysteria, reflect the character of an era.

Hysteria and BPD, although fundamentally the same, do not appear to be precisely equivalent syndromes. The most salient difference is in the form of presentation. Janine Stevenson and her colleagues (2011) point out that depression is the most common presentation for BPD. Those with hysteria attracted the attention of the medical community by more spectacular means, with bodily symptoms currently termed *conversion disorders* but which are better called *somatoform dissociation* (Nijenhuis, 2000; Nijenhuis et al., 1999; Van der Hart et al., 2006a). Cultural differences explain these differing forms of presentation. In the current era, dominated by biological psychiatry, there is a heavy emphasis on depression and its pharmacotherapy. The heyday of hysteria was concurrent with a widespread interest in exotic phenomena such as séances and automatic writing. Influential figures such as William James and W. B. Yeats involved themselves in such activities.

The modern scientific approach to hysteria may be considered to begin with Briquet's *Traité clinique et thérapeutique de l'hystérie*, published in 1859, the same year as Darwin's *Origin of Species*, which launched the modern era of biological science. Briquet's monograph is a dispassionate investigation, performed without preconceptions. It catalogues the details and symptoms of 430 patients diagnosed with hysteria, finding that they present with an enormous range of bodily disorders. Briquet concluded, against the traditional theory of its sexual origin, "that hysteria was caused by the effect of violent emotions, protracted sorrows, family conflicts, and frustrated love, upon predisposed and hypersensitive persons" (Ellenberger, 1970, p. 142). This conclusion is not unlike the ideas concerning the traumatic origins of BPD that followed evidence of the abusive developmental background of most of these patients (Herman et al., 1989; Ludolph et al., 1990; Zanarini et al., 1989).

15

CHARCOT AND HYSTERIA AS A SUBJECT OF SCIENTIFIC INQUIRY

The main studies on the nature of hysteria occurred later in the 19th century during a period of the greatest scientific creativity in the history of humanity. In the half century or so before the outbreak of World War I, the intellectual foundations of the technological revolution of the 20th century were laid down in their first forms or as patents. The germinal center, out of which came the observations forming a new understanding of hysteria, was Paris, which Matthew Arnold (1864) saw as the capital of a new aliveness in European culture. At the ancient hospital of Salpêtrière the charismatic figure of Jean-Martin Charcot (1825–1893), one of the great neurologists of Europe, ruled over a pioneering enterprise: the investigation of mental states for which there were no known scientific bases.

Charcot lived like a prince and treated the royal houses of Europe. His patrician and autocratic style earned him the title "Napoleon of the Neuroses." The fame of Charcot's theatrical lectures attracted students from afar. They included, in 1885–86, a young Viennese neurologist, Sigmund Freud, then 29 years old.

Some months before Freud arrived at Salpêtrière in October, 1885, Charcot made the following observation:

> An idea, a coherent group of associated ideas settle themselves in the mind in the fashion of parasites, remaining isolated from the rest of the mind and expressing themselves outwardly through corresponding motor phenomena. . . . The group of suggested ideas finds itself isolated and cut off from the control of that large collection of personal ideas accumulated and organized from a long time, which constitutes consciousness proper, that is the Ego. (as cited in Ellenberger, 1970, p. 149)

This parasitic form of psychic life operates, in large part, unconsciously. Writing in later life Freud noted the great effect of

Charcot's demonstrations upon him: "I received the profoundest impression of the possibility that there would be powerful mental processes which nevertheless remained hidden from the consciousness of men" (Freud, 1925, p. 17).

Charcot's observation is fundamental. He describes, in its first form, the unconscious traumatic memory system that is repetitively triggered in BPD, intruding upon, even taking over, what he called "consciousness proper."

Charcot's reputation in the field of neurology gave weight to his findings in the study of hysteria, a subject generally regarded as beyond the pale of respectable inquiry. One of his most important and influential discoveries was that certain paralyses following trauma have a psychological origin and are not the result of a lesion in the nervous system. Moreover, he showed that these paralyses could be reproduced by means of hypnotism, thereby suggesting that both phenomena arise in the basis of the same mechanism (Ellenberger, 1970, p. 91). This implication of his finding gains support from recent neuroimaging studies of "conversion disorders" (Marshall et al., 1997).

JANET AND THE THEORY OF DÉSAGRÉGATION PSYCHOLOGIQUE

Charcot's studies reflected the prevailing mood of the time, which was humanistic. It gave value to the ordinary sense of personal existing, that state of mind Winnicott called "going-on-being" (Winnicott, 1971). The essence of this mood was reflected in the work of the two great philosophers of this brief era: Henri Bergson and William James (Honderich, 2005, p. 999). Their ideas were remarkably similar. In Paris, Bergson was enormously influential and a hugely popular lecturer. Photographs show people craning their necks, standing on tiptoe, and using scaling ladders to climb to the window ledges, where they stood to listen outside the lecture hall of the Collège de France (Richardson, 2007, p. 426). For both of these men, the primary datum of philosophy is human experience, which, rather than logic, is the means toward reality and truth. They saw the fundamental unit of reality as the experience of the present moment in which there is, paradoxically, a sense of the movement of time, which Bergson called *"durée."*

As a student Bergson had a colleague at the École Normale Supérieure who became a philosopher but who then trained as a psychiatrist in order to understand better the nature of personal existence. His name was Pierre Janet. Bergson later defended Janet's candidacy for the Collége de France at the assembly of its professors (Ellenberger, 1970, p. 354). Janet attracted the attention of Charcot when the latter chaired a meeting in 1885 at which some of Janet's early data on unconscious mental processing in hysteria and hypnosis were presented. These findings were the bases of Janet's *L'automatisme Psychologique* (*Psychological Automatism*, 1889), which was immediately hailed as "a classic of the psychological sciences" (Ellenberger, 1970, p. 361).

Janet came to Salpêtrière in 1890, where Charcot created for him a laboratory of experimental psychology. The fundamental ideas upon which Janet's approach to mental illness was built were very like those of Bergson and James. For Janet, an understanding of the essential experience of human existing is necessary to the task of formulating the origins of mental illness. Existence, he believed, is found in the present moment. He called it the *"fonction du réel"* (function of the real), a concept very like Bergson's *"attention de la vie"* (attention to life; Ellenberger, 1970, p. 354). The moment was conceived according to a hierarchy of consciousness, a notion that is at the heart of the approach to BPD developed in this book. A full sense of the present moment depends upon the creation of a state of mind in a process Janet called *"présentification."* The process is complex, involving a synthesis of the multiplicities of awareness, both inner and outer, with tendencies to action. It consists of "making present a state of mind and a group of phenomena" (Ellenberger, 1970, p. 376).

The function of the real is the "most difficult mental operation, since it is the one which disappears first and most frequently" (Ellenberger, 1970, p. 376). Loss of *présentification* results in the individual's functioning at a lower level on a hierarchy of consciousness, which Janet conceived in terms of multiple "tendencies," or propensities, for action. This hierarchical descent is essentially the state of dissociation, the centerpiece of Janet's theory of hysteria. In this state, the sense of self shrinks, and what is present in consciousness is diminished, made up of a more limited grouping of phenomena. This grouping is relatively lacking in unity.

Predecessors of Janet who formulated a conception of mind that was hierarchical included Maine de Biran and Moreau de Tours. Maine de Biran (1766–1824), author of *Essays on the Fundamentals of Psychology* (1812), saw self as developing through three phases, the earliest being *vie animale*, which was largely sensory, then the *vie humaine*, and finally *vie de l'esprit*. His ideas influenced Moreau de Tours (1845/1973) who, Ellenberger believes (1970, p. 290), was probably the first person to use the concepts of evolution and regression to understand the genesis of mental illness. In turn, Moreau's notion of psychological dissolution influenced Janet, who always insisted that his theory of *désagrégation psychologiques* was derived from Moreau. Janet's most significant predecessor, however, was John Hughlings Jackson (1835–1911), whose hierarchical concept of self, as MacLeod (1993) has pointed out, influenced Putnam (1898), among others, to understand the psychological consequences of trauma as a regression down a hierarchy of mental function.

As it was for James and Bergson, "the nature of the synthetic unity of consciousness" (James, 1895/1968, p. 152) was an issue of central importance for Janet. He believed that we begin life with the elements of consciousness relatively disconnected. Maturation is the process of integration. This process, however, is never completed but a persisting goal toward which the personality has a "tendency" (Seigel, 2005, pp. 514–515).

Janet's *The Mental State of Hystericals* appeared, with a recommendation from Charcot, in 1893. It is the distillation of meticulous observations of 120 patients. Janet's principal conclusion was that the basic deficit in hysteria is a disconnection of personal synthesis. Those afflicted with the disorder, he said, show "a want of mental unity" (Janet, 1901, p. 222). This was the explanation, he believed, of the basic instability of the psychic function of these patients. "The character is mobile and contradictory," he wrote. "The patient does not remain long in one and the same moral condition. She passes every moment from affection to indifference, from gladness to sadness, from hope to despair" (Janet, 1901, p. 222). This description is remarkably like the affective instability and dysregulation that are cardinal features of borderline personality disorder. In this book, a main thesis is that a fragmentation of self underlies the characteristic instability in BPD patients, and this fragmentation affects not only mood but also relating.

FREUD AND JANET

Breuer and Freud published their *Studies in Hysteria* in 1895, soon after Janet's *The Mental State of Hystericals*. Their text included five case histories. Their main conclusion resembled, in some respects, that of Janet. They wrote that "the splitting of consciousness, so striking in the familiar classical cases of double consciousness, exists rudimentarily in every hysteria, and that the tendency to this dissociation, and with it the appearance of abnormal states of consciousness which we comprise as 'hypnoid,' is the basic phenomenon of this neurosis" (Breuer & Freud, 1895, p. 8). Their understanding, however, of the basis of "this dissociation" contradicted Janet's conceptualization. Their objection to Janet's viewpoint is most clearly stated in a chapter written by Breuer, which amplified Freud's position stated earlier in the book (p. 75). Breuer wrote that "Janet's view, that the disposition to hysteria is based on psychic weakness, is untenable" (p. 179). "We would like to formulate our own view as follows. The splitting of consciousness does not occur because the patients are weak-minded, but the patients seem weak-minded because their psychic activity is divided" (p. 172).

Breuer and Freud (1895) believed that Janet considered this weakness to be a consequence of "hereditary degeneration" (p. 76). I could not find this term in my reading of Janet's (1901) *Mental State of Hystericals*. Rather, he suggested that the diminution of personal synthesis at the core of hysteria is equivalent to a failure of maturation: "This defect of synthesis, this instability, this naïve selfishness, accompanied by jealousy and anger, are found exactly in a state which is in no wise sickly, namely, in childhood" (p. 221). In a later edition of his 1893 work he stated that in these cases it seemed that development at some point "has definitively stopped" (Janet, 1911, p. 532), implying a developmental rather than a congenital disturbance.

Janet's position was that "pathological heredity" had a major role in the genesis of hysteria "as in all other mental maladies" (Janet, 1901, p. 526). "Hereditary influences" result in "a mind predisposed" (p. 527) to be affected by a range of environmental events that "weaken the organism" (p. 526), thus leading to the disturbance of "personal synthesis." This viewpoint resembles an emergent understanding of BPD at the present time.

The environmental events Janet believed to be pathogenic included debilitating diseases and intoxications. He also noted that "certain organic diseases of the nervous system" could act as "provocative agents." This observation has also been made in modern times, most notably by Whitlock (1967), who found that a large number of patients diagnosed with hysteria in a hospital setting had histories suggestive of cerebral pathology.

Janet emphasized, particularly in later publications, the pathogenic effect of "shocks" and "painful emotions, and especially a succession of that sort of emotion the effects of which are cumulative" (Janet, 1901, p. 526). Each shock has the effect of "exhaustion." In a later work, explaining his difference from Freud, he wrote that "dissociation, this migration of certain psychological phenomena into a special group, seemed to me connected with the exhaustion brought on by various causes, and in particular by emotion" (Janet, 1924, p. 40). He rejected the role of "inhibition" in creating the characteristic pathology of the syndrome (Janet, 1901, p. 26), whereas an inhibitory mechanism, repression, was central to the Freudian argument.

The joust between Janet and Freud is considered again in Chapter 7. Recent neurophysiological data suggest that both viewpoints were right, in different ways.

At the beginning of the 20th century, Janet and Freud were seen by others, and by themselves, as rivals, contenders for the dominant position Charcot had occupied. They had both achieved an international reputation. When the American Psychopathological Association was founded in 1910, five honorary members from Europe were nominated: Janet, Freud, Jung, Forel, and Claparède. At first Janet seemed the most likely to found a major school. Although 3 years younger than Freud, he had gained the patronage of Charcot and had produced an impressive list of original works before Freud's run had properly begun. However, as the First World War approached, the tide began to turn toward Freud. During this period the main ideas dominating the intellectual life of the West changed quite suddenly and drastically; 1913 was the watershed year.

NINETEEN THIRTEEN:
THE BEHAVIORIST-POSITIVIST REVOLUTION

Nineteen thirteen was the year of Watson's behaviorist manifesto, of Ford's production line in which human functioned as part of a machine, of the first forms of an architecture in which cultural memory was abolished, and of an art in which the human was depicted as a machine. This new imagery was apparent most famously in the works of Duchamp and Picabia, who were stars of the Armory Show in New York in 1913, one of the most important and influential art exhibitions held in the United States in the 20th century.

Emblematic of the change in the sphere of philosophy was the split between two authors of *Principia Mathematica* (1910–1913), A. N. Whitehead and Bertrand Russell, the former representing holistic views of reality, whereas the latter's approach, which now became dominant, was logical and analytic. Believing it to be more logical, Russell retranslated the *cogito* as "It thinks in me" (Russell, 1921). The *it* in this sentence encapsulates the impersonal, even mechanistic, conceptions of human existing which came into vogue following World War I. Curiously resonant with traumatic consequences of the war, Russell's conception, in separating thought "it" from "me," depicted a traumatic state in which memory of the abusive other recurs as a traumatic experience alien to self. The subject talks of the "it" within him or her.

This new zeitgeist was at odds with the cast of mind evident in the works of James and Bergson, which were now regarded as anachronisms. Concepts of self as a peculiarly human form of reflective consciousness, or "inner life," as William James viewed it, were swept aside by more positivist and behaviorist strands of psychological science. This approach culminated in the philosophical attitude exemplified by Gilbert Ryle's work of 1949, *The Concept of Mind*. Ryle sought to deride the notion of an interior life and the metaphor of "the mind's eye." Although the humanistic approach of those such as James was kept alive by some more existentially inclined philosophers and psychiatrists, the viewpoint summed up by Ryle was paramount for more than a generation. This cultural shift was reflected also in the psychological sciences.

In psychology, the positivist influence led to gross restrictions in conceptualization. Phenomena central to ordinary experience were disregarded. They included, for example, the most human of the various forms of memory, currently called *episodic* and *autobiographical*. Memory now became only that function which psychologists could measure.

The state of the psychological sciences in the years between the wars reflected changes in all walks of life and forms of human expression. Totalizing systems came to dominate the intellectual life of Europe. A relative loss of humanistic values was reflected not only in a darkening political landscape but also in the treatment of the mentally ill. Asylum buildings of the late 19th century, which had seemed then to symbolize an enlightened approach, had become places of degradation, even horror. Of particular relevance to the ideas in this book was the treatment of those who had been psychologically traumatized. The effect of trauma was a main theme in Janet's theorizing. Janet described a total of 591 patients and reported a traumatic origin of the psychopathology in 257 (Crocq & De Verbizier, 1989).

During World War I the consequences of psychological trauma were clearly evident and termed *shell shock*. Influential contributors to an understanding and treatment of this condition were W. H. R. Rivers, C. S. Myers, and William McDougall. These men were friends before the war. In 1899 they had taken part in a celebrated ethological expedition to Torres Strait. After the war their influence faded. Shell shock was understood as a form of hysteria—not a "real" illness. The effects of frontline experience began to be minimized, or even denied, in administrative and official circles, leading to the publicly expressed disgust of Rivers's most famous patient, the poet Siegfried Sassoon, who handed back to the nation the medals he had been awarded for valor during conflict.

In the years that followed, an awareness of the pathogenic significance of trauma was, to a large extent, lost to psychiatry. In addition, as William McDougall wrote as professor of psychology, first at Harvard and then at Duke University, the "functional nervous diseases fell between . . . organic neurologists and organic psychiatrists . . . in a despised no-man's land, neglected by all, with a few distinguished exceptions, such as Dr Morton Prince in this country and Dr Pierre Janet in France" (McDougall, 1926, p. 34).

During this period, interest in understanding hysteria waned. Moreover, its incidence seemed to decline. Authorities pondered the reasons for its demise, some suggesting that the disorder was simply an iatrogenic artefact; that these patients had enjoyed, for example, being the stars of Charcot's spectacular demonstrations. Suggestion, however, was an insufficient explanation for the intractable condition of Janet's "sad, despairing" patients (Janet, 1901, p. 213).

By the 1950s, Janet had become merely a footnote in psychiatric textbooks, his main theory of the origin of hysteria forgotten and his diagnostic approach no longer used. The resulting diagnostic disarray led to the death knell of the term *hysteria*, sounded by Eliot Slater (1965). In an influential paper he reported on a follow-up of patients given the diagnosis of hysteria at the National Hospital of Neurological Diseases in London. He found that after 10 years, a third of these patients had an organic diagnosis such as disseminated sclerosis; another third already had such a diagnosis so that the additional diagnosis of hysteria seemed gratuitous; the remainder had a variety of psychiatric illnesses. Since the diagnosis fragmented over time, Slater pronounced hysteria not only a "delusion but also a snare." His view was that hysteria did not exist.

A FALTERING REVIVAL

Toward 1970 the zeitgeist began to change again with a revival of something like the humanistic spirit of the 1880s and 1890s.

The students rioting in the streets of Paris and on American college campuses in 1968 were harbingers of a changed view of humankind and society. The rights and grievances of minority groups began to be recognized, and feminism resurged in various forms. Left-wing governments were elected during the 1970s in the United States, Great Britain, Canada, and Australia. Large changes were taking place in the world of psychoanalysis. John Bowlby's *Attachment* (1969) developed a principal argument, based on ethological data and on observations of children, that much mental illness could be understood in terms of disruption to the bonds of affection a child has with parents. Bowlby's ideas have profoundly influenced current conceptions of BPD. It was in this atmosphere that the concept of "self" began to reappear, although in etiolated form.

In a revolutionary vein, Kohut (1971) proposed a psychology of self, but so successful had been what Harter (1983) called the "radical behaviourist purge" earlier in the century, he was unable to define it (Kohut, 1977, pp. 310–311). The intellectual background out of which the concept might be formulated had been largely diminished. Nevertheless, the memory, which is part of this experience, was rediscovered, in 1972, by the neuropsychologist Endel Tulving. His aim, as he told me, was to reintroduce the concepts of William James, who distinguished between two kinds of memory. One of them had been lost to psychology following World War I. Tulving (1972) called this form of memory *episodic*: It is peculiarly personal. Episodes from one's past can be viewed again, as it were, in the mind's eye. *Semantic* memory is more public, involving facts garnered from these episodes.

Tulving's distinction between episodic and semantic memory is crucial to an understanding of traumatic memory, which once again became a matter of clinical concern, not only as a result of the Vietnam war, but also due to a growing awareness of the significance of sexual abuse, which, during the mid century when the West averted its gaze from the effects of combat trauma, the psychiatric profession disregarded and grossly underestimated.

In parallel with a renewed awareness of the pathogenic significance of trauma, interest in the work of Janet was revived, particularly by Henri Ellenberger in his great book *The Discovery of the Unconscious* (1970). A study using the diagnostic criteria of Janet showed, contrary to Slater's findings, that hysteria is a stable condition with the diagnosis unchanged after 4 years (Meares & Horvath, 1972). Janet's diagnostic approach followed Charcot, who had found that symptoms that mimicked epilepsy could be distinguished by the presence of the so-called "stigmata." He characterized constriction of the field of vision and disturbances of skin sensitivity, occurring together, as the physical stigmata of hysteria (Veith, 1965, p. 232). Periodic sensitivity of the skin to pain is also found in borderline patients, as Bohus and his colleagues have demonstrated (Ludascher et al., 2007). It is of interest that the infamous *Malleus Maleficarum* (*The Hammer of Witches*; 1494), a handbook for hunting witches, recommended pricking witches on the skin in order to find areas of skin insensitivity. The figure of the witch, it seems, was ancestor to both hysterical and borderline patients, each being a member of a stigmatized group. The origin of the word *stigmatize* is the Greek *stigma*, "a pricked mark" (Partridge, 1983, p. 667).

The list of stigmata given by Charcot and Janet (Janet, 1901, pp. 3–22) extended beyond tunnel vision and anaesthesia to include amnesias, blindness, and pareses. Modifying "stigmata" (Meares & Horvath, 1972), we used symptoms involving loss of only neurological function (i.e., conversion disorder) to diagnose our patients. Two main syndromes were identified. One, termed *acute hysteria*, followed severe trauma. In this case the conversion rapidly remitted. In the second grouping, which we called *chronic hysteria*, the symptomatology of the patients was prolonged and associated with an extended history of various illnesses, symptoms, and operations. This syndrome had been documented by

Briquet, whose account was the basis of an inventory of symptoms used by Perley and Guze (1962) in an attempt to systematize the diagnosis of hysteria. This method was flawed in several ways. It failed to incorporate the diagnostic methods of Charcot and Janet and to acknowledge that "chronic hysteria" is essentially a personality disorder. Our patients with "chronic hysteria" showed, in general, profound disturbances in their main relationships. Moreover, most had suffered deprivation of parental care and other disruptions of early development. One patient, for example, had been hospitalized from ages 2 to 4, largely cut off from parents. Another, with tuberculosis of the spine, had spent the years between 7 and 16 in a provincial Eastern European hospital 150 miles from impoverished parents, encased in a plaster cast. This group of people would now be given the diagnosis of BPD.

In a second paper concerning this group, we proposed a hypothesis about its basis. The patients with "chronic hysteria" showed failure of habituation to irrelevant stimuli equivalent to certain patients suffering schizophrenia (Horvath, Friedman, & Meares, 1980). This finding was consistent with Janet's observation that the attention is deficient in hysteria. He wrote: "With hystericals, attention is altogether the most difficult thing to fix, and . . . but a few can succeed in directing it" (Janet, 1901, p. 22; see also pp. 127–137). In recent times, Michael Posner has proposed a basis for borderline personality, which has as its central feature a disturbance of attention (Posner et al., 2002). Habituation also fails to occur in borderline patients (Meares, Melkonian, et al., 2005).

We suggested that failure of habituation in hysteria is a consequence of deficient higher-order inhibitory mechanisms, whereas habituation failure in schizophrenia is explained by a different mechanism: namely, a disturbance of the matching process that compares the events occurring in the environment with records of similar events in the past, stored in memory (Horvath & Meares,

1979). In this book, the same hypothesis about hysteria applies to BPD.

During this period, around 1970, borderline personality began to emerge as a mainstream construct. Before this, interest in the concept was meager. As Knight observed, writing in 1953, the term *borderline* appeared in the indices of few textbooks. Although Adolph Stern is now seen as the first main descriptor of BPD, in 1938, he must have been a lone voice. As Knight (1953) points out: "The term 'borderline state' has achieved almost no official status in psychiatric nomenclature, and conveys no diagnostic illumination of a case other than the implication that the patient is quite sick but not frankly psychotic" (p. 1). The term *borderline*, as remarked in the previous chapter, implies a mystery, referring to a condition for which no diagnostic category exists.

Stimulation of interest in the borderline concept came from Otto Kernberg's (1967) paper on "Borderline Personality Organization." In this seminal work, a similarity between hysteria and BPD was suggested by the inclusion, among the main features of the borderline organization, symptoms that Charcot and Janet had designated as "stigmata" of hysteria. Kernberg described, as aspects of a "polysymptomatic neurosis":

> multiple elaborate, or bizarre conversion symptoms, especially if they are chronic, or even a monosymptomatic conversion reaction of a severe kind extending over many years duration; also conversion symptoms of an elaborate kind, bordering on bodily hallucinations or involving complex sensations or sequences of movements of bizarre quality. (p. 648)

In addition, he observed dissociative reactions, "especially hysterical 'twilight states' and fugues, and amnesia accompanied by disturbances of consciousness" (p. 648). These phenomena, however, were overlooked in the first formal recognition of borderline personality as a diagnostic entity in 1980.

Kernberg also found identity diffusion and splitting to be among the main intrapsychic characteristics of borderline personality organization. These features are seen, in this book, as the core of BPD and as reflections of dissociation.

In the year following Kernberg's paper, Grinker and his colleagues undertook the first systematic study of what clinicians called borderline at that time. They concluded that "the borderline is not a regressive process but a developmental defect. . . . The aetiological factors for this arrest are not known, and the age or phase represented by the fixation has yet to be delineated" (Grinker et al., 1968, p. 22). This conclusion echoed that of Janet, who wrote of his patients that it is "as if their personality has definitively stopped at a certain point, and cannot enlarge any more by the addition, or assimilation of new elements" (Janet, 1911, p. 532).

These views are resonant with the theory of the borderline disorder outlined in this book, in which the major defect is seen as a failure of maturation of self, as James defined it. This inadequate maturation is seen as a consequence of not only a failure of the caregiving environment to provide for the child appropriate forms of responsiveness but also the effect of traumata, particularly those that can be seen as "attacks upon value" (Meares, 2004a). Such impacts upon the developing personality may be conceived as narcissistic injury. Once again, Grinker and his colleagues (1968) seem to anticipate this formulation: "The so-called structural defect of the ego due to some sort of narcissistic trauma produces a deficiency in the processes of identifications which are maintained at the infantile level of memory and do not reach the secondary level characterized by confidence, independence and the development of regulating structures" (p. 22).

Increasingly sophisticated explorations of a putative borderline condition followed these early works. Gunderson and his colleagues, following a widely cited review of the main features of the condition (Gunderson & Singer, 1975), developed a semistructured instrument, the Diagnostic Interview for Borderlines (DIB), which reliably assessed 29 descriptive characteristics (Gunderson et al., 1981). A discriminant function analysis of a sample of 33 patients with BPD identified by DIB found seven criteria that could differentiate them from comparison groups with 81% success (Gunderson & Kolb, 1978).

Despite these advances, queries remained. Certain authorities suspected that the borderline condition was not a distinct entity but part of a schizophreniform spectrum of illnesses. They included Hoch, who, with Polatin, had called it *pseudoneurotic schizophrenia* (1949). Spitzer, Endicott, and Gibbon (1979) seemed to settle the argument with a large study involving two factor analyses, first on 808 patients with BPD and second on 808 patients with BPD and a similar number of control patients. They were able to distinguish two groups of subjects. The first they called *borderline personality disorder* and the second, *schizotypal personality disorder*.

The 1980 DSM-III catalogue of diagnostic criteria for BPD made the syndrome of BPD, for the first time, a formal diagnosis rather than a mere adjective. The criteria derived particularly from Gunderson's work together with additions from Grinker and Kernberg.

Inclusion of posttraumatic stress disorder (PTSD) among other new diagnoses introduced in 1980 was an equally important event. It gave recognition to a renewed and growing awareness of the potential for traumatic experience to create malign psychological consequences. This new awareness prompted a revival of interest in Janet and his concept of dissociation (e.g., Van der Kolk & Van der Hart, 1989). Evidence soon emerged showing dissociation associated with the borderline diagnosis, particularly in the more severe cases (Shearer, 1994).

A third major change in psychiatric nosology executed by DSM-III was the abolition of the stigmatizing term of *hysteria*, the etymology of which was absurd and the manner of the diagnosis of which bordered on the dangerous, as Slater (1965) pointed out. The syndrome Janet had described was split apart into its main components of (1) a personality disorder, (2) a polysymptomatic disorder now called *somatization disorder*, (3) conversion disorders, and (4) dissociative phenomena.

Despite such nosological reform, the stigmatizing view of *hysteria* was allowed to live on under a different guise with the renaming of "hysterical personality disorder" as "histrionic personality disorder." DSM-IV continued the stereotype, including this as a diagnostic criterion: "Interaction with others is often characterized by inappropriate sexually seductive and provocative behavior" (American Psychiatric Association, 1994, p. 657). Janet discounted medical folklore concerning "coquetry" in hysteria. "When coquetry exists," he wrote, "it is rather connected with that vanity, that selfishness, which we have pointed out as characteristic, than with the erotic properly called" (Janet, 1901, p. 216). His viewpoint seems to be supported by Bakkevig and Karterud (2010), who found that the diagnosis of histrionic personality disorder has little construct validity and concluded that the term should be removed from DSM. However, they also believed that the phenomenon of attention-seeking had clinical significance. The new edition of DSM that emerged in 1994 edged toward a reconstitution of the old syndrome. Conversion disorders were deemed necessary to the diagnosis of somatization disorder; dissociative and paranoid phenomena became a new diagnostic criterion for BPD.

In 1992, Judith Herman pointed out that borderline personality disorder, somatization disorder, and dissociative identity "were once subsumed under the now obsolete name hysteria" (1994, p. 23). These diagnoses overlap to a substantial degree so that a central group of patients can be given all three. Since people suffering from these disorders are frequently survivors of childhood abuse, Herman suggested that these "three disorders might perhaps be best understood as variants of complex post traumatic stress disorder, each deriving its characteristic features from one form of adaption to the traumatic environment" (p. 126). The proposal of Herman and Van der Kolk (Herman, 1994; Herman, Perry, & Van der Kolk, 1989), which gained support from Gunderson and Sabo (1993), has the value of seeing these disorders not only as specific "diseases," but as manifestations of a systematic disturbance in which the individual is conceived not as an isolated organism but as part of a larger organism that includes the social environment. The need of the individual to shore up a sense of personal existing elicits particular adaptations to the social environment. For example, many of the manifestations of somatization disorder can be understood as "care eliciting behavior" (Henderson, 1974).

The concept of complex PTSD has incited controversy and so is not yet recognized as a formal diagnostic entity (Lewis & Grenyer, 2009). The way forward may be an attempt to discover the core feature or features that these disorders have in common and which they share with PTSD. The hypothesis put forward here is that this core may be the fragmentation of being, the disturbance of "personal synthesis" described by Janet.

Chapter 3

SELF DISTURBANCE
AS THE CORE OF BORDERLINE
PERSONALITY DISORDER

ADOLPH STERN, the first main descriptor of borderline personality disorder (BPD; Stern, 1938), gave a sketch of the syndrome that is sensitive and insightful. The DSM-IV catalogue of diagnostic criteria, however, barely overlaps with the phenomena he described. Nevertheless, clinicians who work in the field would see both versions of the syndrome as accurate. This apparent discrepancy between authoritative accounts of the disorder raises a significant question about the diagnosis of BPD: Is it merely a term used to refer to a number of more or less unrelated patterns of symptomatology occurring in difficult patients who do not fit traditional diagnostic molds, or is it, on the other hand, a distinct entity manifest in a variety of ways? The former interpretation is seemingly supported by the way in which BPD is identified in DSM-IV. Nine criteria are given for the specification of the syndrome, but only five are required for the diagnosis. Two people, both diagnosed as suffering from BPD, may therefore have only one criterion in common. This polythetic method allows for the BPD diagnosis to be made by 256 different combinations of DSM-IV symptoms (Lewis & Grenyer, 2009). The method implies that there is no single unifying pattern, no core symptom, or complex of symptoms, which is a particular marker of the condition.

Tyrer (2009) has recently put forward a view that encompasses both interpretations of the protean character of BPD. Describing the term *borderline* and its place in psychiatric nosology, he wrote: "I suggest that it does not belong anywhere; it should be abolished as it is a passport to heterogeneity. Unless it is redefined and reformulated, it will remain a condition that undoubtedly exists but will do so in so many forms that it defies predictions about treatment and prognosis" (p. 94). The sense of clinicians who work in the field is not only that BPD "undoubtedly exists" but also, despite its elusive nature, that it has a phenomenal core, not as yet agreed upon.

As Tyrer (2009) implies, identification of the core of BPD is essential if progress is to be made in developing more effective means of treatment, which must be primarily directed at what is most fundamental among the many phenomena associated with the diagnosis. A number of suggestions have been made about the nature of this notional core. These suggestions, in the main, concern individual phenomena such as a particular affect, a style of relatedness, a form of consciousness, or characteristic way of behaving. Such phenomena, however, cannot stand alone. An affect is always part of a form of consciousness, which in turn is part of a system that involves a particular relationship, whether external or internal. The phenomena are collectively linked to a way of behaving. Each phenomenon is part of a larger dynamism that includes the other people. An investigation, then, into the nature of the core pathology of BPD necessarily focuses on appropriate groupings of symptoms.

A STUDY OF CORE DEFINED BY ENDURANCE

Groupings of symptoms and other phenomena that can be considered as the nucleus, or core, of BPD are those that persist over time, since the cardinal feature of personality disorder, as Tyrer (2009) points out, is *endurance*. In the study outlined in this chapter, the quality of endurance is taken as the criterion of "coreness."

Groupings of phenomena can be discerned by means of factor analysis. The best known and most influential of such studies came from Clarkin, Hull, and Hurt in 1993. In an exploratory factor analysis involving 75 hospitalized female patients with borderline features, they found three main factors of DSM-III-R criteria that have been labeled as *I self*, *II affect*, and *III impulsivity*. Factor I loaded most strongly on emptiness/boredom, identity problems, fear of abandonment, and unstable relationships. The second factor comprised suicidality, anger, and labile affect and was considered to reflect emotional dysregulation. Factor III loaded heavily on impulsivity. Clarkin and his colleagues saw this factor as standing alone as a separate dimension in borderline pathology. Other exploratory factor analyses producing a three-factor structure have come from Blais et al. (1997), Sanislow et al. (2000), and Taylor and Reeves (2007).

Confirmatory factor analysis tends to favor a unidimensional structure (Feske et al., 2007; Fossati et al., 2006; Grilo & McGlashan, 2000; Johansen et al., 2004; Sanislow et al., 2000). A multifactorial structure, however, seems plausible as evidenced by the apparent separateness of the impulsivity criterion, which has a distinct natural history (Stevenson, Meares, & Comerford, 2003), a fact remarked upon by Aggen et al. (2009). A reasonable interpretation of these findings might be that the conflict between them is only apparent, and that both are valid. BPD can be conceived as a unitary disorder made up of several groupings of phenomena that are both distinguishable and related. It is on this assumption that we have used the Clarkin et al. factor analysis in our study. Furthermore, our data were collected using DSM-III-R, which Clarkin et al. (1993) had used.

The Clarkin three-factor structure neatly separates out the two main viewpoints about the core of BPD. The prevailing viewpoint is that affect dysregulation (Factor II), perhaps combined with impulsivity (Factor III), constitutes such a core. The most prominent proponent of affect dysregulation is Linehan (1993) who receives influential support (Lieb et al., 2004; Nica & Links, 2009; Silk, 2000). Links and his colleagues propose impulsivity as the core symptom (Links et al., 1999).

On the other hand, without, in general, using the term *self*, pioneers of the BPD concept proposed nuclear features of the disorder that correspond to three of the four DSM criteria making up Clarkin's "self" factor—that is, Factor I. Adler and Buie (Adler, 1985; Adler & Buie, 1979), Stern (1938), Masterson (1972), and Gunderson (1984) noted the centrality of abandonment fears. Adler and Buie also spoke of the significance of emptiness. They wrote: "We have observed a core experiential state of intensely painful aloneness. This feeling state often includes a sense of inner emptiness together with increasing panic and despair. . . . At these times the patient often states that he has no fantasies at all" (Adler & Buie, 1979, p. 357).

Kernberg found what DSM calls "identity disturbance" to be central to BPD. Following Erikson (1956), Kernberg (1967) called it "identity diffusion; namely, the lack of an integrated self concept and an integrated and stable concept of total objects in relationship with the self. Actually, identity diffusion is a typical syndrome of the borderline personality organization, which is not seen in less severe character pathology and neurotic patients" (p. 677).

A more recent formulation, from Bateman and Fonagy (2004), is also congruent with the "self-identity" criterion. They see a failure of "mentalization" as the central deficit of BPD. *Mentalization* refers to the awareness of mental states, one's own and those of others. This is a cardinal characteristic of a self system in the concept derived from the descriptions of William James (Meares, 1993a, 2005).

In 1993, I proposed that the central disturbance of BPD is a deficit in the self system, represented in DSM by the triad of cri-

teria of self-identity problems, fears of abandonment, and emptiness. This complex of criteria was theoretically derived, based on
the idea that the sense of self depends upon, and arises with, a
sense of the other. Where self is fragile, so also is the sense of the
other. When the sense of self is lost entirely, "emptiness" remains
(Meares, 1993a, p. 196; 2005, pp. 222–223).

Method

Our group tested the hypothesis that a deficit in the self system is the core disturbance in BPD. Endurance was used as the
index of coreness. A cohort of 29 patients with BPD (mean age,
27.9 years; 12 males, 17 females) treated by the Conversational
Model (CM) for 1 year, were compared, in terms of the endurance of Clarkin's three factors, with another cohort of 31 patients
with BPD (mean age, 29.7 years; 15 males, 16 females), who
continued treatment with their referring practitioners for 1 year
(treatment as usual or TAU). In addition, a similar comparison
was made on the outcome of three theoretically derived complexes:

- Complex I consisted of the triad of criteria of the self system
  referred to above.
- Complex II is comprised of the criteria relating to affect dysregulation in Clarkin's Factor II; it also included "unstable relationships," which loads on both Factors I and II in Clarkin's
  study.
- Complex III consisted of the single criterion of "impulsivity."

The data came from the replication (Korner et al., 2006) of our
earlier outcome study of the treatment of patients with BPD
(Meares, Stevenson, & Comerford, 1999; Stevenson & Meares,
1992; Stevenson, Meares, & D'Angelo, 2005).

A second aspect of our investigation focused on the "core
dysphoria" that a number of authorities distinguish from typical
unipolar depression (e.g., Westen, 1992). In our study the Zung

Self-Rating Depression Scale, a measure of typical depression, was used in order to judge whether or not it is related to that grouping of BPD phenomena that shows endurance—that is, the "core."

The participants in this study were allocated to either CM or TAU by a method of naturalistic randomization. Entry into the CM group depended on the chance event of a therapist being available at the time of referral. Allocation to the different groups by standard means of randomization, such as random number sheets, and so forth, was not acceptable to the hospital administration, to ourselves, to the patients, and to their referring physicians, since the clinic at the time was the only one in the state. In terms of the demographic variables of age, marital status, and occupational and educational status, there were no statistically significant differences between the CM and TAU groups. With respect to symptom measures, there were no significant differences between the study and control groups at baseline.

All subjects were scored at an assessment interview with the Westmead Severity Scale (WSS) for BPD. This scale was constructed from the 27 items making up the diagnostic criteria. In scoring the scale, the presence or absence of each item is elicited by means of a semistructured interview, involving a series of probe questions. These questions require a dichotomous response. An affirmative response receives a score of 1. The weighted kappa, used to test the interrater reliability, was satisfactory, with a kappa + 0.81 for the total scale. Further details are given in previous publications (Korner et al., 2006; Stevenson, Meares, & D'Angelo, 1999; 2005). The other main measure, the Zung Self-Rating Depression Scale, correlates well with Beck Depression Inventory (BDI; Biggs et al., 1978). As a self-rating scale, the Zung is likely to reflect the patient's internal perception of dominant affective experience more closely than an observer-rated scale.

The scores on the Westmead Severity Scale were used to identify the factors and complexes described above.

Results and Discussion

The statistical analysis and detailed results are reported elsewhere (Meares, et al., 2011). The essential features of the results are shown in Figures 3.1 and 3.2, which display the outcome for both the BPD factors and complexes after 1 year of treatment.

The grouping of DSM criteria making up Clarkin et al.'s Factor I, which concerns "self," endured with unchanged severity over a period of 1 year in a TAU cohort of patients with BPD. On the other hand, Factors II and III improved significantly over the period of a year. Factor II reflects emotional dysregulation, whereas Factor III measures impulsivity.

Treatment with CM produced a different outcome picture for this cohort of patients. Factor I (self) improved significantly over a year. Factor II (affect dysregulation) also improved significantly, and significantly more, than those in the TAU cohort. Factor III (impulsivity) improved significantly but not significantly more than those in the TAU cohort.

The theoretically derived complexes of BPD criteria provided outcomes indistinguishable from Clarkin's factors. Accordingly, the discussion is confined to those groupings of BPD phenomena created by factor analysis.

The TAU findings suggest that a measure reflecting a disturbance of self is the enduring aspect of the DSM diagnosis of BPD. They give support to the view that a constellation of phenomena related to such a disturbance is at the core of borderline pathology. The other groupings of DSM criteria that do not persist in severity over 1 year mainly describe disturbances of emotion and impulse regulation. This distinction between two groupings of phenomena, based on their relative endurance, gives rise to a demarcation between two zones of BPD symptomatology: one relating to self and the other to regulation. Such a division resonates with the two-component conception of Livesley (2008).

The second aspect of this study concerned the chronic dysphoria that characteristically accompanies the diagnosis of BPD. As Westen, Moses, and Silk (1992) demonstrated, this dysphoria has a number of different facets, including emptiness, loneliness, desperation in relation to attachment figures, and a labile, diffuse negative affectivity. Our findings, although not clear-cut, support the supposition that typical depression is not at the core of BPD. Change in the Zung score over the year of treatment was not significantly related to such changes in any of the three factors in the TAU group. There were moderately significant changes in the CM group, with the strongest correlation found between change in the impulsivity factor and change in the Zung score. If the dysphoria of BPD is like typical depression, it should have correlated with the factor that endured, that is, the self factor.

Overall, the Zung depression score improved significantly in the CM group. This improvement is of note in relation to reports by a number of investigators that the depressive affect in BPD is relatively resistant to treatment (e.g., Linehan et al., 1993). Our data seem consistent with the view of many clinicians that the affect of BPD often comprises not only atypical but also typical features.

Although our findings suggest that the core of BPD is the self factor, they must be considered preliminary, requiring the support of future research, which should involve diagnostic criteria that more adequately describe those criteria which cannot be defined in behavioral terms. The subjectively evaluated criteria of emptiness and "identity disturbance" need elaboration in order to determine their importance among the phenomena of BPD, as illustrated by the account of Adele in Chapter 1.

The nature of the phenomena subsumed under the DSM criterion of "identity disturbance" requires consideration. The term is ambiguous in that it is described as if *identity* and *self* are synonyms. They are not. In the simplest terms, the distinction between identity and self can be seen as the difference between the individual's public reality (identity) and private experience (self).

In ordinary healthy living, self and identity are seamlessly connected, though they metaphorically face, Janus-like, in opposite directions. Identity concerns the individual's relationship with his or her world. It involves a sense of place within family, profession, religion, and other social groups, and it is composed of roles, personal attributes, and conceptions of who one is in relation to others. Self, as William James (1890) described it, is categorically different. It is that flux of images, sensations, feelings, memories, imaginings, and so forth, which James likened to a stream. Here the focus is inward. The cardinal feature of self is a reflective awareness of inner events. The reflective process, James wrote, enables us "to think ourselves as thinkers" (James, 1890, I, p. 296.). It brings with it a conception of "innerness" from which we derive a realization that certain experiences are uniquely our own.

The self aspect of the self–identity complex might be the more fundamental. The philosopher Owen Flanagan, for example, states that "the senses of identity, direction, agency and life plan are all grounded in the memorable connections of the stream" (Flanagan, 1992, pp. 166–167).

Having previously tackled, with his colleagues, the problem of defining the negative affect associated with BPD (Westen, 1992; Westen et al, 1992), Drew Westen, with Tess Wilkinson-Ryan, has more recently turned his attention to the nature of the self–identity complex in BPD (Wilkinson-Ryan & Westen, 2000). Focusing on the concept of identity, these researchers collated items from a number of authoritative sources (Erikson, 1963, 1968; Kernberg, 1975, 1984; Marcia, 1987, 1993), including Westen's own work (1985, 1992), in order to reach a definition of identity in BPD. From these items they constructed an instrument containing 35 indicators of identity disturbance. Patient groups composed of patients with BPD ($n = 34$), those having another personality disorder ($n = 20$), and those with no personality disorder ($n = 41$) were scored on these items. A factor analysis was then conducted on these scores. It produced four main factors: (1) role absorption, (2) painful incoherence, (3) inconsistency, and (4) lack of commitment. These four factors were used to distinguish between subjects with BPD and those without BPD There were important differences between the predictive powers of the four factors. The investigators noted:

> The weakest of the four factors in predicting borderline personality was the fourth, lack of commitment. This may be an important finding given the heavy emphasis most identity research (as well as DSM-IV) has placed on this construct. For example, DSM-IV describes identity disturbance in borderline personality disorder as being "characterized by shifting goals, values, and vocational aspirations." (Wilkinson-Ryan & Westen, 2000, p. 651)

The data of Wilkinson-Ryan and Westen (2000) showed that although this factor is a central component of identity disturbance, it does not distinguish borderline personality disorder from other types of psychopathology. "Painful incoherence" was strongly related to borderline personality after controlling for both histrionic features and a history of sexual abuse. Sexual abuse was largely uncorrelated with the other three identity factors.

The findings of this study tend to suggest that, rather than disturbance of identity as usually defined, what is central to borderline personality is a disturbance of *self*, manifest as a painful sense of personal incoherence. Westen's painful incoherence factor is very like an expanded version of Clarkin et al.'s self factor. The Westen factor is comprised of emptiness; a fear that personal existence would end if a close relationship were lost; and a number of items relating to experience of self (unreality, lack of continuity and an indeterminate sense of "who your self is"). Unreality and lack of personal continuity are cardinal features of the dissociative taxon of Waller, Putnam, and Carlson (1996). *Painful inco-*

herence is, perhaps, the best description we have of the core of BPD. The term encompasses psychic pain and implies a fragmentation of personal existing which can be seen as the fundamental form of the dissociative experience (Meares, 1999a). The personality fragmentation, resembling dissociation, of BPD has also been demonstrated as a central feature (Wildgoose et al., 2000).

Our study must be considered preliminary for a second reason. We began to collect the data just before the emergence of DSM-IV. We used, instead, the criteria of DSM-III-R, as had Clarkin and his colleagues. Our analysis, therefore, does not include the ninth factor concerning dissociation and paranoid features, introduced in DSM-IV. A future study is required in order to test the hypothesis that this ninth criterion is one of those that make up the grouping of BPD features that endure over time and which can be considered the core of BPD.

The influential review of Gunderson and Singer (1975) suggested that the dissociative phenomena of depersonalization and derealization and micropsychotic episodes are central features of the borderline syndrome. Zanarini and her colleagues note (Zanarini et al., 2008) that a number of investigators reported these experiences in BPD following this review (Chopra & Beatson, 1986; Conte et al., 1980; Gunderson, 1977; Gunderson, Carpenter, & Strauss, 1975; Koenigsberg, 1982; Links, Steiner, & Mitton, 1989; Nurnberg, 1988; Perry & Klerman, 1980; Sheehy, Goldsmith, & Charles, 1980; Silk et al., 1989; Soloff, 1981; Zanarini, Gunderson, & Frankenberg, 1990). Overall, this evidence suggested that such phenomena were common in BPD. They also had a discriminative value, given that BPD had higher mean scores than other Axis II disorders on the absorption, depersonalization, and amnesia factors of the Dissociative Experiences Scale (DES; Zanarini et al., 2000; Zweig-Frank, Paris, & Guzder, 1994). Skodol et al. (2002) note that the addition of the ninth criterion to the DSM criteria of BPD in DSM-IV (American Psychiatric Association, 1994)—dissociative symptoms and paranoid ideation—have "excellent specifity, i.e. rarely occur in other diagnostic groups" (p. 937).

In their 2008 study, Zanarini and her colleagues showed that the mean scores on the three DES factors in BPD patients were 2½–3 times larger than Axis II comparison subjects. They also showed that the dissociative factors improved over the 10-year period of the study. Ninety percent of the subjects in both the BPD and the comparison groups were in psychotherapy and taking psychotropic medication at baseline, and about 70% were receiving both of these forms of treatment at each follow-up point in the study. The "coreness" or otherwise of dissociative phenomena in BPD could not, therefore, be judged, where this quality is defined by the endurance of symptoms not being treated by methods specifically designed to approach BPD.

A further difficulty is posed by the suggestion that a grouping of features around "self" is the core of the BPD syndrome. Without the dysregulation features, BPD cannot be diagnosed. Dysregulation is an essential part of the BPD picture. A resolution of the difficulty might be achieved in the following way.

It may be that a failure of self sets off, or triggers, excessive dysregulation in individuals who are genetically predisposed. It is generally supposed that the dysregulation features are more genetically determined than the self features, as suggested by a number of authorities, including Siever et al. (2002). The neurophysiology, however, of dysregulation goes beyond genetic influences. Disruption of the self system is likely to lead, in itself, to a failure of higher-order, prefrontally connected inhibitory mechanisms (see Chapter 5). This effect would likely exacerbate a preexisting tendency to disinhibition and dysregulation. This formulation has the self component as the primary deficiency in BPD, with dysregulation conceived as secondary. The matter is further discussed in Chapter 11.

Fragmentation, or what Janet called a failure of personal synthesis, was central to his concept of dissociation. In essence, Janet was putting forward a "disintegration" theory (1924, p. 40). The modern concept of dissociation, however, is more complex, consisting of two main states, what I am calling *primary* and *secondary dissociation* (see Chapter 7). Fragmentation is the main feature of primary dissociation.

The issue of fragmentation leads us to a consideration of the form of relatedness making up the fourth element of the "self" factor in the Clarkin analysis: namely, "unstable relations." At first sight this item seems somewhat outside the scope of the self concept. It is, however, entirely consistent with it. The concept of fragmentation implies a number of shifting self states in BPD. Each one is necessarily part of the experience of relationship. This idea suggests that in BPD forms of relatedness are relatively unintegrated, so that the individual shifts between various forms of relatedness in an unstable manner. The kinds of relationship that are an aspect of a fragmented self system are multiple, extending beyond those involving abandonment fears. Studies of the relationships represented in the memories of patients with BPD usually involve the child–victim pole of the relationship, leaving implicit the characteristics of the other. Using the notion of schemata (Young et al., 2003) in a study with 30 patients with BPD, Johnson et al. (2009) found that the "angry and impulsive child" and "abandoned and abused child" modes uniquely predicted dissociation scores, consistent with the concept of fragmentation. Other characterizations of the typical forms of relatedness in people with BPD include "anaclitic relatedness" and "self-criticism" (Blatt & Auerbach, 1988; Levy, Edell, & McGlashan, 2007) and "hostile–helpless" (Lyons-Ruth, Melnick, et al., 2007).

Finally, despite the drawbacks of this study (Meares et al., 2011b) the main finding seems clear. Two groupings of DSM criteria, one relating to self and the other to dysregulation, are distinguished in terms of their endurance, leading to the inference that the self system is the more fundamental disturbance of the two. Such an inference has significant implications for the refinement and elaboration of current approaches to the treatment of BPD, which are touched upon briefly in the final chapter.

Chapter 4

"LE MOI EST UNE CO-ORDINATION"

Evidence presented in the previous chapter suggested that the core of BPD is a constellation of features that can broadly be subsumed under the banner of *self*. In exploring the nature of disturbances of the self in BPD, Wilkinson-Ryan and Westen (2000) found that "painful incoherence" is its central characteristic. This is in accord with Heinz Kohut's clinical appraisal of the central pathology of BPD. He saw it as a failure of the development of a "cohesive self" leading to "fragmentation of the body–mind–self and of the self-object" (Kohut, 1971, pp. 31–32). *Fragmentation* is not unlike the identity diffusion of Kernberg (1967), nor is it dissimilar to the broken-up, shifting states of being described by Janet.

The observations of Wilkinson-Ryan and Westen (2000) suggest that in order to discover the basis of BPD, we must find the cause, or causes, of "painful incoherence." Such an investigation demands a more extended concept of self than has so far been given, as well as an understanding of its development. The theories of Hughlings Jackson are helpful in these respects. His definition of self is clear. He also makes a proposal about the way an experience arises in terms of brain function. His proposal is sufficiently precise for a hypothesis concerning the basis of fragmentation to be formulated and tested. Chapter 5 reports on the outcome of such a test. This chapter gives the background to the hypothesis, beginning with an outline of Jackson's concept of self, interwoven with Jamesian ideas. James fully subscribed to Jackson's hierarchical model of mind (James, 1890, I, p. 29; II, pp. 125–126), and his psychological descriptions are complementary to Jackson's evolutionary and neurological approach.

THE JACKSONIAN MODEL OF SELF

John Hughlings Jackson (1835–1911) is often spoken of as "the father of British neurology," yet he once considered a career in philosophy (Taylor, 1925). His abiding interest in notions of mind, or "self," led him to explore the problem of mental illness. His writings on this subject make up much of his opus but remain largely neglected in the fields of psychiatry and psychology. His main theory, derived from meticulous observation of the smallest changes in the mental and neurological functioning of patients with aphasia and epilepsy, and organized by evolutionary ideas, is "particularly modern—so much so, in fact, that his ideas are receiving more serious consideration today than they did in his own time" (Kolb & Whishaw, 1990, p. 338).

Jackson's colleagues considered him a genius. He pioneered the concept of the lateralization of hemispheric function (Jackson, 1958, II, pp. 129–145), anticipated the notion of the triune brain (Jackson, 1958, II, pp. 41–42, 45–75; MacLean, 1990), and suggested that sensory data are integrated during sleep (Jackson, 1958, p. 71). Jacksonian theory provides a preliminary framework for understanding the ongoing state of mind in patients with BPD and also for the syndrome of dissociation that is a central feature of BPD.

Jackson's approach to mental illness was highly logical. He understood it to be a manifestation of a disruption of mind, or self. This being so, it was necessary to begin a study of mental illness with a definition of what *self* might be. He believed himself to be the first person in the medical literature to use this term. He was certainly the first to develop a plausible neural model of self, preceding, and in certain fundamental aspects, compatible with, the important and influential account of Damasio (1996, 1999), formulated over 100 years later.

Jackson's definition of self is condensed, deceptively simple, but philosophically sophisticated. He considered that self is identified by, but not the same as, a reflective consciousness of inner events, which he called "object consciousness." By this he meant that seeing an object such as a brick is not unlike thinking of a brick. "My assertion is that both the seeing and the thinking of are states of object consciousness, that they are but different (compound) degrees of objectification" (Jackson, 1958, II, p. 92).

Self, although a unified state, is double when conceived in an abstract way. Jackson wrote: "It is impossible to speak of objective states without implying subject consciousness. In every proposition, subject and object consciousness are indicated." In his examples of "I see a brick" and "I think of a brick," "subject consciousness is symbolized by 'I,' and objective consciousness by 'brick.' Each by itself is nothing; each 'is only half itself.'" Jackson notes that this duality is expressed in popular psychology with statements such as "Ideas *come into* consciousness." In his view the correct statement is "ideas *come out* of subject consciousness and then constitute object consciousness" (Jackson, 1958, II, p. 93). This concept is important and discussed in more detail in the following chapters. On the basis of his observations, Jackson inferred that the state of mind he labeled *self* is the outcome of evolutionary history, which is reflected in a hierarchical organization of the brain. He conceived the course of evolution laying down successive levels of neural structure, which he termed "lowest, middle and highest" (p. 41), noting that the terms were figurative, a "simplification," since all so-called levels work together.

Jackson built up his model from what he considered the small-est elements of the central nervous system. They are reflexive, simple sensorimotor units. Each unit has a representing func-tion; that is, it has a memory of some kind. This proposal was made before Sherrington introduced the term *synapse* in 1895 and well before Kandel's (1976) demonstration that the synapse has a kind of memory.

The earliest level of the system consists of the basic units oper-ating relatively independently. Movements from an earlier to a later state of evolution come about not through the introduction of any new form of neural tissue but as a consequence of an in-creased coordination between units of neural function. "The whole nervous system," he wrote, "is a sensori-motor mecha-nism, a co-ordinating system from top to bottom" (Jackson, 1958, II, p. 41). The highest level of the brain–mind system, which gives rise to the experience of self, is achieved through greater coordination between brain elements brought about by the evolutionary elaboration of existing structures, most impor-tantly the prefrontal cortex (p. 399). As Jackson put it, quoting his follower Ribot, "*Le moi est une co-ordination*" (Jackson, 1958, II, p. 82). The significance of prefrontal functions, particularly the orbitofrontal cortex in the creation of the experience of self, is a main feature of Damasio's (1996) thesis.

Each stage of enhanced coordination between the elements of the central nervous system (CNS) brings with it states of mind and function that show an increased complexity that is allied to a multiplicity of representation. More recent levels of evolution do not involve the introduction of new representations. Rather, there is re-representation, then *re-re*-representation. In addition, evolution brings greater voluntary control over the contents of consciousness and systems of response. This control includes en-hanced inhibition of earlier evolved "levels."

In essence, Jackson proposed a hierarchy of consciousness. Hi-erarchy is a basic feature of the structure of biological systems

(Smith, 1978) but not in the sense of a unidirectional system of dominance, a command tree found, for example, in military organization. Rather, the coordination of which Jackson speaks is not only across "levels" but also between them. Each level is coordinated with other levels and depends upon them. Switching between levels is related to adaptive needs and environmental circumstances. Fight and flight are dominant and adaptive states of mind in specific situations. *The highest level is not a single level but comes into being through a coordination of lower levels, which creates a larger system that now "contains" all levels.*

This hierarchical organization can be illustrated by the development of memory in an individual life. Early memory systems are sensory and motor. The first sensorimotor memory system involves simple recognition of fragments of the sensory environment; for example, the baby perceives eyes rather than a face. This form of memory, "perceptual representation," is atomized, inflexible, and very accurate (Tulving & Schacter, 1990). Memory for motor repertoires—called *procedural memory*—also emerges early. Tulving calls these early memory systems *"anoetic,"* a neologism derived from the Greek *noesis,* meaning *mind.*

The second "level" of memorial capacity is achieved when the child has the capacity to recall facts of its sensory environment. This achievement, which comes toward the end of the first year of life (Nelson, 1992), heralds the onset of what Tulving (1972, 1983) called *"semantic memory."* It is *"noetic."*

The third level of memory comes considerably later, at about 4 years of age (Nelson, 1992), when the experience of self is discovered. This discovery comes with the child's new sense of an awareness of inner events, shown by the attainment of the concept of secrecy (Meares & Orlay, 1988). This new memory is an aspect of the capacity for introspection. It is *autonoetic.* Tulving called it *"episodic"* (1972, 1983). The child is now able to conjure up, as if in "the mind's eye," episodes from its past. This form of awareness was once called *insight* (Oxford English Dictionary,

1971). It is accompanied by the capacity for some kind of insight into the world of others, a realization that, just as one has a private and unique personal reality, so others have wishes, feelings, imaginings, and so forth, which are their own and different from those of oneself. The child at this stage moves beyond the capacity for sympathy and gains, in addition, the faculty of empathy. This is an important point in the development of the so-called "theory of mind."

Remote episodic memory is now generally termed *autobiographical*. Tulving called the reflective form of consciousness, of which autobiographical memory is an essential part, "autonoetic." This state of mind is larger than earlier states. The individual is now able, figuratively, to roam around in the mind through scenes brought up at will in memory and imagination in a process Tulving likes to call "mental time travel" (Tulving, 2001, 2005; Wheeler, Stuss, & Tulving, 1997).

Although Jackson's hierarchy is described in terms of consciousness, it implies a more extended hierarchy. Consciousness is not a single, isolated phenomenon. It necessarily arises from a brain state determined by the interplay between the sensory environment and the brain–mind system that is constantly taking place. In terms of self, the interplay, or forms of relatedness, with the social world, whether outer or inner, is particularly important. It is mediated by conversation and always accompanied by emotion.

Seen in this way, a hierarchy of consciousness necessarily comprises forms of relatedness, language, and emotion, in addition to forms of consciousness. Forms of consciousness are made up of characteristics including cohesion, continuity, value, and the senses of time, space, ownership, and boundedness. Jackson (1958) did not attempt to enlarge his sketch of the hierarchy, although he did point out that mentation involves emotion and that the highest emotions are compounded out of the lower. All aspects of the highest level of the hierarchy are disturbed in BPD, which is seen here as a manifestation of the failure of development of self, an overarching concept that includes all the features of higher-order consciousness (Armstrong, 1981). How this failure might come about is suggested by a consideration of Jackson's concept of "dissolution," which in turn gives us a way of understanding "fragmentation."

DISSOLUTION AND A FAILURE OF COHERENCE

Dissolution is a reversal of the trajectory of the brain's evolution. An insult to the brain–mind system causes a retreat down a hierarchy of function, which evolution decreed and development followed. Since it is the functions that emerged last in evolution that are affected first, the initial "level" of disturbance is particularly in the fine-tuning and voluntary control of brain mechanisms underpinning those aspects of attention, memory, and affect that together contribute to the experience of self.

Jackson did not include psychological traumata in his list of possible insults. His proposal, however, suggests that this may be the case. He believed that "dissolution" followed excessive excitation of neuronal tissue, which resulted in its exhaustion, or "fatigue," a word repeatedly used by Janet as a synonym of psychological trauma. Temporary failure of function was seen as a consequence not of the excitation but of the exhaustion. Jackson gave an example of dissolution as manifest in memory:

> One of Jackson's patients, a doctor, reported an occasion when he was called to see a patient with a respiratory complaint. While beginning to examine him, the doctor became aware that he was going to have a slight fit and he turned away from the people in the room so they would not notice. "Coming to" some time later, he found himself writing out the diagnosis of pneumonia of the left base. The patient was no longer in the room and had presumably been sent to bed. Nobody seemed to have noticed anything strange about the doctor's behavior.

Feeling the need to check his diagnosis, he re-examined his patient. He found, as he wrote, "that my conscious diagnosis was the same as my unconscious" (Meares, 1999a, summarizing Jackson, 1958, I, p. 405)

The doctor was behaving in a manner that nobody saw as strange. He was conscious and working in a very sophisticated way, using a memory of the facts of his medical training. However, he was unable to remember anything of what he had done; no memory of the event remained. Episodic memory was lost. He was operating at the level of noetic consciousness. In diagnostic terms, he was dissociated. Dissolution is a model of dissociation (see Chapter 7).

In this state there are no imaginings, no memories of past events, and no narrative. The experience is one of the immediate present, in which there is a constriction of consciousness. Jackson's hypothesis predicts that "self" will be lost under noxious circumstances, resulting in a diminution in the sense of "meness" and a feeling of personal estrangement. A story from the British writer Rebecca West (1971) suggests that this state will involve a sense of personal disintegration, presumably mirroring a disconnectedness among brain elements, and a disturbance of the normal inhibitory activity necessary to selective inattention.

Holidaying in a remote village in Cornwall, in the era before antibiotics, Rebecca West became ill with "blood poisoning." In the following days she fell into a "curious state," in which a failure to select out redundant sensory data and modify the intensity of sensory input seemed to be related to discontinuity of psychic life. She wrote:

I lost my power of suppressing irrelevant impressions and co-ordinating those that remained. I felt obliged to watch the trees outside my window and their behaviour in the sunshine and the wind, to note the characteristics of every person who spoke to me, with a quite disagreeable intensity, and I was so

55

fatigued by this constant effort of apprehension that there was no continuity in the working of my brain. Every moment of consciousness was distinct and unrelated to every other moment. Instead of being a stream my mental life was a string of disparate beads. (1971, p. 52)

The disturbance in the continuity of mental life continued for some days even after her temperature had fallen to normal. Just before her discharge from the nursing home, she was allowed to take a walk beyond the grounds. She chose to climb a small hill from which she had heard there was a fine view. When she got there, as she said:

I could not see the view. I could see it in bits, but not as a whole. It was like trying to take a photograph with a non panoramic camera. And what I saw seemed like meaningless painting on glass. The patchwork of colours carried no suggestion of textures and contours. I had to work hard to interpret it; to see, for example, that that spattered rhomboidal patch was a cornfield. (West, 1971, pp. 52–53)

The disconnectedness of psychic life was accompanied, as it had been earlier in her convalescence, by an unpleasant sense of intrusion into consciousness of the stimuli of the internal world. Two miners and their dogs also came to look at the view. Even though she knew that it was unreasonable, that her "mechanism was hopelessly out of gear," "she felt irritable and uncomfortable," as if being "jostled by a dense crowd" (West, 1971, p. 53).

Rebecca West's state of "fragmentation" and failure of adequate inhibitory control over sensory input was extreme. Her description may illustrate what those with BPD experience, in a minor and subtle way, as an ongoing state of existing.

Jackson's "dissolution" hypothesis suggests that the typical childhood of people with BPD, involving multiple and cumulative traumata that excite high levels of arousal associated with negative affects that produce repeated "fatigues," will constantly demolish emergent states of "higher-order consciousness," so impeding its maturation. This idea, not developed by Jackson, was put forward by Janet (1911, pp. 531–532).

Maturation might also be impeded in a second way. The "facilitatory environment" which the mother and other caregivers normally create may not be provided. Jackson did not contemplate such matters, although he did intimate that achievement of psychic maturation is not inevitable. He wrote: "We develop as we must, that is, according to what we are by inheritance; and also as we can, that is, according to external conditions" (Jackson, 1958, p. 71). The unsuitable "external conditions," beyond active trauma, experienced by the typical patient with BPD, are touched upon in later chapters.

P3, REENTRANT PROCESSING, AND SELF

A neo-Jacksonian hypothesis concerning the brain basis of BPD can be tested by studying a major component of the event-related potential (ERP), the P3 or P300.

A typical activation task used to elicit P3 in human subjects is the "oddball" paradigm, in which task-related oddball (or target) stimuli occur randomly among other "background" (or nontarget) stimuli. Using light and sound stimuli, Sutton and his colleagues (1965) first observed that a positive ERP component arises about 300 milliseconds (ms) after the presentation of the oddball stimulus. By contrast to the earlier components, which relate closely to the physical parameters of the stimulus, the appearance of P3 is determined more by the subject's expectancy concerning an event and the information provided by the event, than by the physical characteristics of the stimulus that signals the event.

In the years that followed the research by Sutton et al., P300 has demonstrated considerable utility as an assessment of human mental function in basic and clinical studies. Although P3 appears in average ERPs as a large, monophasic waveform, as if it were the product of a single source, there is general agreement that P3 is not a unitary brain potential but is the result of activity from widely distributed areas in the brain (Johnson, 1993). There is also a generally accepted distinction between an earlier positive potential, called P3a, and the later P3b peak (Squires et al., 1975). The P3a reflects novelty detection (Soltani & Knight, 2000) and orienting (Barcelo et al., 2002), whereas the P3b (classical P300) is less clearly understood. Verleger and his colleagues (2005) suggest that it is akin to a response set. Soltani and Knight (2000) propose that P3a is an automatic response whereas P3b is a more volitional response. Dissolution theory predicts that the coordination between the neural generators will fail relatively, following an insult to the CNS, so that a monophasic wave will be replaced by a biphasic one.

In a very interesting paper, Rolf Verleger and his colleagues (2005) suggest that the P3 represents more than stimulus processing, which is the way in which it is traditionally portrayed as an aspect of attentional function (reviews by Donchin & Coles, 1988; Verleger, 1988). On the basis of their studies, the Verleger group considers P3 to be a measure of response processing. Most importantly, they see it as a manifestation of some aspect of cooperation between brain areas, integrating stimulus and response. They assume that this binding together of stimulus and response takes place in subcortical regions and in the frontal cortex.

In addition to the proposal that P3 is the outcome of integrating stimulus and response, Verleger and colleagues speculatively link it to the notion of reentrant processing. This concept is based on studies, of which Libet is a pioneer (Libet et al., 1983), which demonstrate that a stimulus has to be processed more than once by the CNS for it to be consciously perceived. This idea is supported by more recent work (Di Lollo, Enns, & Rensink, 2000). Libet's observations suggested that the primary processing occurs earlier than 150 ms. At this stage there is sensory detection resembling "blindsight" (Libet et al., 1991). Blindsight is the phenomenon in which an individual, blinded by damage to the visual cortex, is able to locate objects in the environment when asked to guess their position (Weiskrantz, 1986). The concept of reentry has been extended to propose that relevant stimuli will undergo several passes of processing, involving multiple brain areas, before the stimuli can be perceived (Olson, Chun, & Allison, 2001; Woldorff et al., 2002). Verleger and colleagues speculate that this secondary processing triggers P3.

The linking of reentrant interactions to the generation of P3 is intriguing. Edelman (1992) has put forward the view that higher-order consciousness, which involves self, as defined by William James, is brought into being through the reentrant activity of the brain. Bringing the speculations of Verleger and Edelman together, we find that P3, in some way, becomes a reflection of self.

Reentrant interactions as the basis for the necessary integration of self are consistent with the view of the generation of self that is briefly touched upon in Chapter 16 and outlined in more detail elsewhere (Meares, 2000, 2004b, 2005). It depends upon an "analogical relatedness" (Meares & Jones, 2009) between the child and the caregiver in which the response of the latter shows the "shape" of the baby's experience in her face and voice. An analogue, in its original meaning, is something that has a similar shape to another thing. This particular kind of mother–child relationship, then, might be seen as an interplay of patternings, each one resembling the next, but without replication, as if reentrant activity were going on in the world. It is tempting to suppose that this may be another example of the Janet–Baldwin proposal, taken up by Vygotsky, that those functions we sense as "inner" in adult life had their first forms in the outer world as activities (van der Veer & Valsiner, 1988), particularly between people.

Edelman considers that the reentrant activity of the brain brings forth "analogical abilities" necessary to pattern recognition (2004, p.147). With his colleague Giulio Tononi, Edelman demonstrated how reentry "can account for our ability to discern a shape in a display of moving dots, based on interactions between brain areas for visual movement and shape" (Edelman & Tononi, 2000, p. 86). This capacity for the discernment of pattern and shape is a manifestation of one of the two main modes of thought that are available to us, and which are evident in language, as Vygotsky (1962) pointed out. Edelman calls this mode of thought, which I term *analogical*, "selectionism (or pattern recognition)." The other mode is logic.

Reentry is to be distinguished from feedback. Negative feedback is productive of homeostasis. Reentry has a very different outcome. The difference between the two mechanisms is emphasized by Edelman and Tononi (2000):

> It is important to emphasize that reentry is not feedback. Feedback occurs along a *single* fixed loop made of reciprocal connections using previous *instructionally* derived information for control and correction, such as an error signal. In contrast, reentry occurs in selectional systems across *multiple* parallel paths where information is not prespecified. . . . A key anatomical pre-condition for reentry is the remarkable massively parallel reciprocal connectivity of brain areas. (p. 85)

Reciprocal is a crucial term. *Reentry* refers to a dynamic interplay between reciprocally connected areas of the brain that "lead to the synchronization of the activity of neuronal groups in different brain maps binding them into circuits capable of temporarily coherent output. Reentry is thus the central mechanism by which the spatiotemporal co-ordination of diverse sensory and motor events takes place" (Edelman & Tononi, 2000, p. 85). Re-entry, then, may be the means by which the coordination occurs that is necessary, in the Jacksonian thesis, for the experience of self to arise.

Verleger (2002) suggests that the temporoparietal junction (TPJ) is critically involved in reentrant processing. This proposal is a plausible one in view of the strategic location of the TPJ, particularly at the angular gyrus. The angular gyrus is situated where the borders of the occipital, parietal, and temporal lobes meet each other, facilitating linkages that would allow (1) coordination between visual and auditory inputs and (2) functions involving language and the "shaping" of sensory data.

Since such coordination is necessary to the moment-to-moment experience of self, it would be anticipated that disruption of a main aspect of the coordinating system would lead to a disturbance of self, at least in some way. This disturbance is manifest in disruptions of the function relating to the TPJ, for example, in epilepsy. The coordination and integration of various aspects of the bodily component of self-experience are apparently lost, leading to an out-of-body experience (Blanke et al., 2004). A growing literature on the role of the TPJ in the creation of the neural network underpinning self is briefly considered in Chapter 6.

It would also be predicted that disruption of the TPJ area would result in disturbance of P3, since this waveform is the outcome of coordination between different sites of neural activity. Verleger remarks that "re-entrant processing is precisely what is damaged in patients with lesions to the temporoparietal junction" (2002, p. 23). This observation is supported by reports that those with lesions in the TPJ area have more severe reductions of P3 than patients with other cortical lesions (Knight et al., 1989; Yamaguchi & Knight, 1991; Verleger et al., 1994; Hagoort, Brown, & Swaab, 1996).

Finally, these various arguments lead to the view that self is the outcome of a coordination between brain areas that is the result of reentrant processes. P3 is the product of the same process as that involved in the generation of self. Seen in this way, P3 is a neural marker of a fundamental feature of self, making it a suitable focus of a neo-Jacksonian hypothesis concerning the brain basis of the ongoing sense of personal being. An outline of a study designed to test this hypothesis is presented in the next chapter.

Chapter 5

A FAILURE OF NEURAL CO-ORDINATION IN BPD
A Study of P3a and P3b

THE ARGUMENT SO FAR is that the central disturbance in BPD is an incoherence of self, a "broken-up-ness" or fragmentation of psychic life, which I am calling *primary dissociation*. Self is conceived according to the hierarchical model of Jackson, laid down through evolutionary history and, in an individual life, the maturational process. Failure in the emergence of self, according to the hypothesis (Meares et al., 1999), is largely due to the characteristic developmental history of abuse and/or neglect in BPD (Zanarini, 2000), impeding such maturation through an inadequate provision of the "sociogenic" component necessary to it (Vygotsky & Luria, 1994).

THE HYPOTHESIS

I am proposing that disturbance of the self is underpinned by a parallel and "concomitant" maturational failure of prefrontally connected neural networks involved in the coordination of different sites of brain activity. P3, as outlined in the previous chapter, provides a means of testing this aspect of the hypothesis, which gives rise to four main predictions. They are that the cerebral functions of those suffering from BPD will exhibit:

1. Diminished coordination (i.e., disconnection) between areas of brain activity that usually operate together
2. A relative failure of higher-order inhibitory systems
3. A relative hypoactivity of prefrontal systems
4. Evidence of maturational arrest

A background to each of these predictions is as follows.

THE FIRST PREDICTION: DISCONNECTION

Some of the background to this prediction was intimated in the previous chapter. P3 is composed of two distinct components: an earlier component, called P3a, and a later component, called P3b. Convergent evidence links P3a with prefrontal-dependent cortical mechanisms of automatic attention, whereas P3b has been distinguished by more goal-directed types of attentional and memorial operations supported by more posterior neural sources (Ford et al., 1994; Soltani & Knight, 2000). Functional relationships between systems producing P3a and P3b appear to reflect coordinated activities in the prefrontal and posterior cortical areas that drive the switching and updating of task sets in working memory (Barcelo et al, 2002).

The idea that P3 is created by the coordination of different generators is relatively recent. Following its discovery by Sutton and coworkers in 1965, it was thought, for some time, to be a monolithic component of the cortical-evoked potential. Two influential experiments (Courchesne et al., 1975; Squires et al., 1975), however, changed the prevailing view. These researchers found that a distinctly deviant, irrelevant stimulus produced an element of P3 that was different from one induced by a relevant stimulus (i.e., a target).

Evidence concerning the areas involved in the different networks responsible for P3a and P3b is provided by the studies of Halgren, Baudena, and their colleagues (Baudena et al., 1995; Halgren et al., 1995a, 1995b). These studies involved the implantation of depth electrodes in the brains of 36 to 39 patients suffering from epilepsy. Recordings were made at 991 to 1,221 sites of responses to target and rare (nontarget) auditory stimuli. The findings were complex, suggesting that the networks underpinning both waveforms depended upon the coordination of multiple brain areas. The networks, however, were clearly different. P3a was particularly related to frontal field activity. Baudena and his coworkers, noting that this activity was distributed in all frontal areas (i.e., dorsolateral, medial, ventral, and pericentral), supposed that they may be localized to small regions within each field, in a "mosaic" fashion. Other sites that appeared to be involved in the P3a network were the posterior cingulate gyrus and the supramarginal gyrus (Baudena et al., 1995) and the superior temporal gyrus (Opitz et al., 1999). The generation of P3b was found to be more focal, mainly parietal and most prominently hippocampal. The superior temporal sulcus was also involved.

Lesion studies also demonstrate the essential difference between the neurocircuits reflected in P3a and P3b. P3b is largely unaffected by prefrontal damage (Soltani & Knight, 2000) whereas P3a is enlarged (Rule, Shimamura, & Knight, 2002).

The hypothesis regarding the brain basis of BPD predicts that the two systems of neural generation reflected in P3a and P3b will no longer properly coordinate. As a consequence, the correlation between P3a and P3b will be diminished or lost, and the monolithic structure of P3 will no longer be displayed. Rather, two peaks will appear.

SECOND AND THIRD PREDICTIONS: DISINHIBITION AND HYPOFRONTALITY

According to a neo-Jacksonian approach, failure of the self system to develop adequately is associated with diminished higher-order neuroinhibition. Polich (2007) has suggested neuroinhibition as an "overarching theoretical mechanism of P300." Inhibitory activity is necessarily recruited in the switching of attention from one event to another. This inhibitory function is reflected in the amplitude of P3a and in its habituation (Friedman & Simpson, 1994). P3a is underpinned by dopaminergic pathways, whereas P3b depends upon norepinephrenic neurotransmission (Barcelo et al., 2002). Subjects with parkinsonian syndrome, who are relatively dopamine depleted, have difficulty in switching attention and exhibit impaired habituation of P3a (Hozumi et al., 2000). There is now a large literature on the role of the prefrontal cortex in neuroinhibition. It particularly focuses on the orbitofrontal cortex (OFC; e.g., Rule et al., 2002). Since BPD characteristically involves disinhibition, as reflected in dysregulation of affective expression and impulse, it has been suggested that deficient function of the OFC may lead to the manifestation of BPD phenomena (e.g., Berlin, Rolls, & Iversen, 2005).

Since failure of inhibition will manifest in P3a in a large amplitude that does not habituate, the second prediction is that this enlargement of P3a will be shown in those with BPD. Since P3a has a mainly prefrontal origin, the prediction is consistent with the view that the disturbance of BPD is particularly prefrontal.

The fourth prediction, concerning maturation, involves a separate study that is addressed later in the chapter.

THE STUDY

When first devised, the ERP seemed to offer great possibilities for the development of our understanding of brain function, since it appeared to show the millisecond-by-millisecond passage of the nervous impulse through the brain. It has, however, proved a disappointing measure with little capacity to distinguish between psychiatric conditions. This is largely a consequence of the standard method of deriving the ERP,, in which numerous stimuli are presented and the electroencephalographic (EEG) responses averaged. The averaging results in "smearing" the data such that crucial detail is lost. What is required is a means of isolating the EEG response to a single stimulus. This is the method used in our study.

P3a and P3b were determined using a single-trial analytic method devised by Dmitri Melkonian and called "fragmentary decomposition" (Melkonian et al., 2003; Melkonian et al., 2001). The data were elicited by means of two oddball tasks—that is, tasks in which the subject is required to respond to unusual stimuli. When elicited in this way, P3a cannot be distinguished from the waveform evoked by infrequent stimuli presented in the context of three oddball tasks, termed the *novelty–P3* (Simons et al., 2001).

The BPD sample consisted of 17 patients who were unmedicated on presentation (Meares, Melkonian, et al., 2005). Such a sample is only gathered slowly and with difficulty, since those with BPD are almost universally highly medicated by the time they reach specialized BPD care. There were 4 men and 13 women with a mean age of 32 (range 20–44 years). The patients were compared with 17 control subjects who had no psychiatric illness and who were matched for age and sex (4 men, 13 women of mean age 34, range 20–47 years) (Meares, Melkonian, et al., 2005).

The subjects were asked to respond "as fast and accurately as possible" to a target tone, presented at 1,500 Hz and comprising 15% of the tones presented, with the background 85% sounded at 1,000 Hz. The method is described in detail in other studies (Lagopoulos et al., 1998; Melkonian et al., 2001; Williams, Brammer, et al., 2000). EEG responses to each target tone were analyzed by the method of fragmentary decomposition, which allows P3a and P3b to be identified in the response to a single stimulus. The responses appear in the latency windows following stimulus presentation of 240–299 ms for P3a and 300–360 ms for P3b (see Figure 5.1).

The findings were in line with the first three predictions derived from the hypothesis, as follows:

1. Disconnection between P3a and P3b was shown by a loss of temporal synchronicity between them. The results of simultaneous correlation analysis indicated statistically significant time locking of P3a and P3b for normal study participants; in contrast, low and nonsignificant degrees of P3a and P3b synchronicity were shown in patients with BPD. These findings suggest a relative failure of coordination between the neural generators of P3a and P3b in these patients. The effect, in the raw data, is to produce a P3 that has two peaks rather than the monophasic form of the normal controls (see Figure 5.2). The statistical method and detailed results are presented in Meares, Melkonian, et al. (2005).

2. The second prediction is supported by the large amplitude of P3a, which suggests a deficiency in higher-order inhibitory activity. Comparisons between the amplitudes of P3a and P3b in the patients with BPD and the control group are shown in Table 5.1.

TABLE 5.1

0	1 PG	2 CG	3 1 vs. 2
P3a, *A*	16.2 (9.14)	12.8 (6.73)	***
P3a, *L*	268 (17.3)	269 (17.6)	ns
P3a, *O*	242 (19.7)	245 (19.5)	*
P3b, *A*	14.9 (8.36)	14.8 (7.5)	ns
P3b, *L*	328 (16.8)	328 (16.5)	ns
P3b, *O*	303 (20.7)	301 (20.7)	ns

Columns 1 and 2 show the mean (SD) of parameters A (peak amplitude, μV), L (peak latency, ms), and O (onset time, ms) listed in column 0 for P3a and P3b. Column 3 shows intergroup comparisons: patient group (PG) vs. control group (CG), respectively. Significance levels: $*p<0/05$; $***p<0.001$; ns – nonsignificant.

The highly significant finding regarding the enlargement of P3a in the right side in patients with BPD compared with control subjects is in contrast to the comparison on the left, which yields no significant difference. The finding is of great interest because it gives support to a proposal, put forward in Chapter 15, that BPD may be a particularly right-hemispheric disorder.

The inference that the large P3a in BPD reflects relative inhibitory failure is further suggested by the absence of P3a habituation in patients with BPD, in contrast to the controls who habituated normally. The supposition that such a deficiency in inhibitory activity is the basis, at least in part, of emotional dysregulation in BPD is approached in a later chapter.

3. The disturbance in the functions reflected by P3 in BPD is manifest in P3a rather than P3b. Since P3a is underpinned by prefrontally connected neurocircuitry, whereas P3b is connected most prominently to parietal regions, the prediction that disturbance of brain function will be most marked in prefrontal activity is supported.

FOURTH PREDICTION: A MATURATIONAL FAILURE

Does the disturbance of brain function shown by patients with BPD have a basis in a maturational failure? A response to this question depended upon a study of P3a in a large normative sample.

The sample was composed of 50 men and 50 women between the ages of 18 and 70 years. There were 10 men and 10 women at each age from 18 to 30, 31 to 40, 41 to 50, 51 to 61, and 61 to 70. Regression analyses of P3a and P3b amplitudes, with age as an independent variable, revealed highly significant rates of decrease with age for both components, with P3b decreasing more slowly. A comparison of these data and those from the patients with BPD suggests that the P3a component in these subjects is abnormally large. Given that the mean age of patients with BPD was 31.6 years, the regression line in Figure 5.3 indicated 12.3 µV as a normative value of P3a peak amplitude in this cohort. The actual mean value was 16.2 µV, which is the amplitude that might be expected in a 13-year-old. (See Figure 5.3.)

These normative data give support to the notion that the manifestations of BPD reflect, at least in part, a certain kind of maturational failure. They are consistent with related current findings that show increasing capacity for response inhibition in subjects ranging from 8 to 20 years of age (Tamm, Menon, & Reiss, 2002) and increasing inhibition and task-switching capability in children 4–13 years old (Davidson et al., 2006). These studies, however, concerned young people only. An impressive study from Lea Williams and her coworkers (Williams, Brown, et al., 2006), covering seven decades, showed that during life there is a "shift towards greater medial prefrontal cortical control over negative emotional input" (p. 6422). Houston et al. (2005) found that the amplitude of P300 diminished in girls between 14 and 19, but this diminishment did not occur in subjects with BPD.

"Specific Circuit" for the Pathophysiology of BPD

The evidence of this study suggests that there is a relative failure of integration of brain function in patients with BPD. Such disconnectedness among neural systems that usually operate together is a plausible basis for the "fragmentation" that is a main feature of psychic life in BPD, and which is an aspect of the "painful incoherence" Wilkinson-Ryan and Westen (2000) found to be the principal disturbance of BPD selfhood.

The findings also suggest that those with BPD live with a persisting failure of higher-order inhibitory activity, which may be the basis, at least in part, of emotional dysregulation in BPD. Since the two disturbances of neurophysiological function are related, the possibility arises that the self-disturbance and emotional dysregulation in BPD are aspects of disruption of the same system. A relationship between the failure of the sense of personal cohesion and deficient sensory and emotional regulation is given experiential support by Rebecca West's story of her psychic mechanism being "hopelessly out of gear." The two disturbances were linked in her sensitive account of her postpyrexial condition. The neurophysiological data also seem consistent with Livesley's (2008) view of the fundamental nature of BPD. He sees a core of self-fragmentation being related, in a complex and systematic way, to emotional dysregulation.

The idea that BPD is manifest as two main disturbances that reflect the activity of a single system of neurocircuitry has some resonance with the proposal of Michael Posner and his colleagues (2002). They suggested that a "specific circuit" underlies the symptomatology of BPD, with an attentional deficit being the basis to the disorder. Janet had also remarked that disturbance of attention was a central feature of hysteria. He indicated that the disturbance to the sense of self-cohesion is related to attentional incompetence. Attention is an aspect of, and cannot be separated from, the capacity to create coherence from the multitude of sensory impressions impinging upon us at any moment. One of his patients, for example, could not dance and look at the other dancers' costumes at the same time. She had a diminished capacity to coordinate sensory expressions with movement in the creation of "personal synthesis" (pp. 148–149). Another example showed a more complex failure of coordination. His subject could read aloud a passage from a newspaper when asked to, but could not afterwards relate an understanding of it (p. 29). Whereas Janet related attention deficit in hysteria to a failure of "personal synthesis," Posner and his colleagues related a failure of attentional control to a disturbance of the emotion regulating system.

The possibility that emotion regulation is related to attentional processing is suggested by neuroanatomy. The prefrontal cortex can be seen as consisting of two main regions: the dorsolateral and the ventromedial areas. As Williams and her colleagues (Williams, Phillips, et al., 2001) remark, the latter is part of a medial processing system that is concerned with "feeling," whereas the former is an element of a lateral system dealing with "facts."

The medial processing system is concerned not only with emotion but with attention. As we have seen, the ventromedial and orbitofrontal prefrontal cortices are part of the attentional processing reflected in P3a. These regions are part of a frontostriatal circuit that has strong connections to the amygdala, to other parts of the limbic system, and the autonomic nervous system. The orienting response, as a consequence of this connection, is manifest not only in the P3a but in autonomic responses, notably the electrodermal response. They may be considered, together with the P3a, "as constituting different parts of an overall organismic orienting complex evoked by stimuli that merit further evaluation" (Halgren, 1995a, p. 215). The connections made by this neurocircuitry are anatomically well suited to the integration of affective and nonaffective information and to regulation of response to this information (Happaney et al., 2004). Damage to the orbitofrontal cortex results not only in attentional disturbance, as reflected in P3a, but also in affective disturbances such as emotional lability and decreased impulse control (Knight et al., 1995). Damage in this area may also be the basis of autonomic disturbance in BPD, a possibility that is considered in Chapter 13. The medial system necessarily functions in coordination with the lateral system, which has more cognitive functions.

The relationship between attentional and emotional processing systems has implications larger than the particulars of this relationship alone, because it is involved in the creation of those fundamental experiences of meaning that are central to what we call *self*. The orienting response is not simply made on the basis of a cognitive judgment; feeling is necessary to this judgment. The attribution of familiar or strange to a particular stimulus comes with the *feeling* of familiarity or strangeness. The matching process upon which the orienting depends is an aspect of a continuing activity, necessary to everyday existence, in which events of the present are compared with models of similar event experiences in the past. Out of this comparison comes a large and complex array of emotions that gives rise to specific meanings. The hippocampus is necessary to this matching process (Kumaran & Maguire, 2007; Vinogradova, 2001).

The notion that attention, emotion, and self share aspects of a common circuitry of midline brain structures is consistent with the view of the so-called "materialist" philosopher David Armstrong, who pointed out that self cannot be considered as one among a range of mental states and activities but as the totality of the functions and experiences that make up mental life (Armstrong, 1981, p. 65). Under such circumstances, disturbances in primary functions such as attention and emotional regulation will necessarily be associated with self, seen as the ongoing, moment-to-moment sense of personal existing. The relationship between the experience of self and cortical midline structures is discussed in the following chapter.

These remarks lead us back to the proposal of Posner and his colleagues (2002) that a "specific circuit" underpins BPD pathology. Something of the nature of this specific circuit might be inferred from the results of our ERP study. Comparison between the ERP profiles of subjects with BPD and controls showed no significant difference in any of the components apart from P3a. In particular, P3b was unaffected. The exception to this generalization was N2, the component preceding P3a to which it is closely linked. The elicitation of N2–P3a occurs at the stage when the initial processing of sensory information is followed by the detection of the stimulus attributes (Polich, 2004). The particularity of disturbance in our ERP data suggests that large P3a amplitudes may be a marker of Posner et al.'s specific circuit and that its phase of activity during sensory processing is reflected in the time window of 240–300 ms poststimulus, which is when P3a appears.

Role of the Orbitofrontal Cortex

The results of our study (Meares, Melkonian, et al., 2005) suggest that brain function, as reflected in the P3 (mainly in P3a), has gone awry in BPD. The studies of Robert Knight and his colleagues implicate dysfunction of the orbitofrontal cortex (OFC) in this disturbance (Rule et al., 2002). As Elliott, Dolan, and Frith (2000) point out, the OFC has dissociable and opposing functions. It has both excitatory and inhibitory, or orienting and suppressive, functions that generated in different parts of the OFC. It is apparent from the P3a data that the inhibitory aspect is defective in BPD, resulting in the excitatory system showing hyperactivity. The large amplitude of P3a is consistent with the hypervigilance characteristic of the traumatized individual.

The OFC is generally defined as the area of cortex on the ventral surface of the frontal cortex, overlying the roof of the orbit. This region includes Brodmann's areas (BA) 11, 12, and 47. The studies of Knight and his group focused on BA11, the area directly overlying the roof of the orbit. They found that lesions in this area produced enhanced P3 waveforms that did not habituate to the presentation of repeated stimuli (Rule et al., 2002). Thus, OFC damage reproduces the disturbances in P3a demonstrated in a group of patients suffering from BPD (Meares, Melkonian, et al., 2005).

As Rule et al. (2002) point out, Damasio (1998) refers to the OFC as the prefrontal ventromedial cortex (PFC). His studies have stimulated an interest in the role of the orbitofrontal and prefrontal cortices in the neurocircuitry necessary to the experience of self. Damasio uses the example of Phineas Gage, a 19th-century railway worker injured in an accident with explosives. A reconstruction of his injury suggested that the prefrontal ventromedial cortex had been damaged whereas the lateral aspects of the prefrontal cortex were preserved (Damasio et al., 1996). Gage displayed symptoms consistent with a loss of inhibitory control: that is, emotional outbursts, impulsivity, and socially inappropriate behavior.

Without, in the usual case, mentioning the sense of self, a number of investigators have highlighted the significance of the role of the OFC, together with the anterior cingulate (ACC), in the genesis of BPD. The volumetric study of Tebartz van Elst (2003) showed 24% reduction of the left OFC and a 26% reduction of the right ACC in those with BPD. Hazlett et al. (2005) also found a reduction in ACC volume in those with BPD at BA24. Minzenberg et al. (2008) reported a volume reduction in the subgenual cingulate. Lyoo et al. (1998) found smaller frontal volumes in those with BPD compared with healthy comparison subjects. Vollm et al. (2009) found gray matter deficits in prefrontal areas in those with BPD.

Functional studies are consistent with the possibility that areas of volume reduction are a consequence of relative inactivity of these sites of brain activity. Soloff et al. (2003), for example, in a positron emission tomography (PET) study of BPD found that subjects suffering from the disorder were hypometabolic bilaterally in the medial orbitofrontal cortex, including BA9, 10, and 11. Schmahl, Vermetten, et al. (2004) recorded the brain blood flow by means of PET in traumatized women with BPD, who, during the recording, listened to scripts describing traumatic events. Compared to women without BPD, the subjects with BPD failed to activate the OFC and the anterior cingulate cortex. Earlier PET studies also showed hypometabolism in the frontal cortex in BPD (De La Fuente et al., 1997; Goyer et al., 1994). In the latter study the areas affected were the premotor and prefrontal cortex, the ACC, and the caudate and lenticular nuclei.

Data of a different kind, based on psychological tests, led Blair (2004) and Berlin et al. (2005) to propose a specific disturbance of brain function related to the OFC as a basis for certain symptomatology of BPD, particularly to do with dysregulation. Blair's work indicated that reactive aggression is associated with orbitofrontal damage.

A TWO-STAGE GENESIS OF BPD PHENOMENA?

The clarity, however, of the evidence concerning the origins of BPD in dysfunction of the OFC is clouded by the findings of magnetic resonance imaging (MRI) studies, which suggest that other areas of the brain are also likely to play a part in the neurocircuitry that functions deficiently in BPD. Volume reductions have been reported in the amygdala (Driessen et al., 2000; Rusch et al., 2003; Tebartz van Elst et al., 2003); the hippocampus (Brambilla et al., 2004; Driessen et al., 2000; Irle et al., 2005; Schmahl et al., 2003; Tebartz van Elst, 2003); the frontal, temporal, and parietal cortices in men with BPD (Vollm et al., 2009), and the parietal cortex in women with BPD (Irle et al., 2005). A difficulty in interpreting the significance of these various findings is that in those suffering from BPD, the (1) duration and effects of the illness and (2) its consequences in terms of treatment, overdoses, cumulative traumata, and co-occurrence of other mental disorders may have confounding effects on brain morphology. In order to overcome these possible confounding effects, Andrew Chanen and his colleagues (2007) conducted a study on first-presentation teenage subjects. Twenty patients with BPD were compared with 20 healthy controls. The BPD group had right-sided gray matter loss in the OFC but no changes were found in amygdaloid or hippocampal volumes.

A study of a similar kind, with 60 female adolescents, also showed no volumetric change in the hippocampal or amygdaloid areas (Brunner et al., 2010). As Chanen and his colleagues had found, reductions in the gray matter of the OFC were evident. In Brunner et al.'s study, however, the changes were left-sided. Although this possibility was not discussed by these investigators, the difference in lateralization might be explained by difference in the composition of the two samples in terms of gender. This idea is given some support from a small study from Tranel et al. (2005). They had previously concluded that the right-sided prefrontal ventromedial cortices were critical for emotional procession and decision making, whereas the left side appeared to play a less important role (Tranel et al., 2002). The sample for this study was almost entirely male. In their follow-up study in 2005, the investigators included women in their sample. They concluded that the situation in males was reversed in females. The defects in function for women followed left-sided damage. The Chanen sample and adolescents, made up of 15 females and 5 males, differed from the sample of 60 females in the Brunner study. Although the number of males in Chanen's cohort was small, the hypothesis arises that their inclusion altered the lateralization of the findings. Our sample of patients with BPD had a ratio of female to male (13:4) similar to the Chanen cohort. Our findings of a right-sided functional deficit mirror the structural changes they had found.

In a later study from the Melbourne group (Whittle et al., 2009), a smaller left ACC was found in 15 adolescent girls with BPD. This finding is given support by the findings of Goodman et al. (2010), which showed diminished volume of the ACC (BA24) in a group of adolescents with BPD. BA24 is particularly implicated in the ability to suppress pain and painful emotion. It is activated, for example, during pain reduction following use of placebo (Petrovic et al., 2005). It has connections with both the OFC and the amygdala (Bush et al., 2000). Goodman et al. (2010), referring to Vogt et al. (1992), note that BA24 has a principal attentional function which concerns the significance of sensory data and their regulation.

The difference between early and late structural changes in BPD suggests the possibility of a two-stage genesis of the disorder. This possibility can be considered in the light of our own findings, particularly the loss of significant correlation between the onset times of P3a and P3b in BPD. This difference from healthy controls can be understood as a failure of coordination between two systems of neurocircuitry that usually function together. One of these has a large prefrontal contribution, whereas the other is particularly parietal. The hippocampus is its main generator. Usually, but not always, the activity of the earlier prefrontal generation, shown as P3a, is followed by the parietal–hippocampal P3b. If, however, the connection between them is lost, it may be that the appearance of P3b is triggered less frequently than normal. Our preliminary evidence, from an article in preparation, suggests that this may be so. Relative inactivity may cause the hippocampal system to atrophy.

The notion that diminished hippocampal volumes in BPD may be the result of relative underactivity must be considered in relation to reports suggesting a toxic cause, derived from observations that severe stress caused hippocampal damage in monkeys. This damage was believed to be the effect of prolonged glucocorticoid exposure (Sapolsky et al., 1990). Bremner and his colleagues (1997) proposed that this is the basis of diminished hippocampal volumes found in those with PTSD. The explanation, however, of hippocampal atrophy and its relationship to "stress" is not yet clear (Lupien et al., 2009). Why, for example, is the hippocampus particularly vulnerable? And why is hippocampal atrophy not found in children and adolescents who suffer from PTSD following maltreatment (Jackowski et al., 2009; Mehta et al., 2009; Woon & Hedges, 2008)? In contrast, as McCrory, De Brito, and Viding (2010) note in their review of the issue, reduced volume of the hippocampus has generally been reported for adults who have experienced maltreatment as children (Vermetten et al., 2006; Vythilingam et al., 2002; Woon & Hedges, 2008).

The two-stage hypothesis depends upon the following speculations:

- The main proposal is that the volumetric changes are the result of relative inactivity in the affected areas. In the first stage this may be the result of a failure of connection that is "external"—that is, between the child and the caregivers. This possibility is discussed briefly in Chapter 16.
- In the second stage of BPD genesis the disconnection is seen as internal, due to the effect of the first stage in disrupting the maturation of the neurocircuitry involving that prefrontal connections necessary to the neural circuitry of the attentional and emotional processes that give rise to the experience of self.

The volumetric losses in cerebral tissue following maltreatment in children are different from the changes in adults. No adequate explanation for these differences is currently available. The outstanding difference is that whereas maltreatment is associated with smaller hippocampal volume in adults, the most salient finding in children is a decrease in the corpus callosum (De Bellis et al., 1999, 2002; De Bellis & Kuchibhatla, 2006; Jackowski et al., 2008; Teicher et al., 2004), consistent with a relative failure of interhemispheric connection. Although it is not consistently replicated (Zanetti et al., 2007), this finding of diminished corpus callosum thickness is also demonstrated in adult patients with BPD (Reisch et al., 2008). Takahashi and colleagues (2009) remark that this finding "further implicates the role of impaired hemispheric connectivity in the neurobiology of BPD" (p. 842). Their study demonstrated another kind of apparent disconnection between hemispheres: The adhesio interthalamica, a midline structure connecting the medial surfaces of the thalami, was significantly shorter in teenagers with BPD than in controls.

A history of maltreatment as a child cannot be equated to BPD. Nevertheless, since they are related, the data concerning maltreated children are relevant. In addition to the corpus callosum changes, maltreated children and adolescents have decreased cerebellar volumes (Carrion, 2009; De Bellis & Kuchibhatla, 2006).

Findings for prefrontal changes in maltreated children are equivocal (McCrory et al., 2010). The differences in volumetric changes in brain tissues between maltreated children and adults who were once maltreated are explained, at least in part, by children's immature prefrontal function. This immature development may lead to somewhat different connections in the neurocircuitry underpinning the perceptual and emotional processing.

THE EFFECT OF DISCONNECTION ON AMYGDALOID ACTIVITY

Data regarding the structure and function of the amygdala have played a large part in an emergent disconnection theory of BPD that is particularly focused on the frontolimbic system. An influential study by Sabine Herpertz and her colleagues (2001) provided evidence in this regard. Their findings showed overactivation of the amygdala in six patients with BPD, as compared with six controls, in response to standardized aversive slides. This finding has been replicated a number of times. A possible explanation for these observations is that the inhibitory activity of the PFC, which controls the amygdala, is ineffective in those with BPD.

The inhibitory aspect of prefrontal function has been particularly linked to the OFC (i.e., the ventral aspect of the PFC) at BA11. The amygdala and the OFC are anatomically and functionally related (Amaral & Price, 1984). The OFC has a central role in modulating limbic response to threat (Davidson et al., 2000). As previously noted, Damasio has shown that damage to the OFC is associated with poor emotional and impulse control (Damasio, 1996). Subjects with BPD who have poor control of aggression have been shown to exhibit exaggerated amygdaloid reactivity and diminished OFC activation to faces expressing anger (Coccaro et al., 2007).

Despite the general conclusion regarding the overactivity of the amygdala in BPD, the structural and functional findings are not entirely consistent. In terms of volumetric change, the most common finding is a reduction in the size of the amygdala (Driessen et al., 2000; Schmahl et al., 2003; Tebartz van Elst et al., 2003). On the other hand, Brambilla et al. (2004) found no evidence of decreased amygdaloid volume in those with BPD. Furthermore, Minzenberg et al. (2008) found an increase in gray matter concentration in the amygdala in those with BPD. Like Herpertz et al. (2001) and Donegan et al. (2003), they had previously found exaggerated responses to social and emotional stimuli in the amygdalas of people with BPD (Minzenberg et al., 2007).

Findings regarding loss of cerebral tissue are not unique to BPD. Volumetric reduction in the hippocampus is also found in people with PTSD (Karl et al., 2006; Smith, 2005). Meta-analysis also revealed minor size reductions of the left amygdala in patients with PTSD, but no amygdala size reduction in trauma-exposed patients without PTSD (Karl et al., 2006; Smith, 2005). Reduced hippocampal size has also been found in major depression (e.g., Bremner et al., 2000; Frodl et al., 2002; Lange & Irle, 2004; MacQueen et al., 2003; Mervaala et al., 2000; Shah et al., 1998., Sheline et al., 1996, 1999) but not generally in bipolar I disorder (e.g., Altshuler et al., 1998; Hauser et al., 2000; Pearlson et al., 1997; Strakowski et al., 1999). Amygdaloid volumes are reported as both normal in depression (Mervaala et al., 2000; Sheline et al., 1999) and as enlarged (Bremner et al., 2000; Lange & Irle, 2004).

IS THE DISCONNECTION BETWEEN P3A AND P3B RELATED TO DISSOCIATION?

The consistent finding emerging from this data concerns hippocampal size reduction. A meta-analysis suggests that the reduction is likely to be greater when BPD coexists with PTSD (Rodrigues et al., 2010). The possibility arises, then, that what is common to these disorders is one effect of trauma—and this effect may be dissociation. We tested the hypothesis that the finding of neural disconnection, evident in P3a and P3b in people with BPD, would be also be exhibited in a group of patients who dissociate. Twenty-five patients with PTSD and low dissociation scores were compared with another group of 16 patients with PTSD who scored high in a measure of dissociation using the same methods as were used in the study of patients with BPD described earlier in the chapter. Those patients who scored high on dissociation showed the same failure of coordination in onset times of P3a and P3b as those with BPD. They also had enlarged P3a amplitudes that did habituate, replicating the findings in BPD (Meares, Melkonian et al., 2011).

This finding—that dissociative patients show the same electrophysiological stigmata, at least as concerns P3a and P3b, as those with BPD—suggests that this disturbance reflects an aspect of the pathophysiology of dissociation. Unfortunately, dissociation scores in our patients with BPD were not available.

SUMMARY

This chapter has considered the possibility that the "painful incoherence" or disconnectedness among the elements of psychic life identified by Tess Wilkinson-Ryan and Drew Westen (2000) as the main feature of self-identity disturbance in BPD is underpinned by "concomitant" disconnection between brain systems that usually function together. This hypothesis was tested using an innovative method of analysis of single trials of ERPs, in particular, that aspect of the response appearing about 300 ms following stimulus presentation (i.e., P3). This waveform is generated by two main generators that produce the two parts of the waveform that are usually coordinated to give a single output.

The hypothesis predicted that in BPD the two generators do not function together. The hypothesis was confirmed. The onset times of P3a and P3b were not significantly correlated, in contrast to a control group whose onset times were correlated.

A related hypothesis was also tested. Neo-Jacksonian theory predicts that failure of coordination among brain systems will be associated with a deficiency of higher-order inhibitory control, which is an aspect of prefrontal hypofunction. The amplitude of P3a provides a way of testing this hypothesis since large amplitudes reflect inhibitory inactivity, if this is supported by habituation failure of P3a. Those with BPD showed significantly larger P3a amplitudes than controls, and those larger amplitudes did not habituate, in contrast to controls. A prefrontal origin of this disturbance is suggested by the fact that P3a depends upon prefrontally connected circuitry whereas P3b is parietally connected.

P3a is an important reflection of the attentional system. It is the cortical component of an overall organismic orienting reflex. The circuitry underpinning this system necessarily overlaps with that involved in the emotion processing that is central to the experience of selfhood, the matrix of which may depend upon the same midline structures as those necessary to attentional and emotional processing (Chapter 6).

The discussion focuses on the possibility that the main deficit in the production of a large and nonhabituating P3a is centered on the PFC, particularly BA11. A failure in this area, Damasio has suggested, fundamentally disrupts the development of self. Our data suggest that this disturbance might be particularly right-hemispheric, since our subjects with BPD showed a difference from controls in P3a only on the right side. This matter is further considered in Chapter 15.

Our findings appear to be resonant with those from Chanen et al. (2007). Whereas we found a right-sided deficiency of the prefrontal–orbitofrontal neurocircuitry productive of P3a, they found volumetric deficits in the right prefrontal–orbitofrontal cortices of young patients with BPD. Older patients with BPD, however, have more widespread deficits, including hippocampal shrinkage. The difference between older and younger groups gives rise to the proposal that the genesis of BPD is a two-stage affair. The first stage involves an external disconnection, in which a crucial form of responsiveness, which I term "analogical relatedness" (see Chapter 16), is not provided by caregivers. The second stage is one of inner disconnectedness, in which a maturation failure of specific neurocircuitry involving the PFC and OFC, and also BA24 of the ACC, results in connection failure among brain systems, which, in normal individuals, are connected and coordinated in function.

This idea implies a maturational hypothesis for the origins of BPD. This hypothesis was also tested in our *NeuroReport* study (Meares, Melkonian, et al., 2005). We found that the P3a in subjects with BPD had an amplitude similar to that of a preadolescent child, giving support to the hypothesis.

Finally, since I am suggesting that the subtle disturbances of brain function in BPD are reflected in the phenomenon of dissociation, it was necessary to consider whether these characteristic disturbances were associated with scores for dissociation. Since this information was not available from our subjects, a separate study was performed. A comparison was made between subjects with PTSD judged as dissociators and subjects with PTSD who did not dissociate. Those who dissociated showed the same disturbances of P3a and P3b coordination and enlarged P3a as did patients with BPD.

Chapter 6

A NEURAL NETWORK FOR THE MATRIX OF SELF

In the previous chapters the proposal has been put forward that the core of BPD is a sense of discontinuity in personal being, a feeling of "painful incoherence," a state arising from a form of brain activity in which the usual coordination between areas of neural function is diminished. In common parlance, those affected with BPD lack a cohesive self. This idea, however, provokes a question: How can the notion of the fragmentation of self be conceived, first of all in an experiential sense, and secondly in terms of neural function? The question, then, has two parts. The attempted answer is also necessarily double, leading to a division of this chapter into two main themes.

SUBJECT AND OBJECT CONSCIOUSNESS

One way of answering the first part of the question depends upon a description of personal experience. In order to begin this consideration, we must return to the descriptions of our ongoing sense of personal existence given by William James, and to those of his predecessor, Hughlings Jackson.

James's background was unusual for a philosopher/psychologist. His first professional appointment was as a physiologist. One of his initiatives, upon being appointed professor of psychology at Harvard in 1875, was to set up the first physiological psychology laboratory in the world. His view that self is an effect of brain function, which was by no means universal in those days, presumably led him to the writings of Hughlings Jackson. We cannot know the extent of Jackson's influence upon James. Nevertheless, James's "duplex self" seems, at first reading, to be a more complex and better described version of Jackson's double self. Jackson was very struck by the notion of the duality in higher-order consciousness, noting, for example, that humor typically reflects the manifestation of such duality (Jackson, 1958, II, pp. 359–364). Seen in this way, humor is a sign of maturity, of the emergence of selfhood.

William James had corresponded with Jackson, met him, and quoted him extensively in his major work of 1890. He added experiential flesh to Jackson's skeletal model of self. There was, however, a subtle and important difference between them. The doubleness of which Jackson wrote was slightly but significantly changed in James's description of a "duplex self," which was composed of an "I" and a "me." James wrote:

> Whatever I may be thinking of I am always at the same time more or less aware of myself, of my personal existence. At the same time, it is I who am aware; so that the total self of me, being as it were duplex, partly known and partly knower, partly object and partly subject, must have two aspects discriminated in it, of which for shortness we may call one the Me and the other I. (James, 1892, p. 176)

There is no "me" in Jackson's definition.

A problem now arises in the Jamesian concept. In his description of self, James has two different kinds of "me." The first is inner, the "stream of our personal consciousness" (1890, I, p. 296), which is "identified with the self more than any outward thing" (1890, I, p. 297). The other is outer, "a man's social self," "the recognition which he gets from his mates" (1890, I, p. 293) who "carry an image of him in their mind" (1890, I, p. 294). Together they make up the Janus-faced nature of personal reality, contained, as it were, by the body, which is recognized by the world and in which is figuratively located the flow of feelings, ideas, memories, imaginings, and so forth, which make up the flux of inner life.

Just as there are two main aspects of "me," which in ordinary existence are seamlessly connected, so also there must be two main states of the "I" that are necessarily coordinated. The difference between the two states of "me" is evident in the lives of those suffering from BPD in whom the inner aspect is characteristically ill developed. These individuals complain of a sense of hollowness in living, an emptiness, a feeling that nothing is happening, and that in some way, difficult to formulate, an element of selfhood is lacking. At the same time, they may maintain, sometimes to the point of desperation, a way of being seen by others which, for them, is adaptive, providing some form of compensation for this lack.

James did not contemplate the significance of his distinction between different kinds of "me" in evolutionary or developmental terms. Nor did he consider the idea that, since "I" and "me" are irrevocably linked together, not only must there be at least two main kinds of "me," there must also be a similar number of "I" forms. The difficulty of conceiving multiple "I's" can be approached by means of the Jacksonian hierarchy.

In talking of such a hierarchy, it is convenient to use the three-tiered concept of brain organization used by both Jackson and Maclean, while recognizing, as they did, that it is a simplification. The brain hierarchy gives rise to a hierarchy of consciousness that can also be envisioned as three-tiered, as Tulving did. Each level of consciousness is an aspect of a form of relatedness with the environment when this concerns others. The relatedness and interplay are mediated by language, which is, at first, merely a language of signs. This sign language grows into a language in which symbols are used and a syntax develops and in which "I" and "me" are spoken. Before this stage they might be understood as implicit.

A baby has an "I," as a system of awareness, at birth or earlier. The "me," at this stage, is sensorimotor. Babies presumably know, in some way, that the hands they see moving before them are theirs. Beyond the bodily "me" is a social "me," which becomes manifest at about 18–24 months, when, as a number of experiments have shown, the child can point to a figure in a photograph or a mirror and say, "That's me" (Amsterdam, 1972; Lewis & Brooks-Gunn, 1979). An enlarged and more complex relationship with others emerges that involves emotions such as shame and embarrassment (Lewis, 1992). The child is now vulnerable to the pain of public exposure.

The social emotions are not entirely new. Rather, they are "compounded," to use Jackson's word, with earlier, more fundamental states of pain and distress so that the pain of humiliation is not to be understood as merely "psychic" but as containing the original feeling of "physical" pain (Eisenberger, Lieberman, & Williams, 2003). The "me" and the "I" are also compounded, containing the basic sensorimotor reality. The child at this stage, however, does not use the word *I*.

The third tier of the "I–me" system emerges rather late, at about the age of 4, when the child discovers the experience of innerness, manifest in his or her attainment of the concept of secrecy (Meares & Orlay, 1988). The child can say "I know a secret," using "I" in a statement implying an awareness of a personal zone that is distinct from the public world and the sense that certain experiences are uniquely one's own. The vulnerability to exposure now extends to include that which is sensed as private.

The compounding of "me" becomes more complex with the emergence of a sense of an inner life. There is, beyond an ongoing bodily reality and the "me" that is "who-one-is-in-the-world," a third experience that relates to that which is inner. It is implicit in the following statement in which *myself* is another form of *me*: "I was not myself when you saw me last" (for a further discussion, see Meares, 2000). The sense of the public "me" who appears to the world is usually called *identity*. The composite term *self–identity* suitably describes the compounded nature of personal reality, which is both public and private life.

The three-tiered schema of personal reality suggests three main aspects of "me," which in ordinary existence are seamlessly connected. There must also be three main states of the "I" that are necessarily coordinated with "me" states. Jackson's approach to this complexity is, at first sight, contradictory but on further reflection, intriguing. First of all, as noted in Chapter 4, he identified self by the capacity for introspection—which is, in his terminology, a particular kind of object consciousness.

The concept of object consciousness resembles some accounts of Franz Brentano's concept of "intentionality," "the direction of the mind on an object." *Intentionality* is a technical term that has "nothing special to do with intentions, though intentions do have intentionality" (Armstrong, 1999, p. 7). A key feature of an intentional state is that it points beyond self; it is "about" something (Armstrong, 1999, p. 139). For Brentano, intentionality was the special mark of the mental realm. But this awareness is not the same as self.

During much of the 20th century intentionality became a cardinal feature of conceptions of personal existing or self. Freud's ego, for example, is an intentional mechanism, as described in his final definition (Freud, 1939, pp. 145–146). Freud had attended Brentano's lectures at the University of Vienna for a couple of years (Jones, 1953, p. 61). Jackson's viewpoint was somewhat revolutionary, moving against a current orthodoxy. He remarked that although object consciousness is what is commonly called consciousness (1958, p. 96), it is insufficient, in itself, as a basis of self. Consciousness in its intentional, or object, mode is not self itself, but a revealing of self (Jackson, 1958, II, p. 96), its realization. An experience of personal existing made up purely of object consciousness would not be a self state. As critics of the ego concept have observed, it leaves no room for self (Rycroft, 1972, p. 149). Personal experience constructed simply of object consciousness would be broken up and atomized, a clutter of successive states directed toward stimuli, either external or internal, without any connection among them. It would be a condition lacking the qualities of cohesion and continuity that are central to the ordinary feeling of existing.

Not all states of mind, however, are intentional. Some are not directed toward, or focused upon, an object but involve a more general awareness, an implicit characteristic of the background state of "going-on-being" that is Jackson's subject consciousness. In Jackson's view, this is the source of self. He describes subject consciousness in the following way:

> Subject consciousness is something deeper than knowledge; it is that by which knowledge is possible. Perhaps we may say that it is an awareness of our existence as individuals, as persons having the object states making up for each, the (his) Universe; it is us in an emphatic sense. Subject consciousness is the comparatively unchanging, the most unchanging. It is thus a constant to object consciousness which is the continually changing. Most unchanging, that to which all more changing is relative, is the same as unchanging. (Jackson, 1958, II, p. 96)

This passage leads us to the intriguing, even mysterious, difference from the Jamesian "duplex self." Subject consciousness seems to be analogous to the "stream of consciousness" that James called "me." Jackson, however, has it symbolized by "I." Yet the "I" is also necessary to object consciousness. Jackson presents a paradox, seeming to make the "I" an aspect of both object and subject consciousness. He implies, perhaps, that something within subject consciousness grasps an aspect of it in the creation of object consciousness. Despite its difficulty, Jackson's concept of subject consciousness as the fundamental form of self gives us a way of conceiving personal fragmentation or failure of cohesion.

James's writings are very much in the spirit of the Jacksonian concept, but the impression remains that he did not resolve the logical problem of conceiving as duplex a unitary state of personal existing. Nevertheless, he wrote about the implausibility of a personal reality depending upon an intentional stance alone by making an analogy between the passage of states of consciousness and going for a walk. His language is amusing, as if he is enjoying himself, which adds to the pleasure of reading him. He wrote: "Now the most general way of contrasting my view of knowledge with the popular view (which is also the view of most epistemologists) is to call my view ambulatory, and the other view saltatory" (James, 1909/1996, p. 139). *Saltate* is a rare verb meaning "to leap, jump, or skip." James suggests, consistent with his stream metaphor, that although we may focus on successive objects or ideas, reality is not made up of a series of jumps with nothing between them, but rather includes "the intermediaries which in their concrete particularity form a bridge" (1909/1996, p. 143) linking individual perceptions and ideas, and which are part of, and contribute to, the reality of the foci. "My thesis is that the knowing here is *made* by the ambulation through the intervening experiences" (James, 1909/1996, p. 141).

The saltatory argument is a consequence of the view that "the anatomy of the world is logical" (James, 1909/1996, p. 58). James wanted to replace this view with a way of understanding living processes, including human reality, which was more organic and influenced by evolutionary thought. His contemplations on the intervening experiences through which the mind ambles between specific perceptions and ideas were consistent with his pluralistic view of reality. His description suggests that consciousness is not singular but comprised of at least two kinds, one of which is intentional. His description mirrors Jackson's more explicit concept of consciousness as the coordination of subject and object modes, which have different forms. James was saying that it is the form of consciousness discovered through an "ambulatory" attitude that is fundamental, and which resembles the Jacksonian subject consciousness.

It is implicit in the descriptions of the two forms of consciousness given by Jackson and James that it is subject consciousness that is continuing and cohesive. It is the basis of our feeling that, although our mental states are constantly shifting, there remains the sense that we are the selfsame person who endures from day to day. The origin of states of fragmentation, it might be supposed, is to be understood in terms of a disturbance in subject consciousness.

In the next section I propose that the two different kinds of consciousness are manifest as different language forms that reflect two qualitatively different states of mind. I call the ongoing and enduring form of consciousness *analogical*. Jackson made the tentative suggestion that subject consciousness depends upon the right hemisphere. This proposal has important implications for understanding the basis of BPD and is approached later in this book, where I suggest that the unifying factor in the coherence of personal being is an analogical mode of thinking (Meares & Jones, 2009) and that this mode of thought is based in right-hemispheric function.

TWO MODES OF THOUGHT AND LANGUAGE

Human speech has two main forms, both described by Piaget (1959) and Vygotsky (1962). They derived their descriptions from observations of child language. The most salient speech form is language of intentionality, which Piaget called "directed-thought":

> Direct thought is conscious, that is, it pursues an aim which is present to the mind of the thinker, it is intelligent, which means that it is adapted to reality and tries to influence it, it admits of being true or false (empirically or logically true) and it can be communicated by language. (Piaget, 1959, p. 43)

This kind of speech is social. It has a communicative purpose and is intelligible. Depending upon syntax, its form is linear, and the connections between its elements are relatively clear. It reflects a state of mind that can be called logical.

The second form of verbal expression Vygotsky (1962) called "inner speech." He wrote: "Our experiments convinced us that inner speech must be regarded, not as speech minus sound, but as an entirely separate speech function. Its main distinguishing trait is its peculiar language. Compared with external speech, inner speech appears disconnected and incomplete" (pp. 138–139). Inner speech might be conceived, somewhat paradoxically, as right-hemispheric language. The right hemisphere is usually considered to have no place in speech production. Damage to the right half of the brain does not interfere with the capacity for speech, whereas left-hemispheric damage may render the subject mute. Nevertheless, there remains a capacity for brief, automatic, and emotional utterances. The subject may be able to sing or to express him- or herself tonally, (Jackson, 1958, II, pp. 129–145). Right-hemispheric damage may involve loss of the musical qualities of language, the use of tones, and the way that words are inflected.

The clear distinctions made between the function of the right and left hemispheres are somewhat artificial, since they are based on pathological situations such as cerebral damage and section of the corpus callosum, whereas ordinary function involves the whole brain working in a coordinated way. Nevertheless, a distinction made in terms of musicality seems to involve the right hemisphere in a fundamental way. Daniel Levitin (2007), writing about the neurological basis of music, states: "We've found lateralization in the brain basis of music as well. The overall contour of melody—simply its melodic shape, while ignoring intervals—is processed in the right hemisphere, as is making discriminations of tones that are close together in pitch" (p. 125). He further noted: "Isabelle Peretz discussed that the right hemisphere of the brain contains a contour analyser that in effect draws an outline of a melody and analyzes it for later recognition" (p. 173). The "shaping" function of the right hemisphere gives "inner speech" its peculiar characteristic—the way in which its elements are connected.

Inner speech is found in relatively pure form in the language of the child during symbolic play, which goes on from time to time in that period of life that Winnicott (1971) called "transitional." The chattering that accompanies this activity seems, at first sight, disconnected. Whereas social speech involves connections that are intelligible, in that one thing follows another as things are connected in the world (i.e., in succession), in "inner speech" the connections are not immediately clear because they are typically made by analogy and other associations. The discovery of analogy depends upon the discernment of resemblance, particularly of shape. An analogy, as mentioned earlier in the book, is a thing that has a shape, or proportion, similar to another thing. The analogical mode of thought that is the basis of "inner speech" is reflected in the objects the child chooses in symbolic play to represent the little story that is being told. A tumbler lying on its side, for example, is a rabbit burrow, and a rolled-up ball of white paper is the rabbit.

Analogical and logical modes of thought can operate relatively independently in early life but become coordinated at about the time that the experience of self is discovered—that is, between 3½ and 5½ years of age. Ordinary language now comprises two different speech forms that are seamlessly integrated. The linear form of social speech is the vehicle for another, nonlinear language form, which is more particularly related to the zone of the personal (Meares, 1993a). The difference between logical and analogical modes of thought are reviewed in Chapter 16 in relation to the treatment of BPD.

The way in which language arises from its double basis must be a matter of conjecture, to some extent at least,. Nevertheless, both Jackson and Damasio agree that "the process of verbalizing is dual: the second half of it being speech" (Jackson, 1958, II, p. 164). This is not the place to make a detailed comparison between Jackson and Damasio, but it is intriguing to note briefly some parallels in their thought.

Both see the brain as a complex representational system, with mind arising from these representations. Both consider that the experience of mind or self is not produced by any specific part of the brain but by the whole brain working in a coordinated manner. As Damasio puts it, "mind derives from the entire organism as an ensemble" (1996, p. 225). The representations concern the body. Damasio understands the emergence of mind as dependent upon neural circuits that represent the organism continuously monitoring its interplay with environment. "The basic topic" of those representations "are anchored in the body" (1996, p. 226). Using different language, Jackson seems to say something similar: "A man, physically regarded, is a sensori-motor mechanism. I particularly wish to insist that the highest centres—physical basis of mind or consciousness—have this kind of constitution that they represent innumerable different impressions and movements of all parts of the body, although very indirectly" (Jackson, 1958, II, p. 63). Jackson gives greater emphasis to the representation of movement than does Damasio, who focuses mainly on topographically organized sensory maps that can become images.

In consideration of the double process that gives rise to speech, Jackson spoke of "the right half of the brain as being the part during the activity of which the most nearly unconscious and most automatic service of words begins, of the left as the half during activity of which there is that sequent verbal action which is speech" (p. 169). Damasio (1996) says something similar. He considers that "images are probably the main content of our thoughts" (p. 107) and that of "most of the words we use in our inner speech, before speaking or writing a sentence, exist as auditory or visual images in our consciousness," although this consciousness may be fleeting (p. 106).

Inner speech might be understood as the first part of the verbalizing process. It is not really speech at all but something more akin to a symbolic process, dependent upon images. In the context of symbolic play Vygotsky saw it as relatively wordless: "In inner speech words die as they bring forth thought." He distinguished between what he termed "thought" and words. In the "transitional" child, existing in a zone that is neither inner nor outer but both, "inner speech" is a "dynamic, shifting, unstable thing, fluttering between word and thought, the two more or less stable, more or less firmly delineated components of verbal thought" (Vygotsky, 1962, p. 149).

The struggle to translate the first part of the verbalizing process into what Jackson called "propositional speech"—to make logical and linear what was analogical and non-linear—is often considerable. Although Jackson does not remark on the resemblance between his formulation of the two parts of speech and that of the two parts of consciousness, subject and object, a parallelism between the two processes seems to be evident. The former process involves the same principles, on a smaller scale, as the latter, like a microcosm in relation to a macrocosm. A concept resembling "inner speech," or more theoretically, a wordless system of analogically connected imagery, makes comprehensible the somewhat enigmatic description of self as made of two halves ("each is only half itself") labeled subject and object consciousness. Jackson wrote that we should not then use an expression such as "Ideas come into consciousness." Instead, "it should be ideas come out of subject consciousness and then constitute object consciousness" (Jackson, 1958, II, p. 93), rather as language emerges from a basis of imagery, thus constituting speech. "Using the word 'self' for once we may say that what is commonly called consciousness (object consciousness) is 'a revealing of self'" (Jackson, 1958, II, p. 96).

Using a background that includes the work of Jackson, James Damasio, Edelman, Vygotsky, and others, I conceive of self as arising from two partly overlapping systems of neurocircuitry, which are the bases of two different kinds of thought and means of processing sensory data. The coordinated activity of both systems is fundamental. One of the two systems underlies an *analogical mode* of thinking whereas the other system produces *logical* or *intentional* thought. The hypothesis in this book is that the basis of BPD symptomatology is an inadequate development of the analogical mode, which Edelman calls "selectionism" and which Jackson called subject consciousness. The more primary disturbance has the secondary effect of disrupting the proper emergence of object consciousness.

THE DEFAULT MODEL NETWORK: THE BASIS OF SUBJECT CONSCIOUSNESS

An understanding of the mode of consciousness that Jackson called "unchanging," which is cohesive and continuous, may be the means of conceiving the relative failure of cohesion and continuity characteristic of the psychic life of those with BPD. Until very recently, little interest has been shown in the persisting background to mental life. The greater value given in Western culture to logical and intentional forms of consciousness has led to neglect, in scientific terms, of this other mode of thought. Neuroscientific research has largely focused on the kinds of brain function that are exhibited by the organism that can be conceived as adaptive and which are activated during the performance of a specific task. In the last few years, however, a new field of inquiry has arisen concerning the patterns of neural activity evident when the individual is not performing a task—that is, when, apparently, no adaptive function is being fulfilled. This form of brain functioning, termed the "default mode" (Raichle et al., 2001; Gusnard & Raichle, 2001), may be the neural basis of Jackson's subject consciousness.

Particular brain regions have been shown to deactivate during task-oriented experiments (Shulman et al., 1997). The regions involved are very largely cortical midline structures, particularly the ventromedial and dorsomedial PFC and the posterior cingulate/precuneus. These regions are main features, apparently functioning like nodal or seed points (Uddin et al., 2009), in a neural network that is active when the individual is not engaged in a specific task (Greicius et al., 2003). The network also includes the medial, lateral, and inferior parietal cortex, with increasing interest being focused on the temporoparietal junction (TPJ). That this pattern of neural activity is not mere random firing of the system at rest, but a specifically connected network, has been demonstrated in different ways on a number of occasions (e.g., McKiernan et al., 2006; Singh & Fawcett, 2008).

The default mode network (DMN) has been associated with states of introspection and those functions associated with the achievement of selfhood. They include, for example, autobiographical memory (Gusnard et al., 2001; Buckner & Carrol, 2007), "mentalizing" (Frith & Frith, 1999, 2003), and also certain tests of "theory of mind," such as false belief, which are likely to reflect a developed sense of inner life (Gallagher & Frith, 2003; Vogeley et al., 2001). Another association is with "stimulus independent thought" (Gusnard & Raichle, 2001; Mason et al., 2007), a state that is opposite to the characteristic way of thinking of those with BPD, who display "stimulus entrapment" (Meares, 1993a, 2005).

Although default mode function has been understood as reflecting the brain at rest, the evidence concerning brain energy utilization belies such an inference. The brain is only a little less active in the default mode than in the task-oriented condition (Raichle & Gusnard, 2002; Raichle & Mintun, 2006).

The DMN is "anti-correlated," with the network associated with task performance, one growing as the other fades. The individual appears to switch between modes, in an on–off manner. The switch, however, is not complete. In its "off" condition, the DMN is not entirely deactivated. Rather, it persists in an attenuated form as our ongoing sense of personal being. The stream of consciousness remains as a background while our attention is focused on an external object (Eichele et al., 2008; Fransson, 2005; Greicius et al., 2003; Greicius & Menon, 2004). Unsurprisingly, the greater the attentional demand of the external environment, the greater the deactivation of the DMN (McKiernan et al., 2006; Singh & Fawcett, 2008). Also unsurprisingly, deactivation of the DMN is reduced when the task to be performed is self-referential (van Buuren et al., 2010). On the other hand, we might suppose that in situations of extreme threat and traumatic arousal, when the ordinary ongoing sense of personal existence is almost obliterated, the deactivation of the DMN would be almost complete.

Since the task-related network and the DMN are linked together in time, in an anti-correlated manner, it has been suggested that they are different manifestations of a single system, in which an attentional mechanism changes channels, as it were, to either an extrospective or introspective function (Fransson, 2005; Sonuga-Barke & Castellanos, 2007). This proposal offers a preliminary model of Jackson's object and subject consciousness in which each form of consciousness is half of the other. Moreover, the evidence regarding self-related function suggests that the DMN is the primary or more fundamental system, supporting Jackson's view of subject consciousness as the more basic form. Nevertheless, subject and object modes must both be seen as aspects of a system of self.

Disturbance of the Default Network

A plausible basis of psychic fragmentation—that is, a disturbance in the continuing feeling of personal existing—is a disturbance of, or a deviation from, the usual patterning of DMN neurocircuitry. Future research, however, will necessarily involve definition of "usual" and refinements in the accounts of the state of mind during periods of so-called "rest" state, during which recordings of the DMN are made. Rest can involve a multitude of differing states. Ian Gawler and Paul Bedson (2010) point out that there is likely to be a very considerable difference between the rest involving certain meditative states of near objectless thought and another condition in which the rattle of consciousness is merely undirected. It might be supposed, indeed, that there are very many different sorts of default mode.

A certain amount of evidence, including that presented in the previous chapter, suggests that the symptoms of BPD reflect a disturbance in the maturation of particular aspects of brain function. The hypothesis predicts that this disturbance will be particularly evident in the brain basis of the non–task-oriented form of consciousness (i.e., in the DMN). Fair et al. (2007) have demonstrated the main difference between mature and immature individuals in the patterning of DMN circuitry. Young people have diminished connectivity, with connectivity increasing with age. It is minimally present at 2 weeks of age when activity in the posterior node of the DMN is evident, in the posterior cingulate cortex (PCC; Fransson et al., 2007; Gao et al., 2009). The main network structure is apparent in children of 7–9 years, but it is not fully developed (Fair et al., 2008; Supekar et al., 2010). A comparison between the extent of connectivity in children of this age and adults is shown in Figure 6.1. Supekar et al. (2010) observe that the linkage between the medial PFC (MPFC) and the PCC along the cingulum bundle is the most important of the

DMN connections in the maturational changes that occur between childhood and adulthood.

These findings lead to an expectation that the DMN in BPD will be relatively disconnected, in the manner of children. As far as I am aware, such a study has yet to be performed. However, some indication of the likely outcome of such a study is given by the findings in a group of subjects with a traumatic background similar to those with BPD. Seventeen patients with PTSD related to early life trauma were compared with 15 controls in an fMRI procedure during which the participants were asked to let their minds wander. If they found that they "were focusing too long on any one subject," they were instructed to "pull their minds away." The results showed diminished connectivity of the DMN in the traumatized group. Activity in the seed area of the precuneus/ posterior cingulate was more strongly correlated with activity in other areas of the default network in healthy controls than in the patient group. These areas included the medial PFC, lateral parietal cortices, inferior and middle temporal cortices, thalamus, and cerebellum. In the patient cohort there was correlation only between the seed area and right superior frontal gyrus and left ventrolateral thalamus. Greater connectivity with the seed area in the healthy group included the right amygdala, the right hippocampus, and the right insula (Bluhm, Williamson, Osuch, et al., 2009). The authors remarked that the right-hemispheric disturbance may be important "given the suggestion that the early life trauma experienced by the patients with PTSD may have interfered primarily with the development of the right hemisphere," referring to the work of Schore (2002).

The PTSD subjects scored highly on the Dissociative Experiences Scale (DES). Their mean score of 28.5 compared with the mean in the controls of 2.0. These data suggest a fragmentation of brain function in traumatized people who dissociate, and so may provide support for the hypothesis about the neurophysiological origins of the fragmentation of self in BPD. It is possible, however, that the findings merely reflect psychiatric illness in general and are not specific. Against this possibility is evidence reviewed by Broyd et al. (2009) of studies on schizophrenia, depression, Alzheimer's disease, and anxiety. This preliminary evidence suggests that each illness may eventually be found to have a characteristic pattern of disturbance. For example, patients suffering from schizophrenia, and their first-degree relatives, show abnormally high functional connectivity within the default network. Furthermore, these people, in comparison with controls, showed disturbances in the anti-correlations between the DMN and the task-related system, most particularly involving the MPFC. During the performance of a working memory task, patients and their relatives exhibited significantly reduced suppression in MPFC activity (Whitfield-Gabrieli et al., 2009).

Findings in depression are different. A study of 14 patients with depression, who, except for one subject, were medication free, compared them with 15 controls. In contrast to the schizophrenia findings, there were no areas of increased connectivity in the depressed cohort. There was, however, decreased connectivity between the precuneus/posterior cingulate gyrus and the caudate nucleus bilaterally. The investigators noted that these regions are involved in motivation and reward processing (Bluhm, Williamson & Lanius, et al., 2009).

SELF AS SCENE

The main point of trying to discover the brain basis of BPD is that it may be helpful in guiding our efforts to devise more effective treatment for the condition. If an arrested development of the DMN is at the bottom of the borderline patient's troubles, then an important aim of treatment should be to activate this system. Activation of the system must depend upon knowing what function the system serves. The writings of Jackson and Damasio suggest that the matrix of psychic life out of which intentionality arises is made up of imagery, where imagery is understood to refer to "shapes" of both the visual and auditory kind. Elicitation of a particular kind of imagery, involving personal events and having the larger shape of scenes, may potentiate the activity of this system.

Scenes are the main components of autobiographical memory and imagination, which are markers of the experiences of self (Sartre, 1966). Those who write about the DMN link it to autobiographical memory. The creation of scenes in the "mind's eye" may have a significance in the generation of "self" beyond the confines of memory. Scenes are the basic units of narrative. The Jamesian concept of self as the ongoing and enduring experience of personal existing, when translated into speech, resembles a story of a particular kind that we might call *narrative*. It is to be distinguished from tales in the form of *chronicles* and *scripts* in which the manifestations of self are relatively lacking and which resemble much of the conversation of those suffering from BPD (Meares, 1998). In a review of neuroimaging studies of story processing, Raymond Mar (2004) found that the brain areas associated with narration resemble those associated with autobiographical memory and theory of mind.

A coordination of scenes is necessary to the creation of narration. Our lives are experienced in the moment, each moment a scene, and each moment passing seamlessly into the next. Our lives are metaphorical travel stories, as implied in Dante's famous opening lines:

> *Nel mezzo del cammin di nostra vita*
> *mi ritrovai per una selva oscura*
> *ché la diritta via era smarrita.*

> Midway though the journey of life,
> I found myself in a dark wood,
> The right road lost.

Michel de Certeau, a leading French sociologist who died in 1986, has remarked that "narrative structures have the states of spatial syntaxes" (1988, p. 115), an ordering of scenes that always occur in places that can be "mapped," and which are linked to other maps in an overarching map. These ideas are introduced into a consideration of the DMN because they have important therapeutic implications. If the major problem confronting the therapist who is trying to help a patient with BPD is a disunity in the sense of self, then the principal therapeutic endeavor must be directed toward an integration of a sense of self. The way in which self is conceived will determine how the therapy is done. Since we can only experience the present, the scene is not only the basic unit of narrative but also of selfhood. The fostering of selfhood gives a primary therapeutic role to the co-creation of scenes and their connections through the use of words having a picturing function (Meares, 1983). In this way, therapy is conceived not as a primarily verbal but as a visuospatial praxis.

A relationship between the capacity of the mind to create scenes and the DMN is suggested by a most interesting study conducted by Hassabis, Kumaran, and Maguire (2007). Their subjects were given three different tasks: (1) to recall very recent episodic memories; (2) to retrieve fictitious experiences previously constructed in a pre-scan interview 1 week before; and (3) to construct new fictitious experiences during fMRI scanning. The researchers hypothesized that, since each of these experiences, remembered and imagined, depends upon scene construction, they would all share a common neural basis. The investigators noted that scene construction involves more than visualization of a single object. It requires complex coordination of disparate elements into a single coherent whole.

Their results supported that hypothesis. They found an extended neural network associated with scene construction, including the hippocampus. The hippocampus has a system of "place-cells" (O'Keefe & Dostrovsky, 1971) and "grid cells" (Moser et al, 2008) that function together to provide the basis of a form of a spatial mapping, necessary to scene construction. This system is obviously related to our capacity to navigate. (In a now-famous study Maguire and her colleagues [1997] asked London taxi drivers to imagine the routes that would take them to different parts of the city while undergoing PET. As they traveled these routes in their minds, their right hippocampi lit up.)

Hassabis et al. (2007) found that a distributed neural network resembling that activated during navigation, and also in the DMN, was recruited during both the recall of episodic memory and the visualization of fictitious experiences. These investigators found that the default mode system can be "broken down into at least two distinct components with dissociable neural bases: a network centred on the hippocampus responsible for scene construction and a second network involving medial prefrontal cortex and the posterior cingulate gyrus–recuneus mediating self-projection in time, sense of familiarity and self scheme" (p. 14372). They point out that navigation depends mainly upon the hippocampal scene construction network, whereas episodic memory, which depends upon personal experience, requires both.

A report from Spreng, Mar, and Kim (2009) gave support to the proposals of the Maguire group and also of Buckner and Carroll (2007), who suggested that a network similar to the DMN reflected what they called "self projection," which they defined as a shift in perception from the immediate environment to an alternate, imagined environment. Spreng and his colleagues conducted four separate meta-analyses of neuroimaging studies on (1) autobiographical memory, (2) navigation, (3) theory of mind, and (4) the default mode. Their findings favored the idea that within the default network there is a core network of brain areas underpinning autobiographical memory, navigation, and theory of mind, with autobiographical memory being more closely related to DMN than the other two capacities. They also concluded that prospection, or future thinking (i.e., the capacity to imagine ourselves acting in a particular way in the future), is also dependent upon this network. This inference is consistent with earlier proposals that prospection and episodic memory are related and are reflections of the same neural system (Addis et al., 2007; Atance & O'Neill, 2001; Szpunar et al., 2007).

The association with autobiographical memory is evidence in favor of the idea that the DMN is the neural basis of self, or more particularly that aspect of selfhood that is most fundamental and which Hughlings Jackson called *subject consciousness*. Its functions are likely to include the manipulation of imagery and the "shaping" of sensory data, a capacity involved in the "mapping" of experience and in the creation of "scene."

An intriguing study from Lange and Irle (2004) suggests that the capacity for scene production may be diminished in those who dissociate, including in those with BPD who dissociate. They found reduced glucose metabolism in the left PCC–precuneus and right temporal pole/anterior fusiform gyrus in 17 young women with BPD who had pronounced dissociative symptomatology. They noted that the PCC has the highest resting perfusion rate in the human cerebral cortex (Gusnard & Raichle, 2001). Fletcher et al. (1995) have suggested that the precuneus might operate as the metaphorical "mind's eye" that is necessary to mental imagery and to the creation of mental scenes in imagination and in autobiographical memory. We return to the significance of scene in the construction of self in the final chapter in which a consideration is given to the therapy of individuals with BPD.

THE SENSE OF FAMILIARITY

A crucial aspect of the feeling of continuity at the heart of personal existing is the sense of familiarity, of sameness. The word *self* has an ancient alternative meaning of *same* (as in Shakespeare's *Titus Andronicus*: "He is your brother, lords, sensibly fed of that self blood that first gave life to you" [IV, II, 123]). William James put this experience at the core of selfhood. It enables us to say that "I am the same I that I was yesterday" (1890, I, p. 283). It is an aspect of remembering, rather than conceiving, our own states (1890, I, p. 239).

The judgment of familiar versus strange is essential to the process of orientation–habituation, which reflects the function of one of our most basic means of adapting to the world: the capacity to select from the mass of sensory information available to us those percepts that are significant and to selectively ignore those that are not. Although there has been a great deal of research into orientation–habituation, the feeling of familiarity upon which this process depends has been largely neglected and its origins remain unknown. The observations of Hassabis et al. (2007) offer a considerable advance in our understanding.

Hassabis et al. (2007) found significantly greater activation in the precuneus when recall of previously imagined experiences was compared with newly imagined experiences. They inferred that the difference could be explained in terms of familiarity. In the same way, they found that real memories were associated with greater precuneus activation than imaginary ones. The investigators noted that their inference regarding the precuneus was in line with the proposal about the functional significance of this area in recognition memory (Hornberger et al., 2006; Rugg et al., 2002; Wagner et al., 2005; Vincent et al., 2006).

Other parts of the DMN may be involved in the feeling of familiarity. Temporoparietal cortex activation may be necessary to the detection of what is personally familiar rather than a familiarity that does not involve the sense of selfhood, as in the process of recognizing a familiar object, person, or scene (Sugiura et al., 2009). The left TPJ is related to self-representation in children (Lewis & Carmody, 2008), whereas the right TPJ maintains the integrity of bodily feeling that is a cardinal experience of self.

THE "I," P3A, AND THE SWITCHING MECHANISM

The judgment of familiar versus strange underlies the orienting response—of which P3a is the cortical component—and its habituation. The orienting system has long been a subject of psychophysiological research (Sokolov, 1960, p. 5), studied, for example, in electrodermal response, changes in heart rate, and behavioral orientation. It is only in recent years, however, that sophisticated studies of the fundamental phenomenon have been possible. These studies strongly suggest that P3a may embody the cortical component of the orienting response (Halgren et al., 1995a) and the direction of attention. The proposal that P3a reflects the cortical output of the orienting response is supported by the observation that it is only evoked in conjunction with an electrodermal response (Halgren & Marinkovic, 1993). The key neural substrates of orienting and reorienting are still being defined. Orienting involves a widely distributed network that includes prefrontal and hippocampal regions. These areas are particularly implicated in the habituation process (Yamaguchi, 2004).

The responses of the orientation and habituation, excitatory in the former and inhibitory in the latter, reflect a switching mechanism in which the focus of attention is directed and redirected. Sestieri, Shulman, and Corbetta (2010) have recently investigated the neural basis of the switch between intrinsic processing related to the environment and intrinsic activity related to "inner" events. They found that "in memory and perception-related regions a mechanism of reciprocal dynamic competition . . . was related to behavioural performance" (p. 8445).

The report of their findings focused on parietal networks, giving "first evidence for a double dissociation between parietal networks involved in top-down attention to memory and the environment" (p. 8445). The actual networks involved, however, were extensive. Beyond lateral parietal activity, a memory task also evoked activation in midline structures associated with the default mode—that is, the posterior cingulate, precuneus, and retrosplenial cortex. The memory search regions neighbored the perception-related fields of activity but were physiologically distinct from them. Regions activated by perception were deactivated by memory, and vice versa.

The report of Sestieri and his colleagues (2010) considered memory of an impersonal kind, whereas memories of one's own experience are at the heart of self. In a previous study from the same group, on what they called "internally cued" mental activity, which involved affect, it was inferred that "self-referential" mental activity seems to be particularly related to the dorsomedial prefrontal cortex (Gusnard et al., 2001). A study specifically focused on self-related experience during rest, when the midline structures composing the default mode are active, found that this was associated with activation of the ventral and dorsomedial prefrontal cortex and the posterior cingulate cortex (Schneider et al., 2008). These two studies suggest that the dorsomedial prefrontal cortex is necessary to the sense of the self, that curious quality of the personal that Claparéde (1911/1951), in a classic paper, called "me-ness." The absence of activity in this region in subjects who dissociate, reported by Felmingham et al. (2008), is touched upon in Chapter 7. Their finding is consistent with clinical reports that with increasing intensity of trauma and dissociation, the feeling of me-ness dissipates.

A review article from Corbetta, Patel, and Shulman (2008) addresses the extremely complex problem of the switching between outer-directed thought and a focus upon inner events—that is, a shift between object and subject forms of consciousness. Corbetta et al. elaborate a proposal previously made concerning the two main attentional systems involved in this process of orienting and reorienting. One is ventral frontoparietal, the other is dorsal frontoparietal. The former is particularly associated with orientation to a new stimulus, whereas the latter is related to maintenance of focus. Corbetta et al. (2008) proposed that "when attention is re-oriented to a new source of information (stimulus driven re-orienting), output from the ventral network interrupts (as a 'circuit breaker') ongoing selection in the dorsal network" (p. 308). This explanation might imply that the ventral system triggers the goal-oriented, task-related, stimulus-driven form of consciousness, whereas the dorsal system might concern the default mode network. But this is not so. The two modes of thought must be governed by a jointly coordinated system, as Jackson implied in his use of the word *I*.

Corbetta et al. (2008) are intrigued by the recent findings on the role of the right TPJ, the proper function of which seems to be necessary to the integrity of the bodily self. False-belief stories, which perhaps identify self more clearly than other theory-of-mind tasks, activate the right TPJ (Gallagher & Frith, 2003). Theory-of-mind tasks, as mentioned previously, are associated with the default mode network, yet the right TPJ is the posterior core of the ventral attention network, which is stimulus-driven. These data suggest that the network of the stimulus-orienting mechanism appears to be an aspect of the DMN, as, to use Jacksonian language, object and subject consciousness arise from the same system. A conundrum confronts us akin to that posed by the Jacksonian "I": The "switch" is part of that which is switched.

Despite the apparent contradictions, Corbetta and his colleagues consider that good evidence exists to support the hypothesis that the ventral network functions as the switching mechanism between internally and externally directed activities. What then is the role of the dorsal system, which is also activated during reorienting? It seems that the dorsal system may be antagonistic to the default mode, deactivating it during goal-directed tasks (Fox et al., 2006). In the Fox study it is suggested that, although segregation between the dorsal and ventral networks is nearly complete, it is possible that they connect and coordinate, not directly, but through the PFC. This idea suggests that orientation toward something new that appears in the environment depends upon the central and dorsal systems operating in concert but in opposite ways, with the dorsal system deactivating the default mode and the ventral system activating systems of awareness.

Chapter 7

DISSOCIATION IN BORDERLINE PERSONALITY

TWO FORMS OF DISSOCIATION

A WOMAN SUFFERING FROM **BPD** says she lives as if disconnected from things. Her body feels strange, even changing shape at times. She is afflicted with a pervasive feeling of numbness and a sense of unreality. Her memory seems to have gaps in it. According to authoritative criteria for the diagnosis, she exists for much of the time in a state of dissociation—that is, she exhibits the symptoms of derealization, depersonalization, and disturbance of memory (Waller et al., 1996).

Since the main thesis of this book is that BPD has a dissociative core, it is necessary to come to grips with what dissociation might be. This consideration is clouded by the fact that since the waning of the influence of Pierre Janet and his ideas, the concept of dissociation has suffered more than half a century of neglect. Despite a great deal of research in recent years, the concept "continues to be vague, confusing and even controversial" (Dell, 2009, p. 225). Authorities use the term in different ways, impeding clinical discourse and the conduct of scientific study. In a thorough and extensive review of the subject, Emily Holmes and her colleagues (2005) found that these various viewpoints can be collapsed into two main categories, to which they gave the names of "detachment" and "compartmentalization." The main argument of this chapter is that, although dissociation can be seen as having at least two main forms, the fundamental form is one of subtle psychic disintegration, termed "primary dissociation." The state involving compartmentalization I am calling "secondary dissociation."

Disintegration is a cardinal feature of the "official" description of dissociation as given in DSM-IV (American Psychiatric Association, 1994). The essential element of the dissociative disorders, it is remarked, "is a disruption of the usually integrated functions of consciousness, memory, identity and perception of the environment" (p. 477). Disintegration was also central to Janet's theory. What is currently called dissociative amnesia he described "in 1889 under the name of subconsciousness through disintegration" (Janet, 1924, p. 40). The nature of this disintegration remains unclear. An attempt at clarification begins with an examination of Janet's concepts.

JANET AND DISSOCIATION

Although Pierre Janet is seen as the main descriptor of what we now call dissociation, he gave it no overarching name. Instead, he spoke of the various aspects of this complex and heterogeneous phenomenon, giving them descriptive labels such as *abaissement du niveau mental* (lowering of the mental level), restriction or constriction of consciousness, *désagrégation* (disintegration), dissociation, and subconscious fixed idea. Since dissociation is, in Janet's conception, only part of the phenomenon, it is not a suitable name for the whole syndrome. Nevertheless, common usage has decreed that this is what it should be called. Accordingly, I follow this usage, with some misgivings, since the word is somewhat misleading or at least ambiguous.

The theoretical framework provided by Hughlings Jackson is very helpful in understanding Janet's theory. Although one was working psychologically and the other neurologically, there is a close resemblance between their theories. Both depend upon a hierarchical model of mind. Onno van der Hart, an expert on Janet, has told me that he believes that Jackson did not exert a direct influence on Janet. Nevertheless, it would seem likely that there was an indirect influence through Théodule Ribot, one of Janet's principal masters (Janet, 1907, p. 3), the other being Charcot. Ribot was a thoroughgoing Jacksonian and largely responsible for the introduction of Jackson's ideas into France.

The "enormously complex" "words 'I, me'" (Janet, 1901, p. 35) were central to Janet's theorizing. Rather than *self*, he tended to speak of *personality*, which, in the way he described it, was equivalent to the self–identity concept. Late in his career, he declared that human personality is "a construction that tends towards unity but is not certain to arrive at it" (as cited in Seigel, 2005, p. 514). In essence, for Janet, *integration is what self is.*

Janet based his theories on a model of mind, or "personality," which he believed is the outcome of the integration of a hierarchy of "tendencies," this word implying a disposition to action. Janet considered that no state of mind is separable from activity. Even at the lowest level of psychic life there is no sensation without movement (Ellenberger, 1970, p. 361), an idea resonant with Jackson's sensorimotor coordinating machine. The lowest level of the hierarchy is simply sensorimotor without any accompanying sense of self. "Reflective and personal" tendencies are at the highest level, directed toward the establishment of selfhood.

Like Jackson, Janet considered that noxious environmental events cause a regression down the hierarchy. His emphasis was on psychological events of a traumatic kind. Traumatized patients formed a large part of Janet's practice. He described a total of 591 patients and reported a traumatic origin in 257 of them (Crocq & De Verbizier, 1989).

Janet considered that the "vehement emotions" and "shocks" arising from traumatic events cause a retreat down the hierarchy of consciousness, "decomposing" a state of mind. He wrote:

"Emotion has a decomposing action on the mind, reduces its synthesis and makes it, for the moment, wretched. Emotions, especially depressive ones such as fear, disorganize the mental synthesis; their action, so to speak, is analytic, as opposed to that of the will, of attention, of perception, which is synthetic" (Janet, 1889, p. 457).

It is this state that I am taking to be the basic form of dissociation. This kind of disintegration may perhaps be called *désagrégation*, using Janet's language, to distinguish it from a consequence of it, which can be more truly called *dissociation*. Janet used both terms, and the latter cannot be regarded as a translation of the former (Van der Hart & Dorahy, 2006).

Désagrégation will vary in degree. At one extreme, rapid switches in state of mind are evident, and conversation has a disconnected, incoherent quality. At the other end of the spectrum is a diminution in the organization of thought, which is not detectable by an observer but can be demonstrated experimentally. In one such experiment the individual is asked to choose the best match for the top figure from the two lower figures in Figure 7.1.

Frederickson and Branigan (2005) have shown that negative emotion causes the individual to choose the figure on the right, on the basis of similarity to detail. Positive states influence the subject to select the figure on the left, which resembles the overall triangular pattern. This choice, then, is made on the basis of coherence, an awareness of the similarity of shape. A choice of the right figure, on the other hand, is made on the basis of relative fragmentation, of resemblance between parts rather than a global shape. As far as I know, there is no evidence of testing dissociative subjects in this way. Nevertheless, this small experiment illustrates how differences in the sense of coherence can be demonstrated when they cannot be described by the subject. I am suggesting that those with BPD have an ongoing state of subtle psychic disintegration that fluctuates with mood, which in turn depends upon the interplay with the social world. Brandchaft and his colleagues have pointed out that BPD is highly dependent upon the form of relatedness with others and that its manifestations may be perpetuated by unsatisfactory styles of relating, a state which can be seen as co-created (Brandchaft, Doctors, & Sorter, 2010).

In Janet's system the decomposition, or disintegration, of psychic life is accompanied by a "lowering of the mental level" (i.e., "abaissement du niveau mental") to a state of mind lower on a hierarchy of consciousness:

> One of the marks of emotion is that it is accompanied by a decided lowering of the mental level. It brings about not only the loss of synthesis and the reduction to automatism which is so noticeable in the hysteric, but proportionately to its strength it gradually suppresses the higher phenomena and lowers tension to the level of the so-called inferior phenomena. Under the influence of emotion, mental synthesis, attention, the acquisition of new memories, are seen to disappear; with them diminish or disappear all the functions of reality, the feeling of and pleasure in reality, confidence and certitude. In place of these we observe automatic movements. (Janet, 1903, as cited in Jung, 1957, p. 171)

In this passage, Janet suggests that all those functions that make up a state of mind are changed by the effect of traumatically induced emotion. His description includes the main features of dissociation as currently understood—that is, derealization, depersonalization, and disturbance of memory. The description also implies that these phenomena, however, cannot be separated from attention and affect. Emotional numbing and reduced awareness of one's surroundings are aspects of these phenomena. In some circumstances the attentional deficit can be extreme, beyond a reduction in the field of consciousness and difficulty in concentration, to include concentric constriction of the visual field. This curious disturbance is one of the stigmata of hysteria (Janet, 1907, pp. 196–197). For Charcot it was the cardinal diagnostic sign (Veith, 1965). It may be a consequence of acute and severe battle stress (Myers, 1915).

In this 1903 description, Janet is talking particularly of an ongoing personality disorder that resembles BPD. Loss of the "feeling of pleasure of reality" is at the core of BPD and also of the dissociative experience. As the dissociative state increases, the sense of "me-ness" diminishes. There is a growing alienation from the world and from one's own inner life, which may begin to feel false and not one's own. The loss of hedonic tone may be akin to the dysphoria chronically felt by those with BPD, but lesser in degree.

The "reduction to automatism" that Janet observed during a "lowering of the mental level" echoes the language of Jackson in his remarks about certain postepileptic behaviors. In both cases, there is a loss of voluntary control over psychic life that may be slight, for example, shown in the quality of remote episodic or autobiographical memory.

These various phenomena (with the exception, of course, of chronic dysphoria) are part of peritraumatic dissociation—that is, the state of mind and behavior during and immediately following a traumatic event. It is sometimes said that these experiences are protective, shielding the individual from terror or harm. An alternative view is that dissociation is the outcome of the disorganizing effect of intense emotion. Panic is very commonly associated with the traumatic episode (Bryant & Panasetis, 2001; Resnick et al., 1994). Moreover, dissociation is common during panic attacks (Krystal et al., 1991). If peritraumatic dissociation is a defense, it is an ineffective one since a series of prospective studies show that it is a strong predictor of PTSD (Ozer, et al., 2003). The issue of defense is discussed in a later section of this chapter.

Janet's work was focused on the aftereffects of trauma rather than the immediate consequences. A single trauma, or a succession of slight, forgotten shocks, is registered in memory in a particular way, somewhere down the hierarchy, remaining unconscious, at least in part. This organization of memory is complex, and the phenomena associated with it more numerous than the experience of peritraumatic dissociation. Janet called it a "subconscious fixed idea," a constellation of traumatic experience that becomes sequestered, split off from everyday consciousness.

The traumatic memory is stored at the level of the hierarchy of consciousness which was that of the subject at the time of the traumatic event. The more severe the trauma, and the less mature the psychic organization of the subject, the lower in the hierarchy will be the registration of memory. At a lower level on the hierarchy there is a disorganization of mental synthesis, a diminished coordination between the elements of psychic life. This is a state of *désagrégation*, brought on, as in Jackson's system, by exhaustion of neuronal tissue following excessive cerebral excitation. This state of relative disconnection between functional units of the CNS facilitates the "migration of certain psychological phenomena into a special group" (Janet, 1924, p. 40). The separation of this group from ordinary consciousness is what Janet called *dissociation*. Morton Prince believed, with Janet, that the "subconscious fixed idea" is only formed to any great degree when there is underlying vulnerability created by *désagrégation*. He wrote: "The tendency to preserve complexes that have been organized with a certain amount of automatic independence varies greatly from person to person, but it can only be manifested to a high degree when there is a fundamental condition of mental disaggregation" (1911, as cited in Janet, 1925, I, p. 599).

As I read it, *désagrégation*, or disaggregation, is the relative failure of mental synthesis, whereas dissociation is the separation of a certain grouping of psychological phenomena from the rest of consciousness. Janet used the term *dissociation* to refer to compartmentalization. For example, in his Harvard lectures he spoke of "the personality divided into two successive or simultaneous persons, which is again the dissociation of consciousness in the hysteric" (Janet, 1907, p. 4). A schematic representation of the processes of *désagrégation* and dissociation and the formation of the subconscious fixed idea is difficult. An approximation is provided in Figure 7.2.

In this diagram, healthy or everyday consciousness is portrayed with a high degree of coordination among the elements of mental function, both within and between "levels." In traumatic consciousness, this coordination is diminished, allowing the system of traumatic memory to become separable. Reflective or higher-order consciousness is lost so that the memory is stored prereflectively not as a scene or an episode, but as feelings and certain "facts" concerning the felt attributes of the subject, the other, and the form of relatedness at the time of the trauma, wherein the traumatic environment is made up of a person or persons. This constellation also includes bodily experience, sequences of movements, and fragments of perceptual representation. They may be skin sensations, visual flashes, smells, pains, and sounds of various kinds, such as footsteps or spoken words. Further aspects of the system are considered later in the chapter.

Since the traumatic system is stored prereflectively, it cannot be retrieved as episodic memory by the reflective processes. Nevertheless, it has an effect as memory operative in the other memory systems. In this way, there is a compounding of the separation of the system from ordinary consciousness, arising, as Janet saw it, through a relative failure of the synthesis of mental life. There is also a third factor contributing to the sequestration and quasi-independence of the traumatic memory, which we can only infer from Janet's writing.

Janet described treatment of unconscious traumatic memory by "mental liquidation" (Janet, 1925, I, pp. 589–698). This metaphor conveys the idea that the traumatic memory has a form or structure which differs from that of mature consciousness. Consequently, it cannot be "dissolved," as it were, in its stream, and so remains unassimilated. The idea that each kind of memory has a different structure was an aspect of Tulving's descriptions of the "layered" memory concept comprising autonoetic, noetic, and anoetic memory. Although he does not explicably address this problem of unassimilable traumatic complexes, Janet's treatment approach implies that the pathological structure of a traumatic complex must change for it to become integrated into ordinary reflective consciousness. The nature of this pathological structure can be studied by linguistic analysis. Such a study is reported in the following chapter.

The complex of traumatic memory becomes enlarged by "satellites of trauma" (Meares, 2000) that "surround" it. Janet describes at least two (Ellenberger, 1970, p. 368). One he calls a "derivative fixed idea," in which the traumatic memory is extended to include aspects that were not part of the original experience but which become linked to it through association. For example, a woman robbed at gunpoint on a train becomes afraid to travel not only on trains but also more generally.

The other category of fixed idea Janet calls "stratified." As the therapeutic work goes on, another trauma system is discovered, from an earlier period of life, which is apparently unrelated to the presenting trauma. Then, a third trauma system from an earlier time still might become evident. For example, the young woman on the train, who was not physically harmed, was precipitated into a state of depressed and derealized inertia, in which she was no longer able to work. It soon emerged that as a young adolescent she had been repeatedly sexually abused by her mother's brother who lived in the same house and who was intellectually handicapped. After this a third layer of trauma began to appear. It concerned the cold, remote mother who suspected what was going on but did nothing about it.

CHRONIC DISSOCIATIVE DISTURBANCE
OF MEMORY OF BPD

Janet's descriptions of what we now call dissociation reveal a state of mind of great complexity. His concept of *abaissement du niveau mental* implies that in some cases dissociation is more than a transient phenomenon concerning a particular traumatic experience. He remarked upon a "continuous forgetfulness" in his patients (1901, p. 78), noting that Charcot had observed the same phenomenon in those who are "victims of traumatization" (p. 76). If the characteristic state of mind of those suffering from BPD is analogous to a mild and continuous, though fluctuating, dissociation, then memory disturbance should be evident in these patients. This disturbance has been demonstrated in the case of autobiographical memory.

Autobiographical memory for specific events emerges later than general memories. The hypothesis that those with BPD exist in a state of subtle *abaissement du niveau mental* can be tested by a study of autobiographical memory. Jones and colleagues (1999) have conducted such a study. They found that patients suffering from BPD had difficulty in recapturing specific personal memories, particularly as they concerned negative events. They remembered, instead, general memories—for example, "My mother was often critical." The number of general memories correlated with dissociation scores on the DES, consistent with the notion that the greater the disturbances of the self system, as manifest in autobiographical memory, the greater the vulnerability to dissociation. These patients had suffered an *abaissement du niveau mental*.

Williams and his coauthors (2007) have reviewed evidence associating a disturbance in the emergence of autographical memory with a history of trauma, an association that was first documented for adult survivors of childhood sexual abuse by Kuyken and Brewin (1995). These studies, dependent upon self-report, were supported by the findings of an investigation of children who had documented histories of maltreatment (Valentino, Toth, & Cichetti, 2009). These reports, then, support the possibility that trauma, or more particularly *repeated traumata*, have a deleterious effect on the individual's form of consciousness beyond the time of the occurrence of the traumata, inducing a slight retreat down a developmentally formed hierarchy of consciousness as manifested in memory.

The findings of Valentino et al. (2009) are valuable in clarifying the association between overgeneral autobiographical memory and trauma. In particular, their data help to resolve a question about the effect of depression. For a time, depression was seen as the cause of overgeneral autobiographical memory. This assumption derived from the first observations of the phenomenon, which came from J. M. G. Williams. Williams and Broadbent (1986) found, serendipitously, that suicide attempters have difficulty retrieving specific memories. This finding was followed by a study of people with depression, showing that they too had difficulty (Williams & Scott, 1988). Both depression and attempted suicide are associated with BPD. Both, also, may have a background of trauma. In the case of depression, it is those individuals who are resistant to treatment who typically have a history of trauma (Kaplan & Klinetob, 2000).

Valentino and her colleagues (2009) found that the difficulty with retrieving specific personal memories was not mediated by depression, although depression was also associated with overgeneral remembering. In the BPD study of Jones et al. (1999), depression scores did not correlate with overgeneral memories. The principal inference from these studies is that the main cause of overgeneral measures is trauma, but depression may also have an effect. Kuyken et al. (2006), for example, found that adolescents who were depressed and who had a trauma history showed greater overgenerality in their personal memories than depressed adolescents with no trauma history. A difficulty, however, with studies of trauma and depression is that trauma is often simply defined as sexual or physical abuse, whereas the effect of a familial environment that is equally pathogenic, for example, through relentless criticism, may not be recorded as traumatic.

Another important observation of Valentino and colleagues (2009) was that overgeneral memory, although associated with maltreatment, was surprisingly not linked to neglect. This group of investigators had previously found another difference between the outcomes of two forms of failure in the caregiving environment. They found that narratives of physically abused children had extremely negative self and maternal representations (Toth et al., 1997). A further finding from Valentino's study supports the notion that overgeneral personal memory reflects maturational failure. They found that younger children produced more overgeneral memories than older children.

It is not clear at present how overgeneral memory in patients with BPD, which seems to reflect a failure of maturation in this sphere of function, comes about. Jones et al. (1999) suggest that it is a kind of defense, that those afflicted with BPD do not want to remember specific negative events. This idea is consistent with a study from Spinhoven et al. (2007) in which patients with BPD retrieved less specific autobiographical memories in response to cue words that matched highly endorsed attitudes or schemata. Williams et al. (2007) have a more complex theory, proposing that highly active negative self-representations have the effect of "capturing" a memory search at the level of traumatic self-representations. Janet believed that repeated activation of the trauma system prevented the assimilation of new material, thereby impeding maturation.

Perhaps, however, the effect of trauma in impeding maturation might be conceived in terms of the attractor concept, which Lewin explains in the context of discussing Boolean networks (i.e., a set of variables whose state is determined by other variables in the network). They provide a model for the process of ceaseless shifting going on in neural networks:

> The network proceeds through a series of so-called states. At a given instant, each element in the network examines the signals arriving from the links with other elements, and then is active or inactive, according to its rules for reacting to the signals. The network then proceeds to the next state, whereupon the process repeats itself. And so on. Under certain circumstances a network may proceed through all its possible states before repeating any one of them. In practice, however, the network at some point hits a series of states around which it cycles repeatedly. Known as a state cycle, this repeated series of states is in effect an attractor in the system. (Lewin, 1993, p. 27)

Janet does not remark on the tendency to overgeneral memory of events in the distant past in patients with dissociation. He does, however, describe a reduced temporal range of memory in which the patient barely remembers what has happened a few days earlier. Those with BPD also live within a narrowed temporal horizon in which there is little apparent awareness of a future or a past. The conversations of our patients at Westmead Hospital have been studied by the linguist Michael Garbutt (1997). He coded all utterances recorded in randomly chosen audiotapes of 15 sessions with different patients with BPD. The codings identified the temporal domains with which the utterances were concerned. Those domains included the recent past (the last few days), the remote past, and the world of the therapeutic relationship (i.e., the present). Whereas the therapists focused on the last of these domains, the great majority of the patient discourse (57.8%) was about the previous few days. The remote past of childhood was rarely referred to (3.9%). Such patients live as if trapped in the present, with limited access to the past and the future. When the patient with BPD begins to use words indicative of thought beyond the present—for example, through modal auxiliaries such as *could, may, might, will, would, shall, should, must,* and *might,* along with their negative forms—improvement in the condition is signaled (Meares & Sullivan, 2002).

A study from Bremner and colleagues (1995) concerning memory in adult survivors of childhood abuse, including those with BPD, suggested that the deficit is verbal rather than visual. Although they did not discuss this idea, their findings are consistent with the dissolution hypothesis, which posits that those functions that are more recent in evolutionary terms are lost first.

It is not always clear in the therapeutic session whether the limited range of memory evident in the patient's productions represents true amnesia. It often seems as if the patient does not experience episodes from the personal past as aspects of a continuous series. Rather, the patient's response, when a therapist attempts to link a current happening with one in the previous session, suggests that the therapist must have gone mad. The therapist is told, in various ways, that what is occurring now has nothing to do with what happened in the past. Existence seems to be made up of punctate events without connection between them.

EVOCATION OF UNCONSCIOUS TRAUMATIC MEMORY IN BPD

The "subconscious fixed idea" is a second feature of Janet's descriptions of what we call dissociation that needs further elaboration. It is better called a *subconscious* or *unconscious traumatic memory system.* It is a particular form of dissociation that is more complex than peritraumatic dissociation. Further details of this system are given in chapter 9. This section concerns the circumstances of its evocation.

Systems of traumatic memory are repeatedly triggered in the lives of those with BPD. In these states they are dissociated, although to an observer the state may not be detectable. Nor could the subject, for whom it may be almost a habitual state, always describe it in terms used to diagnose dissociation. The triggers include specific stimuli, events, scenes, places, and so forth, which in some way resemble an aspect of the traumatic situation. In the clinical situation, something the clinician does may trigger the system. Very small events—the way something is said or a facial movement—may be a sufficient precipitant. At times, the trigger is internal. Some thought, image, or memory that comes into the patient's mind and that can be connected with the trauma in some way activates the system. Vulnerability to an evocation of traumatic memory, even when it is unconscious, causes the subject to develop a narrowed focus of awareness so as not to be accidentally tripped into the zone of horror and terror that is the traumatic memory. For example, a woman cannot talk about, or even think about, a 13-year-old girl who lives next door because it may remind her of sexual abuse in her own life at that age.

In this case, the woman is aware of her avoidance. Another situation, in which the subject lacked such awareness, concerned a woman whose traumatic past involved repeated devaluation. In her job as personal assistant to a powerful businessman, she would work all hours, to the point of exhaustion and to the detriment of her familial relationships. Her efforts were directed to the avoidance of any criticism. The limitations to the range of consciousness brought about by avoidance—the narrowing of awareness—dulls vitality and diminishes the evolution of personality. Personal experience tends toward deadness and monotony.

Manifestations of the activity of the traumatic memory system in the session vary in severity from shifts in tone of voice, posture, and facial expression to severe disruptions, such as a sudden, chilling screams or fearful crouching behind a chair. In such cases, the traumatic scenario is being reenacted, and the subject experiences in the present what happened in the past. The reexperiencing of the trauma, however, becomes more complex than the original experiencing when the enactment involves those behaviors developed to avoid the trauma or to effect restorations of the sense of selfhood.

In those with BPD, there is a varying degree of vulnerability to the triggering effect of the specific stimuli that might cause the traumatic memory to be evoked. This vulnerability is increased by anything that can disorganize higher cerebral function, which leads to an *abaissement du niveau mental*. Put metaphorically, the subconscious fixed idea is nearer to the surface. Anxiety disrupts an already fragile self system, leading to further enfeeblement, so that "inferior phenomena," to use Janet's expression, are more easily released. Since anxiety is likely at the beginning of a session, the system may be particularly emergent at this time. Something of its nature can be gleaned through careful listening and imagination. For example, the opening of an early session with a middle-aged woman seems incoherent. She speaks in broken, incomplete sentences, her eyes downcast and head hanging down. She seems to make no sense. The therapist offers no responses as he listens, trying to discern what she is trying to say. The pattern is repeated in the following session. This time the therapist begins to sense what is happening. In imagining the circumstances that bring about her behavior, he speculates, to himself, that she believes that he believes that she makes no sense when she speaks. He supposes that his silence, which is not characteristic of him, has reinforced this view. Furthermore, he supposes that this small scene is a repetition, as she experiences it, albeit unconsciously, of similar scenes in early life when she was made to feel a fool by hypercritical parents. Her demeanor, he realizes, is one of shame.

A second example shows the dissociative basis of a session's opening in a more obvious way. The session begins in silence as the therapist waits for his patient, a young man, to speak. The silence is broken suddenly by the patient's voice, which is harsh, deep, and somewhat menacing. "Yes?" he growls, as if to say "What's your problem now?" The therapist pauses for a few seconds before asking quietly, "Was that your voice or was it your father's?" There is a pause and then the reply, in a higher, softer, and younger voice, "I don't know." The patient seems somewhat bewildered.

This is an example of a "reversal" (Meares, 1993b, 1999b) in which the poles of the traumatic script are switched and the subject takes on the role of the abuser, as if inhabited by an alien other. It is a feature of the conversation with those with BPD that is often puzzling, unsettling, and even frightening. The "release" of the unconscious traumatic memory system in this instance appears to be related to the patient's rising anxiety, evoked, as in the previous case, by the therapist's silence.

Disturbance of cerebral function by means other than anxiety—notably, via brain damage or drugs such as alcohol—also create a vulnerability to the emergence of the unconscious traumatic memory system, compounding a preexisting vulnerability. Janet gives an example of a boy whose fugue states were often preceded by bouts of drunkenness (Janet, 1907, p. 51). Those subjects who have such a vulnerability and who are afraid that the traumatic state will recur, learn to refrain from the use of alcohol.

Traumatic brain injury creates another vulnerability, as Eames (1992) has pointed out. Predictably, such a vulnerability is also associated with the development of BPD. Van Reekum and his colleagues (1993) found, in a chart review study of patients with BPD compared to those with other psychiatric illnesses, that 81% of those with BPD had a history of brain injury, and only 22% of the others had such an injury. A later study from this group concerned 43 male veterans with BPD diagnoses: 42% of the patients with BPD had a history of traumatic brain injury whereas only 4% of controls had such a history (Streeter et al., 1995).

Neuropsychological studies repeatedly find poor functioning in patients with BPD, suggesting to Swirsky-Sacchetti et al. (1993) that subtle organic factors may be operative in a subgroup of BPD patients. In a meta-analysis of 10 neuropsychological studies in BPD focusing on six domains of function—attention, cognitive flexibility, learning and memory, planning, speeded processing, and visuospatial abilities—Ruocco (2005) found that the patients with BPD performed poorly in all six domains.

PTSD AND BORDERLINE PERSONALITY

The reactivation of traumatic memory is unconscious in the sense that the subjects are typically unaware that they are in the grip of memory during a reliving of the traumatic event. There are many resemblances between these forms of reactivation of traumatic memory and PTSD. Whether they are reflections of different aspects of a continuum or whether they are categorically different is yet to be determined. One difference may be that PTSD is often the outcome of a single catastrophic event, whereas the unconscious traumatic memory system can be the resultant of cumulative traumata taking place in a developmental atmosphere in which, day after day, the developing individual suffers small inflictions of harm. Another difference may be the degree to which the reactivated memory is experienced consciously. PTSD is typically, but not always, accompanied by memory. The individual, for example, suffers "recurrent and intrusive distressing recollections of the event" (American Psychiatric Association, 1994, p. 28).

Studies show that PTSD can be diagnosed only in a proportion of those with BPD. For example, Zanarini and her colleagues found that 58% of 290 patients with BPD could be given this diagnosis when first seen (Zanarini, Frankenburg, & Hennen et al., 2004). This figure was higher than found in a group suffering from a personality disorder other than BPD, 25% of whom had

PTSD at initial examination. Both figures are much higher than that of the general population, which is about 8% (American Psychiatric Association, 1994). A more recent study found that 56% of patients with BPD also had a PTSD diagnosis (Zlotnick et al., 2008). For Golier and colleagues (2003) the figure was 25%.

The high comorbidity between BPD and PTSD suggests the possibility that the latter is part of the former, and that they are not independent syndromes. The evidence, however, is equivocal. Heffernan and Cloitre (2000) studied two groups of women who had suffered sexual abuse as children. One group suffered from PTSD only ($n = 45$) whereas the other had both PTSD and BPD diagnoses ($n = 26$). The investigators found that the severity and frequency of PTSD symptoms were not affected by the diagnosis of BPD, suggesting that the two diagnoses are "independent symptom constructs." The additional diagnosis of BPD was associated with an early age of abuse and of significantly higher rates of physical and verbal abuse by the mother. Those with BPD scored higher in dissociation, anger, and anxiety than those with PTSD alone. Harned et al. (2010), however, had found that those who had both disorders were more impaired.

A study of Zlotnick et al. (2003) tended to support the conclusion of Heffernan and Cloitre (2000). They found that the additional diagnosis of PTSD in patients with BPD did not increase borderline features in those patients. Axelrod, Morgan, and Southwick (2005), however, came to a somewhat different conclusion. Their report concerned questionnaire responses of 94 veterans of Operation Desert Storm. The questionnaires measured PTSD and features of personality diagnoses 6 months after return from the Gulf. The subjects were asked to score the personality inventory in two ways, "6 months before the war" and "past 6 months." PTSD was also measured 1 month after leaving the Gulf. They showed that BPD features before active service increased the risk of PTSD on return; that soldiers who had been in combat showed more BPD features postwar; and that an increased PTSD symptomatology following the war was related to enhanced severity of postwar BPD features. The investigators concluded that "adult traumatic experiences and post traumatic stress sequelae may contribute to the development of BPD features" (p. 273).

These data were consistent with Gunderson and Sabo's (1993) suggestion that those with BPD have limited reserves for dealing with traumatic events. Such vulnerability might be conceived in terms of a hierarchy of consciousness. A well-developed sense of selfhood is likely to be associated with measures of ego strength and resilience. Those who have suffered an *abaissement du niveau mental* are deprived of a psychological buffer against the impacts of traumata.

A DISINTEGRATIVE BASIS OF DEPERSONALIZATION AND DEREALIZATION

The markers of pathological dissociation, identified by Waller et al. (1996), are amnesia, depersonalization, derealization, and identity alteration. They were derived from a taxometric analysis of the 28-item Dissociative Experiences Scale (DES; Bernstein & Putnam, 1986). The pathological dissociative class (i.e., *taxon)* was made up of eight terms. The item numbers were as follows:

3. Finding themselves in a place . . .
5. Finding new things among belongings . . .
7. Standing next to themselves . . .
8. Do not recognize friends or family . . .
12. Other people or objects are not real . . .
13. Body does not belong to them . . .
22. Act different in different situations . . .
27. Hear voices inside their head . . .

So far in this chapter the discussion concerning dissociation, which began with Janet's concept, has mainly concentrated on only one of the symptoms making up the dissociative taxon: memory disturbance. This section focuses on two of the remaining symptoms, once again developing an argument for their disintegrative basis. Out-of-body experiences (OBEs) provide a good starting point for the consideration of the phenomena of depersonalization and derealization.

In OBE states, people experience themselves as floating out of their bodies, which they watch, typically from above. OBE is commonly reported by sufferers of sexual abuse. This experience is a florid form of depersonalization, which is authoritatively defined as a condition in which "the individual perceives himself to be detached and physically separated from his own body and his own mental activities" (Roth, 2004, p. 247).

Recent neurological evidence suggests that OBE may arise through disturbance of cerebral function at the temporoparietal junction (TPJ). Olaf Blanke and his colleagues (2004) reported on six individuals. Four of them suffered from complex partial seizures, one had hemiplegic migraine, and the sixth patient had severe hypertension. In one of the patients with complex partial seizures, OBE could reliably be reproduced by electrical stimulation at the TPJ. Blanke and his colleagues suggested that OBE is related to a failure to integrate the various cerebral representations of the body provided by proprioception, vision, and skin sensation. C.D. Frith (2004), in a commentary on this report, came to the same conclusion.

A disturbance related to OBE is the experience of an illusory or "shadow" person who moves closely in accord with the subject's position in space (Arzy et al., 2005). This is very like item 7 in the taxon, which also describes OBE: "Some people sometimes have the experience of feeling as though they are standing next to themselves. . . . " Arzy and his colleagues suggest that the shadow illusion may be related to disturbance of the left TPJ, whereas OBE is a consequence of disruption in the right.

A consideration of these findings leads to the view that, at least in terms of depersonalization and derealization, the phenomenon of dissociation might be conceived as the obverse of self. An extreme form of depersonalization, OBE can be understood as a disintegration of the bodily basis of self. Activity of the TPJ, as noted in the previous chapter, is closely connected to the subject's sense of self.

The depersonalization–derealization phenomenon is likely to have multiple etiological bases. The hippocampal comparator system is likely to be involved. The match–mismatch process, in which hippocampal function is a necessary component, produces the judgment, which is fundamentally a feeling of estrangement or otherwise. The mismatching that produces this feeling might come about through disturbance of the comparator system or through a disturbance of the individual's relationship with the environment. This is suggested by the story of Adele. She described a relationship with her father in which her reality, particularly as it concerned her feelings, was, as she said, "not validated." An expression of her emotional states was denied, contradicted, or simply ignored, making more tenuous an already frail sense of personal reality. She was describing an interpersonal disconnection that could be seen as the analogue of her psychic state.

IDENTITY ALTERATION IS RELATED TO DEPERSONALIZATION

Identity alteration, another feature of the taxon, is often clearly related to the depersonalization–derealization phenomenon. For example, this association between depersonalization–derealization and so-called identity disturbance seemed to be evident in the experience of Adele, mentioned in Chapter 1, who said, "When I look in the mirror, I don't see me." This experience is item 11 of the DES: "Some people have the experience of looking in a mirror and not recognizing themselves." Adele related it to the feeling that "I don't know who I am anymore."

A more extensive example of an experience in which the sense of oneself is lost, together with growing alienation from the world and from personal/bodily reality, is the account given by a surgeon who developed a strange state of mind during a period of military duty:

> "One can't go on being frightened for ever, and depersonalization set in. This, again, is difficult to describe to others. One might best illustrate it, perhaps, by saying that it was a feeling of anonymity. I remember that I felt it all the time, and very acutely at some times. It was all so odd, I might be having a conversation with a friend or eating a meal, yet without any sense of my own identity or indeed of any identity. At such moments I sought other human company desperately, for if others recognised me and knew my name and treated me as a person, then I must exist. . . . But the depersonalisation became worse and worse, and there was an acute stage when, after three nights without sleep, a fundamental separation seemed to have taken place from the world that other people inhabited. After that I continued to live, talk, and act, but I felt like a walking ghost. I was in limbo. Everything seemed to happen at one remove." (Lancet, 1952, pp. 85–86)

This man's state continued for months. Although it took a more severe form in his case, he describes the ongoing state of many of those affected with the borderline condition. The sense of being "nobody nowhere" and of being alienated from both personal reality and the reality of the world is characteristic. One very intelligent subject was able to describe a sense of personal hollowness that was experienced in a bodily way, so that when he contemplated leaping from a high building, he wondered if he would ever reach the ground. Such was his feeling of insubstantiality, he imagined being blown away by the breeze. He lived in a state of disconnection from himself and from others, leading to a sense of deadness and what he recognized to be an unreasonable dissatisfaction with his marriage to a wife he saw as a "wonderful woman." As a consequence, he had a wild and turbulent parallel relationship with a woman he, in a way, did not like and who he knew to be disordered. They recognized each other, however, as fellow travelers in the zone of damage.

A further possible linkage between disturbance of self experience and dissociation is suggested by the findings of Felmingham and colleagues (2008) in a study considered in more detail later in the chapter. They found a large reduction in dorsomedial prefrontal activity in people who dissociate. Gusnard, Akbudak, and their colleagues (2001) produced evidence suggesting that activity in this region is associated with the experience of self. They concluded that "the presence of self-referential mental activity appears to be associated with increase from baseline in dorsal medial prefrontal cortex" (p. 4259). We can assume that the opposite relation would also obtain: that diminished activity of the dorsomedial prefrontal cortex would be associated with a diminished experience of self.

HALLUCINOSIS

Another cardinal feature of dissociation, as identified in the taxometric analysis of Waller et al., (1996) is auditory hallucinosis. A nonschizophrenic form of hallucinosis has been considered, for more than a century, to be visual rather than auditory. In the famous study by Sidgwick (1894), "The Report on the Census of Hallucinations," 17,000 subjects were asked whether they had ever experienced hallucinations. The figure was surprisingly high. About 10% of the subjects replied positively, and most of these experiences were visual. The author of the report commented that this was different from the phenomenology of mental illness, in which auditory, rather than visual, hallucinosis is typical. This old saw, however, must be challenged, at least in the case of the dissociative hallucinosis of BPD. A very common finding is a rather characteristic form of auditory hallucinosis in which the subject hears an alien voice, often that of the original abuser, which utters the same or similar derogations, humiliations, and abuse as those of the abuser. They tend to be brief and repetitive; some have the form of command hallucinosis. These phenomena may cause the patient to be misdiagnosed as suffering from schizophrenia. For example, the voice might say "Slut! Useless bitch! Kill yourself!" Although it is also commonly said that hallucinatory phenomena in BPD are transient, lasting only several weeks, in our experience they are persistent in a significant number of patients (Yee et al., 2005). For example, one of the illustrative patients described in our report, a 30-year-old woman, had heard "voices" since high school. They were present 20% of the time, like "a conversation inside my head." They were worse during periods of stress, when she sensed them "take over." They were negative and critical and she felt "under their control." She believed them to "paralyze" her and prevent her from making decisions. She had not told previous doctors or therapists of their existence, fearing the diagnosis of insanity and its consequences.

Hallucinosis is common in BPD. We found that about 30% of 171 patients had this symptom. Zanarini and her colleagues (1990) also found a very high rate and considered that this type of disturbance of thought to be "virtually pathognomonic" for BPD.

Little is known about the basis of the hallucinatory experience in BPD. It is possible, however, that information about the origin of auditory hallucinosis in other conditions might apply to these phenomena in BPD. This approach implies that, although the conditions in which auditory hallucinosis arises differ, they may share a commonality of mechanisms underlying the phenomenon. Investigation in this area has almost entirely focused on schizophrenia. Recently a most intriguing report came from Sommer et al. (2008), in which they found, in a study of 24 people suffering from schizophrenia, that hallucinosis was associated with activation in the right-hemispheric homologue of Broca's area. The right brain is regarded as virtually without language function. The language centers of Broca and Wernicke are left-sided.

As the investigators point out, a study such as theirs is extremely difficult to conduct since patients who are hallucinating are not an easy subject group to manage for neuroimaging purposes. For this reason, studies of this kind are relatively rare. In their study, in order to explore the difference in lateralization between hallucinatory activation and normal language production, the patients not only experienced hallucinatory phenomena during an fMRI scan but also performed silent word generation. During hallucinosis the most extensive activation was found in the right inferior frontal area, including the right insula and the right homologue of Broca's area. Intriguingly Broca's area itself did not show significant activation during hallucinatory periods, but it was active during silent word generation.

The authors noted that they are not the first to have found that auditory hallucinosis is mainly related to right-hemispheric areas whereas speech activates the left (Woodruff et al. 1995; Copolov et al. 2003). Other studies, however, showed activation in Broca's area during hallucinosis (McGuire et al., 1995, 1997; Shergill et al., 2000, 2001, 2003).

Sommer et al. (2008) noted that both Shergill et al. (2000) and Copolov et al. (2003) reported activation in the left (para) hippocampal activity during hallucinosis. Sommer et al. found no such activation. Their results, however, are the more powerful since the sample size was adequate, whereas previous studies concerned only one to eight patients. Furthermore, in the Sommer study more rigorous thresholds for significance were applied in the statistical analysis.

These authors also cast doubt upon the inferences of previous investigators regarding findings that led them to hypothesize that auditory hallucinosis was a consequence of the subject misattributing to an external source events which had arisen internally (David, 2004; McGuire et al., 1995; Seal et al., 2004; Shergill et al., 2004). Sommer and colleagues (2008) point out that it is hard to understand how the silently generated word task was not misattributed whereas the hallucinatory phenomena were.

Overall the data from the Sommer group suggest that the homologue of Broca's area in the right hemisphere is active in auditory hallucinosis and seems to be the source of these phenomena. Although it is often said that the right brain is a non-verbal domain, patients with left-hemispheric damage are able to produce language of an emotional kind, which is brief and relatively without syntax. Jackson (1958), in describing this phenomenon, remarked particularly on the patient's ability to swear. His observations have been confirmed by Strauss and Wada (1983), Van Lancker and Cummings (1999), and Winhuisen et al. (2005).

Can the production of auditory hallucinosis by activation of the right-hemispheric homologue of Broca's area be explained in terms of a disintegration theory? Some support is given to this idea by a report from the Copolov group (Gavrilescu et al., 2010). These investigators compared 13 patients with auditory hallucinosis and another 13 patients who suffered from schizophrenia but who had no auditory hallucinosis. Using fMRI, they found that those patients who hallucinated showed disconnections between right and left hemispheres involving both the primary and secondary auditory cortices.

Data from this study seemed to resonate with the finding of Sommer and colleagues (2008) that when patients were hallucinating, there was no function in Broca's area, only in the Broca homologue. On the other hand, when they were silently thinking, only Broca's area was activated, as if each hemisphere were acting independently, switching on and off between modes of language experience. The hemispheres were no longer coordinated, or integrated, in terms of language function. If it is valid to extrapolate from these findings in schizophrenia to the field of auditory hallucinosis in BPD, they are consistent with a disintegration basis to hallucinatory phenomena.

The hypothesis that auditory hallucinosis in individuals not ordinarily considered psychotic is underpinned by activation of the right-hemispheric homologue of Broca's area was anticipated in a remarkable way by Julian Jaynes (1990). His thesis was based on the differences between the *Iliad* and the *Odyssey*, which he believed must have been written by different people, although both are attributed to Homer. He supposed that the two texts represented different phases of communal consciousness in Greek society, with about a century between them. The *Iliad* is the earlier composition. Jaynes describes the heroes of the *Iliad* in a way that is reminiscent of the more pejorative descriptions of those suffering from BPD: "The characters of the *Iliad* do not sit down and think out what to do. They have no conscious minds such as we say we have, and certainly no introspections" (p. 72). "The picture then is one of strangeness and heartlessness and emptiness. We cannot approach these heroes by inventing mind-spaces behind their fierce eyes as we do with each other" (p. 75). He saw them as lacking interior life. Their actions were directed by the voices of gods, as if they were without volition, acting under the influence of auditory hallucinosis. He proposed that these "hallucinations were indeed organized and heard from the right hemisphere" (p. 353).

IS DISSOCIATION A DEFENSE?

It is a widely accepted view that dissociation is primarily a means of protection (van IJzendoorn & Schuengel, 1996). Personal accounts of the experience, however, suggest that this is not always so. Here is one such account given to me by a colleague, an eminent psychiatrist:

The period of dissociation occurred to me during my late childhood or early adolescence, my exact age escapes me. The context was that of the long summer holidays, which I usually spent up at my grandfather's property in the country in northern New South Wales. The episode occurred on Christmas day. As part of this celebration my family would go to the local church that was in a small town some 20 kilometers from the property. I can remember it being a hot day even for the standards of country NSW, and the church itself, which is an old mock Gothic structure with a very high nave, [was] very hot and stuffy and filled with people. The service would have been the 9 o'clock service, which meant that I would have come to it after opening some presents but having little in the way of breakfast. I was seated in the church on a hard pew next to my family in a bored and contemplative state and feeling a little tired and detached from the service that was going on around me. I can remember the sounds of the service becoming quieter and a feeling of withdrawing from what was about me. I then distinctly remember feeling as if I was detaching from my body and floating. *Floating* is a word I suppose that I use to describe what happened, but feeling as if I was drifting up in the body of the church and looking down upon myself and the congregation. I have no recollection for the period of time over which this occurred, though I suspect it was relatively momentary, nor whether anything had occurred or had been said in the service that could have triggered this one way or the other. I suspect there was little to traumatize me within the Christmas service at this church in a small country town. The sensation overall was one of tiredness and distance both from myself and the proceedings that were occurring around me.

Beyond a change in a sense of time and the sound of what was happening around me, I can't remember any change in the visual input beyond the rather extraordinary feeling of floating out of myself and looking down on the congregation. I seem to remember feeling as if I floated up. However, I did remain attached in some way to myself during this experience.

I "woke" from this experience soon during the service and besides feeling a bit tired, nothing particularly intervened after this and the day continued much the same way as Christmas days always did. I can't remember having any subsequent experience similar to this, nor prior to it.

This man had never had such an experience before and never had one again. The episode might be explained in terms of Janet's concept of "fatigue," brought about by the tiredness, hunger, and the various emotions evoked by the events of this particular day.

OBE is not as uncommon as might be expected. Roberts (1960), for example, collected accounts of OBE after explaining to a group of students what it was like. He provided a questionnaire to 57 students, which allowed those respondents who had had such an experience to describe it. Twenty-three students gave reports of OBE. A typical response was given by a young woman of 19:

> I was in Nottingham with a friend and suddenly, as we were walking along, I seemed to be completely apart from myself. I felt that I was somewhere above looking down on the scene of which I was a part and yet not a part. I was walking and talking, as though automatically. I couldn't feel any movement and yet I knew that I was walking.
>
> Everything appeared to be of little importance any more. The experience on this occasion lasted for at least five minutes, but time as far as I remember passed as usual. We crossed the road, and although my legs moved with the motion, I felt that my brain had gone somewhere else and from there was just watching me. . . .
>
> The experience disappeared as suddenly as it had come and once again I felt complete. (Roberts, 1960, p. 481)

Neither the boy in the church nor the girl walking in the Nottingham street were using OBE as means of defending against unpleasant experience. On the other hand, in those suffering from sexual abuse, depersonalization seems helpful in creating a detachment from what is being inflicted upon them, and in diminishing their fear, pain, and humiliation.

Horowitz and Telch (2007) devised a way of testing whether the dissociative state is a defense, that is, protective against painful experience. They induced dissociation by means of pulsed audiophotic stimulation. This procedure involves steadily flashing lights and pulsing tones delivered to each subject through an eyepiece and an earpiece. A group of undergraduates were compared with a matched cohort of students who listened to music. Both conditions lasted 10 minutes. Those in the audiophotic stimulation group showed significantly greater dissociation than those who listened to the music. This dissociation was evident not only in the total score of the Acute Dissociative Inventory but in particular items of this score indicating gaps in awareness and derealization. Before and after the induction condition all participants underwent a cold pressor test, in which they were instructed to immerse an arm in a tank of near freezing water and to remove it only when the pain became unbearable. The investigators' hypothesis was that induction of dissociation would lead to a greater tolerance of pain. The opposite was the case: There were significantly greater reports of pain in the dissociative group.

The investigators were surprised by their finding, having supposed that dissociative experience would be protective against pain. They wondered how to reconcile their result with data such as that of Bohus et al. (2000), who found an association between dissociation and analgesia. They suggested that there may be different kinds of dissociation—which is the main thesis of this chapter. It is proposed that there are two principal forms of dissociation that have different neurophysiological bases.

The first and fundamental form of dissociation is that predicted by Jackson's "dissolution" concept. The subject's experience is one in which there is a reduced range of awareness and in which there is relative failure of the cohesion of consciousness. In common parlance, the individual is "fragmented." This condition is underpinned, according to Jacksonian theory, by a diminished coordination among areas of brain function and diminished higher-order inhibitory activity. The latter disturbance results in hyperarousal and excitability and a decreased tolerance of pain. This phenomenon is not often remarked upon as a cardinal feature of dissociation, but its description appears in the trauma literature. C. S. Myers (1940), for example, found hyperalgesia in his shell-shocked patients. This formulation makes explicable the pain experience of Horowitz and Telch's (2007) dissociative subjects.

The second form of dissociation is clearly protective. It is demonstrated in studies of dissociation in patients with PTSD in whom the traumatic memory is triggered by traumatic scripts. Lanius and her colleagues (2006), for example, reviewed reports of such experiments and found two subtypes of response: one of hyperarousal and the other "primary dissociative," characterized by "zoning out." In their own work, this second state was associated with a widely distributed pattern of brain activation, including frontal areas (BA9 and BA10) and the anterior cingulate areas (BA24 and BA32) believed to reflect the activity of inhibitory mechanisms diminishing amygdaloid response (Lanius et al., 2002). Activation of BA24 is found during pain reduction following placebo (Petrovic et al., 2005). The Lanius subjects who zoned out also showed activation of the superior and middle temporal gyrus (BA38), inferior frontal cortex (BA47), and right parietal cortex (BA7) relative to controls.

The subjects with the hyperarousal response showed a neurophysiology that in some ways was the opposite of those who zoned out. They had reduced bilateral medial frontal activity (BA10 and BA11) and left anterior cingulate cortex activity (BA32) relative to controls. I conceive of this state indicated by hyperarousal as the basic form of dissociation, whereas the zoning out is secondary and a form of defense. These different states roughly correspond to the conditions Holmes and her colleagues (2005) labeled *detachment* and *compartmentalization*, and which they regarded as qualitatively different.

Felmingham and her colleagues (2008) showed that oscillations between the two kinds of dissociation may occur in the same subjects depending upon their awareness of threat. These researchers examined 23 patients with PTSD, 12 of whom displayed dissociative reactions as judged by a cutoff score greater than 15 on the Clinician Administered Dissociative States Scale (CADSS). The subjects viewed repeated images of individuals showing either fearful or neutral expressions while fMRI recordings were made. Fearful facial expressions are likely to trigger responses akin to the original traumatic experience. The images were exposed for either 500 ms, when they could be consciously perceived, or for 16.7 ms followed by a neutral mask, when they are not consciously perceived. Those people judged as "dissociators" showed enhanced activation in the ventral prefrontal cortex in response to conscious fear compared with the others, presumably indicative of a defense against the emotional effect of the aversive image. However, in the nonconscious condition these individuals showed greater activation in the bilateral amygdala, insula, and left thalamus. The latter response could be explained by the inactivity of a protective inhibitory system, which is triggered by an awareness of threat and is dependent upon prefrontal circuitry.

The systems of defense and avoidance that might figuratively ring the traumatic core are many. They range from the rapid, automatic, and unconscious, as demonstrated in the Felmingham (2008) study, to clearly conscious efforts to avoid those persons, places, and events, which, through their likeness, however distant, might trigger the original trauma. Between the extremes of unconscious and conscious avoidance are intermediate mechanisms, such as the normal capacity for selective inattention, a process involving both "knowing and not knowing." Selective inattention is manifest in the so-called cocktail party phenomenon in which surrounding conversations are unheard until something significant is said (e.g., the mention of one's name). It is important to note that these avoidant mechanisms are not in themselves "dissociation" or "normal dissociation." To speak of them in such a way is to use a faulty syllogism.

Fluctuation between the states of dissociation is shown in the lives of those suffering from BPD, for example, during episodes of self-mutilation. The subject gazes at the bleeding wound in a way that suggests an absence of pain and also a changed sense of the reality of such an experience. This state of mind was replicated, to a degree, in an experimental situation in which there was an expectation of threat via aversive electrical stimulation. In this situation subjects with BPD showed evidence of both dissociation and increased tolerance of pain (Ludascher et al., 2007). Such relative invulnerability to pain is presumably brought about by the triggering of descending neuroinhibition. On the other hand, where no threat is apparent, patients with BPD typically show an opposite physiology of hyperarousal (Ebner-Priemer et al., 2005), suggesting a relative failure of normal inhibitory systems. This failure is consistent with findings in those patients who characteristically exhibit dissociation; that is, those who were once given the diagnosis of hysteria. They were investigated in a situation devoid of threat and showed, unlike other nonpsychotic psychiatric patients, a failure to habituate to a randomly presented and insignificant sound. This finding was replicated only in some forms of schizophrenia (Horvath & Meares, 1979). Moreover, the finding could not be explained in terms of arousal since the comparison group, comprised of people with anxiety disorders, showed significantly higher physiological indices of arousal. It was concluded that those suffering from so-called hysteria have an ongoing vulnerability, a deficiency of sensory processing involving a relative failure of the higher-order inhibitory systems that are necessary to modulate the intensity of sensory input.

This idea creates a paradox. How is it that people able to summon up powerful neuroinhibition, sufficient to diminish pain, have a deficiency of neuroinhibition? An answer arises in the form of a hypothesis that depends upon the notion of hierarchy. Inhibitory activity in the CNS can be conceived as operating at a number of evolutionarily determined levels that are coordinated. The lower level consists of coarse and general activity, whereas the upper or evolutionary new level, following Jackson, is more complex, differentiated, and specialized, subserving the fine-tuning of higher-order function. This so-called *level* is an aspect of the neural networking necessary to the generation of self. The hypothesis postulates that those with deficient higher-order inhibitory systems necessarily use coarser and more general mechanisms in order to control high arousal. Kim Felmingham has told me that she believes that data from the study she conducted with colleagues (Felmingham et al., 2008) gives support to this hypothesis. The investigations found a large reduction in dorsomedial prefrontal activity (in superior frontal and middle frontal gyrus) in the group of subjects with the high CADSS scores. This finding suggests that the neural network usually employed in inhibitory processes is deficient in dissociation. As a consequence, a coarser inhibitory system, lower in a hierarchy of function, is operative when inhibition is required.

Another puzzling issue that confronts us when pondering the notion of dissociation as defense is that the symptoms of dissociation are present in both hyperarousal and neuroinhibitory conditions. For example, in the former case, subjects report feeling "numb," "unreal," and "outside myself" when hyperaroused during panic attacks. Horowitz and Telch (2007) found that the high arousal state they induced through audiophotic stimulation produced feelings of unreality in the experimental cohort.

The latter case, in which neuroinhibition is active during dissociation, has been known for many years. In 1969 Malcolm Lader recorded a very high skin resistance, suggesting low arousal, in a young woman who was feeling "like a robot" and devoid of feeling. Some weeks later she was recorded in her usual anxious state, and this reading showed very high arousal. Lader proposed that "depersonalization is linked to some physiological mechanism for counteracting excess arousal" (1969, p. 60). This proposal is supported by more detailed physiological studies in recent years. Depersonalization has been associated with heightened ventral prefrontal activity (Hollander et al., 1992; Phillips et al., 2001) and diminished activity in emotion-related limbic areas (Phillips et al., 2001).

It is easy to conceive how dissociative phenomena arising from neuroinhibitory activity can have a protective, or defensive, value for the individual. On the other hand, it is quite difficult to see how those dissociative phenomena are protective when occurring in a state of arousal. Nevertheless, states of derealization and depersonalization arising in a state of high arousal may be protective in creating a feeling of "detachment," a sense of disconnectedness from oneself and one's surroundings that enables fear and harm to be borne more easily. It seems possible that some individuals may be able to recreate these states when required, just as some children with epilepsy are able to induce a fit, for example, by repetitively waving a hand across the face, when circumstances of living become intolerable.

CONVERSION DISORDERS

Conversion disorders are comprised of symptoms having the common feature of loss of function—for example, paresis, anaesthesia, or blindness (American Psychiatric Association). They can be understood in terms of the activity of coarse or lower-order inhibitory activity. Seen in this way, they are better conceived as somatic manifestations of "secondary dissociation" rather than as a distinct class of symptoms. A strong argument has been advanced by Nijenhuis (2000) and Van der Hart et al. (2000, 2006) in favor of abandoning the term *conversion* and replacing it with *somatoform dissociation*.

Freud introduced the concept of conversion "into psychopathology in order to account for the leap from mental process to somatic innervation" (Laplanche & Pontalis, 1973, p. 90). The process was regarded as defensive, designed to protect the individual from unacceptable feelings and overwhelming anxiety. The term *conversion* has been widely used and misused, often referring to bodily complaints for which no medical explanation can be given. This practice has led to diagnostic disarray (Slater, 1965). Attempts are now being made to define the phenomenon more precisely.

Nijenhuis (2000) and Van der Hart et al. (2000, 2006) put forward a view of "somatoform dissociation" that is larger than the DSM-IV description of conversion. In their description *somatoform dissociation* refers to three different groups of symptoms. All can be understood as having dissociative bases but the basis, in each case, is somewhat different. The first group is comprised of symptoms that manifest as loss of neurological function; that is, the group of disorders currently called *conversion* by the DSM and identified by deficit. Current evidence suggests that such symptoms are typically associated with activation of the prefrontal cortex, supporting the idea that the loss of function is due to the effect of descending inhibitory mechanisms. Involvement of the orbitofrontal cortex (OFC) and anterior cingulate gyrus was found by Ghaffar et al. (2006) and Marshall et al. (1997). Such studies give support to the inference that activation of medial prefrontal areas accompanies symptoms of conversion, understood as loss of neurological function. This patterning of neural function, however, is likely to be complex (Cantello et al., 2001).

Further studies are required in order to understand the strange features of psychogenic loss of neural function. For example, blindness coming in this way is rather like "blindsight" (Weisk-rantz et al., 1974), in which those with damage to the visual cortex can detect and visually follow an object, but, remarkably, object detection is not accompanied by awareness. A patient with psychogenic blindness, asked to walk across a room where a chair has been placed in the projected pathway, will avoid the chair. Someone feigning blindness bumps into the chair.

Despite the preliminary nature of the evidence, this class of symptoms, which appear to have the aim of "blocking out" a particular aspect of function for defensive purposes, can be understood as a manifestation of a particular kind of neuroinhibition. Perhaps the most common form of "secondary dissociation" in BPD is exhibited during self-mutilation. During episodes of cutting, the subject typically experiences an anesthesia of a kind that is analogous to the loss of function in psychogenic blindness. Pain is reduced or even absent, but feeling in the skin remains, so that the individual is aware of the sensation of the knife cutting the flesh.

A second group of somatoform dissociation symptoms is made up of "positive" movement disorders (e.g., tremor, dystonia, and gait abnormalities) that are likely to be associated with a different pathophysiology than the first group (Voon et al., 2010). Some of these disorders represent an aspect of a traumatic event. Janet (1901) gives an example of a man who:

> was a tiler by trade; two years ago he fell from a scaffolding, which became loose under him, and by sheer miracle he succeeded in catching at a cornice, where he remained suspended by the *right arm*. His comrades were ten minutes in rescuing him. When they took him down, more dead than alive, he trembled in all his body and his teeth chattered terribly. Nothing more natural; only, the accident took place two years ago and he trembles still. This tremor, it is true, has diminished; but it reappears with violence when the patient tries to use his

right arm, and, at this moment, he still experiences fear and anguish; he still fancies that he is falling and expresses it by a terrified gesture; he prefers using his left arm. (pp. 320–321)

This man's tremor and the flailing of his left arm are motor representations of the traumatic event as if they were imprinted in the procedural system of memory. This class of symptoms, involving representation in the body of the traumatic occasion, are discussed further in Chapter 13. Janet called them "accidents" and distinguished them from the "stigmata" that are essentially symptoms of loss of function.

A third group of patients suffer pain that often seems exaggerated. The basis of these symptoms is considered in a later chapter on "somatization" (Chapter 12). In some cases, at least, the pain can be seen as representing a failure of inhibitory mechanisms i.e. as a particular manifestation of primary dissociation.. In this way they are almost the opposite to the first category of symptoms.

FUGUE STATES

The unsatisfactory nature of distinguishing between *dissociation* and *conversion* or between *psychoform* and *somatoform dissociation* is exemplified by the phenomenon of fugue, which is fairly common in BPD, though infrequently reported. In this condition, the psychoform state of amnesia, which is often partial, is combined with the "somatoform" motor component of automatic and apparently purposeless wandering. Direct evidence is obviously unobtainable during a fugue state, so that it is unknown whether its basis is primary or secondary dissociation, or both. In any event, Kopelman (1995) observes that during this state both autobiographical memory and the sense of personal identity are impaired.

The phenomenon of fugue is traditionally understood as a defense of flight from circumstances with which the individual is unable to cope. Stengel's (1939, 1943; Stengel & Vienna, 1941) now classical studies, however, suggest something else. Fugue is not always an escape from an intolerable situation such as the scene of battle. It frequently represents a search for care or solace. The wandering, although apparently purposeless, is vaguely directed toward this end. The care and solace are not specific but are related to memory, for example, of a district where a kindly grandmother had lived, or to something imagined. The basis of these imaginings is suggested by some of Stengel's 36 case histories. Stengel remarked:

> The individual case histories of these patients reveal one characteristic feature. *They are persons during whose development there has occurred a serious disturbance in the child–parent relation, usually of such a nature that relationship to one or both parents was either complete lacking or only partially developed.* [He noted that some patients imagined] that the dead parent was not really dead, but alive, and perhaps to be met in their wanderings. (Stengel, 1939, p. 252, italics in original)

In my experience, those with BPD usually exhibit the latter form of fugue, which is typically brief, lasting hours rather than days. In some cases, the wandering can be understood as "attachment to the trauma" (Meares, 2005, pp. 136–138). For example, a woman wanders at night in an area frequented by prostitutes who are picked up by the passing truck drivers. She has a history of sexual abuse, the abuser being also the only source of care and comfort. Since the source of care had once been traumatic, she seeks it out again, in a situation that might be dangerous.

Shoplifting, which is often included in the catalogue of impulsive behaviors in BPD, may occur in a state of mini-fugue. The individual does not behave like a typical thief. One woman, for example, stared at the shop assistant as she pilfered clothing. When apprehended by security staff, she seemed bewildered.

TERTIARY DISSOCIATION: TRAUMATIC STRUCTURALIZATION OF PERSONALITY

Traumatic memories tend to become hedged about by defensive systems of a kind reflected in neuroinhibitory activity. Traumata that are repeatedly triggered and reenacted lead to disturbances in the development of personality structure. A deformation not uncommon in BPD is a split in which a core of traumatic memory becomes compartmentalized and separated from the rest of the personality. Certain memories, feelings, situations, and thoughts are avoided, having a stunting effect on selfhood. Life is lived through an "apparently normal" personality, to use the term C. S. Myers (1940) introduced following his experiences with shell-shocked soldiers in World War I. From time to time, however, this protective shield fails, often in an explosive way, and what Myers called the "emotional personality" emerges. Myers's observations have been further developed by Van der Hart et al. (2006a).

The "apparently normal" personality resembles the "as if" mode of relating to others described by Deutsch (1942). Kernberg (1967) considered this article fundamental to an understanding of the borderline syndrome.

A more extensive example of the compartmentalization of personality function is dissociative identity disorder, which is typically the result of "chronic and intense sexual, physical, and psychological abuse that started at a very early age" (Van der Kolk, Van der Hart, & Marmar, 1996, p. 308). These investigators conceive such enduring traumatic deformations of personality as "tertiary dissociation." Those with BPD may switch between a condition or state when dissociative identity disorder could be diagnosed and those states, when they are improving (i.e., when the "alters" are much less salient), when dissociative identity disorder would not be diagnosed.

CONCLUSION: PRIMARY, SECONDARY, AND TERTIARY DISSOCIATION

The terms *primary, secondary,* and *tertiary dissociation* have been used here as ways of talking about a complex subject. This triadic classification is taken from an article by Van der Kolk et al. (1996). My use of the term *primary dissociation* broadly corresponds to theirs but differs in several important respects. I understand from Onno Van der Hart that their description of 1996 would now be rewritten.

In my usage, *primary dissociation* refers to a fragmentation or a disintegration of the sense of personal existing. It includes peritraumatic dissociation; states in which an original traumatic memory is reexperienced; and states in childhood, evident during the exhibition of disorganized attachment, when the child appears as if stunned, bewildered, and frightened. The child's bodily expression reflects a state that would be called *dissociated* in an adult. In a series of papers Giovanni Liotti (e.g., 1992, 2004, 2009) has described the relationship between disorganized attachment and primary dissociation, the one mirroring the other.

Secondary dissociation arises out of a state of primary dissociation. As Van der Kolk and his colleagues put it: "Once an individual is in a traumatic (dissociated) state of mind, further disintegration of elements of the personal experience can occur" (1996, p. 307). A sequestration of a complex of psychic life now occurs. This compartmentalization is achieved by the activity of neuroinhibitory mechanisms such as demonstrated in the experiments of Lanius, Felmingham, and their colleagues. The effect of these mechanisms is to reduce the high arousal characteristic of primary dissociation. This state shares with primary dissociation the sense of unreality and a disturbance of the experience of the body and of time, but these symptoms become more profound so that the condition may be noticed by others.

The range of "blocking-out" maneuvers that is involved in the production of secondary dissociation extends from the rapid and unconscious physiological response demonstrated in the experiments of Felmingham et al. (2008) to more conscious strategies. One of these is absorption, one of the three factors that reliably emerge when a pool of dissociation items is examined. The taxometric analysis of Waller et al. (1996) found that those items of the DES that are indicators of absorption (i.e., an intense involvement in imaginative activity and daydreaming) can be distinguished from true, or pathological, dissociation as indicated by amnesia, derealization, depersonalization, and identity alteration. Absorption, then, is a reflection of the normal process of selective inattention that is recruited at the higher levels of intellectual and creative endeavor.

Evidence of absorption used as a defense is provided by Giesbrecht and colleagues (2007). They measured the cortisol responses to stress of 58 students who had been scored on the depersonalization–derealization and absorption subscales of the DES. They found that students who scored high on depersonalization–derealization had more pronounced cortisol responses, where those who scored high on the absorption subscale had attenuated responses. These findings can be seen as consistent with the view that primary dissociation, indicated by depersonalization–derealization, is associated with raised arousal and cannot be considered protective, whereas absorption may be an aspect of secondary dissociation and have a defensive and anxiety reducing function.

The emergence of secondary dissociation out of primary dissociation can be considered in the light of Liotti's vulnerability theory, put forward in 1992. He proposes that an initial vulnerability is established by a disturbance in attachment formation. If subsequent caregiving is suitable and able to facilitate the generation of mature selfhood, this vulnerability is overcome. If, however, a disturbance in the child's relationship continues to the level where it constitutes chronic trauma, the vulnerability is maintained and enhanced so that in early adult life, the person is likely to display symptoms of dissociation.

Tertiary dissociation might be understood as a more or less chronic state of secondary dissociation. The compartmentalization of psychic life undergoing this deformation of personality structure is presumably related to volumetric and other changes in brain structure, the patterns of which have not as yet been elucidated in detail. It should not be supposed that such alterations in brain structure necessarily condemn the individual to a state of incurability. Janet describes the remarkable story of a patient of Dr. Azam, from Bordeaux, who eventually recovered from a state of spectacular compartmentalization. The case, published first in 1860, concerned Felida, first seen when she was 15. She was "reserved, melancholy and timid," suffering from a wide range of disorders, including pains and "diffuse insensibilities." From time to time, however, "she would wake up suddenly, become active and gay, without any anxiety or pain." This oscillation at first lasted only a few hours, but as life went on the second state became progressively longer. Toward the end of her life, the first state had almost disappeared (Janet, 1907, pp. 79–83, 91–92).

The triadic distinction of forms of dissociation is useful as preliminary categorization that will be modified and expanded with increasing understanding of the phenomena that comprise the syndrome. A three-stage concept is limited in that it has no satisfactory place for the "representing" form of symptom that Janet called an "accident" (more on this topic in Chapter 13). States such as fugue and PTSD are only equivocally accommodated. Nor does the three-stage concept readily encompass such phenomena as the remarkable productions of Hélée Smith, who, during the trance-like states of her séances, told stories of herself in other historical eras in which she spoke and wrote strange languages that had their own script and syntactical structure

(Flournoy, 1899). Nevertheless, the sketch of dissociation given here serves as a necessary background to a proposal that BPD has a dissociative basis.

Patients with BPD manifest significantly more dissociation than other psychiatric patients, with the exception of those with dissociative identity disorder with which BPD overlaps diagnostically (Boon & Draijer, 1993; Dell, 1998). I consider them to be different manifestations of the same systematic disturbance as illustrated in the case presented in the following chapter. Nevertheless, about a third of those with BPD cannot be given the diagnosis of dissociation according to standard diagnostic instruments (Korzekwa, Dell, & Pain, 2009). This has led some observers to conclude that dissociation is not an inherent aspect of BPD, although dissociative states are frequently "comorbid" with BPD. Korzekwa, Dell, Links et al. (2009), in concluding a study of a small sample of BPD outpatients ($n = 21$), noted that those patients who could not be given the diagnosis of dissociative disorder according to the protocols they used (which characteristically reflect the more florid aspects of dissociation) "reported a surprising number of dissociative symptoms, but to a milder degree" (p. 363). The average patient with BPD endorsed a wide variety of deeply disturbing dissociative symptoms that were anything but "transient and stress-related."

Janet expressed the view that certain individuals "experience chronic dissociative states" (Waller et al., 1996, p. 315). The proposal being developed in this book is that central to the syndrome of BPD is a disturbance of psychic life that can be called *primary dissociation*. It is a state that can be conceived as the obverse of self, that is, as self broken up. The conception echoes that of Ogawa and colleagues: "Self, in fact, refers to the integration and organization of diverse aspects of experience, and dissociation can be defined as the failure to integrate experience" (1997, p. 856). Such basic disintegration leads to attempts to adapt to the environment by secondary and tertiary dissociation.

Chapter 8

FUSION AND DISCONNECTION
The Paradoxical Structure of Dissociative Experience

THOSE WORKING WITH people suffering from the borderline condition frequently find themselves caught up in a strange and alienating experience. It is shared by both partners in the therapeutic dyad.

There is a curious paradox in this experience. It is illustrated by the story of a young woman whose symptomatology included intractable atypical depression and impulsive, self-destructive behaviors, including frightening suicide attempts. At times during her therapy she would sense her body as changed. She felt shrunken and tiny, so that as she looked out from herself she would see her arms grotesquely large, although they were actually slim and small. Such episodes of depersonalization would often last weeks. After one such prolonged period of dissociation she was able to describe a persisting sense of disconnection from others—from me, her husband, and her children.

The disconnection during sessions was profound. She spoke in a monotonous voice as if I were not in the room, as if she were alone. As she spoke, she stared past me, to the side of me, always in the same direction. What I said seemed to alter her state not at

Written in association with David Butt, Alison Moore, Caroline Henderson-Brooks, and Joan Haliburn.

all, as if she were impervious. The opposite, however, was the case. She showed an extreme sensitivity to my presence, betraying an awareness of the smallest changes in my body, of tone of voice, of posture, and even, I suspected, variations in respiration. It seemed as if, coincident with disconnection, there was no boundary between us, as if the dyad were fused, two people living the same life.

A mood was created of tension, boredom, and alienation. I, too, experienced something of her depersonalized state.

Inferences from such experiences include the fact that the experience of self, including the bodily self—its density, form, and spatiality—is an aspect of the interplay with the environment (Meares, 1980, 1984). The experience of self cannot be distinguished from the kind of interrelatedness in which the individual is engaged at that moment. This leads to the hypothesis that dissociation is a state of mind in which the individual senses others as paradoxically both alienated and fused and in which the psychic condition in some way mirrors the form of relatedness. This hypothesis was tested by means of a linguistic analysis of a therapeutic conversation involving a patient who dissociated during sessions.

Sophisticated analysis of the therapeutic conversation provides a window into the still mysterious phenomenon of dissociation. It gives a view that is not open to procedures such as neuroimaging or even to self-report, since the subject, in the usual case, cannot adequately describe the experience. The linguistic enterprise is based on the idea put forward by Wilhelm von Humboldt (1767–1835) that the structure of language reveals the structure of mind (Humboldt, 1988).

FUSION AND A DISTURBANCE OF THE BOUNDARY

Although *disconnection* is a word frequently used in descriptions of dissociation, *fusion* rarely appears. The state of fusion can be understood as a disturbance of the sense or experience of self-boundary. I have suggested that this disturbance may be a consequence of a deficit in the regulation of the intensity of sensory input (Horvath & Meares, 1979; Meares, 1977, pp. 38–47). The idea is derived from a story told by a man who, as a boy of 9, had suffered bilateral otitis media in the era before antibiotics. He had been deaf for 3 weeks. His deafness was relieved immediately when a doctor pierced his eardrums. Following this, he heard a ticking in his head, and wondered whether the doctor had left a bomb inside it. The voices of his mother and the doctor were booming and ominous. After 20 minutes he realized that the ticking was not in his head but came from the bedside clock. At about the same time, the voices returned to normal. As I reported several decades ago:

> For twenty minutes the boy's capacity to distinguish between inner events and those outside was impaired. One imagines that during the three weeks of deafness some hypothetical "valve" regulating his input of sound was operating at a maximum in order to compensate for his deafness. In the twenty minutes following the restoration of his hearing, it seems likely that the "valve" was readjusting to its previous level, but that during this period the boy was relatively flooded with auditory input. (Meares, 1977, p. 40)

Findings from Malcolm Lader (1969) suggest that, at times, those patients who characteristically dissociate, formerly called *hysterics*, might periodically be afflicted with a sensory overload similar to this boy during the 20 minutes in which his boundary sense was impaired. Lader and Sartorius (1968) investigated a group of people who were diagnosed with "hysteria" and who were still symptomatic at the time of investigation. They exhibited extraordinarily high levels of arousal. Using the rate of spontaneous fluctuation in skin resistance per minute as an index, these researchers showed an average level of arousal about twice that of a group of people with anxiety states. Such arousal might be sufficient to impair one's sense of boundary.

It may have been that during the period in which she was de-personalized, my patient was in a state of anxiety resembling sensory overload. The mechanism for such a state can be inferred from data presented earlier. The system regulating sensory input, necessarily involving inhibitory activity, is relatively deficient in those with BPD.

THE LINGUISTIC APPROACH

A principal difficulty of studying mental states is that they cannot be observed. Progress toward a science of mental life is therefore impeded. The behaviorist project sought to overcome this dif-ficulty by implicitly proposing that thought inevitably involves an action, whether this action is carried out or not. On this as-sumption, behavior, being observable, offers some means toward a scientific approach to that which is "mental." The behavior of conversation, however, which is essential to humankind, has been relatively disregarded in this approach. A study of language as it is used, including its phonology and syntax, and not merely the lexicon, may provide an insight into the intricacies of psychic life. This is not to say, of course, that the lexicon is without sci-entific value. The words that people use to describe their state of dissociation—such as "numb," "unreal," "spacey," "zoned out"— enable us to know the peculiar subjective qualities of this expe-rience. Such qualities, however, do not offer an insight into the structure of the experience. A greater complexity of analysis is required. In a study reported in this chapter, systemic functional linguistics (Halliday, 1975–2007) was used to examine the struc-ture of the conversation employed by a woman who dissociated during a therapeutic session. The hypothesis was advanced that this analysis would show both disconnection and fusion of language elements, fusion being understood as connection between elements not usually connected.

The principal measure used in this study was developed by Ruqaiya Hasan (1984, 1985). It identifies textual coherence as "cohesive harmony." Essentially, cohesive harmony is based on a "picture" (diagram) of word chains and how the separate lexical chains (related words) cross-connect with each other through the repetition of a grammatical role: for example, when a word (token) in one chain acts on a word (token) from another chain through the same grammatical role (i.e., when members of the chains are grammatically linked twice and hence "echoed").

CASE REPORT

The patient, Jennifer, was first seen as an adolescent some 20 years before the session to be examined. She was treated by my colleague Joan Haliburn, who was supervised, on that occasion, by me. Jennifer presented with a severe, atypical form of obsessive–compulsive disorder in which the dominating obsession concerned the evil of sexuality. This forced her, whenever she had a sexual thought, to smash her head against a wall as punishment. Since both food and bathing made her think of sex, she avoided both. She arrived at the emergency department of Westmead Hospital emaciated and filthy, with severe bruising about the forehead.

It emerged that she had suffered this condition for at least a year, during which time she had been treated behaviorally in two other hospitals for several months on each occasion. Her condition on first presentation and its apparently intractable nature suggested that her life was in danger. Under the care of Dr. Haliburn, however, she made a remarkable recovery, even becoming a swimming instructor. She married and had a child.

Relapses occurred as a consequence of stressors, one of which was the breakup of her marriage. On these occasions, she returned to Dr. Haliburn. Different symptomatology now emerged: self-harming behavior, somatization, and alterations in self-perception and self-regulation. Like many of those suffering from BPD Jennifer had received multiple diagnoses before, and in conjunction with, the eventual diagnosis of the disorder. The most recent return to the care of Dr. Haliburn came with a referral from a psychiatric unit where Jennifer had been diagnosed with dissociative identity disorder. She had been an inpatient there for 3 months subsequent to several dissociative episodes followed by a near-fatal overdose. It was during this illness that the session considered in the following material took place. Dr Haliburn describes the background and the nature of this session in the following way:

> Several acute family stressors, followed by a vicious sexual assault by a stranger, had precipitated this disturbance. Jennifer presented with a multiplicity of self states, at one stage reenacting one of several exorcisms she reportedly had undergone, during which time rapid shifts in consciousness were evident, during which she believed she was possessed by Satan who lived in her throat. From time to time her voice changed, as she claimed that I did not really know her, and that "he" had never met me; and from time to time she became a little baby who was "lost" and could not find her way "home." In thrice-weekly long-term psychoanalytic psychotherapy based on the Conversational Model, there were several times when we became triangulated as she experienced me alternately as a perpetrator, victim, and rescuer (Liotti, 1995). This mirrored the fact that she had to cope with disparate images of her father, an often intoxicated caregiver, whom she loved but who often physically and sexually abused her from an early age, until he was removed from the home when she was 7 years of age. Her mother was unavailable, critical, and punitive, and was away at work a lot.
>
> The parent who was the source of her fear was often also

the source of her happiness. She enjoyed the games he played with her, but also accommodated to him because he would severely punish her if she disobeyed. When her father was removed, she grieved for him, but his absence was referred to as "bad" because she missed him. She then ceased doing so and completely accommodated to her mother in order to be seen as pleasing. This inner and outer shift was indeed immensely disorienting and disorganizing for her (Liotti, 1999), as a result, I would suggest, of concurrent or alternating activation and deactivation of the attachment system for her as a child, and repeated in adulthood as she recalled traumatic experiences. It was impossible for her to maintain a stable image in her mind, which created considerable dysregulation in her day-to-day life.

We had come to a point in the therapy when there were signs of integrating, except for the "baby" who often came out; and then she would not give up the baby, which presented time and time again with a very little voice. She symbolically placed the baby beside her, saying to me, "Look at her and feel sorry for her," before she could finally say "It happened to me, it should not have happened to me."

The session (audiorecorded) is in the third year of her therapy. Jennifer looks bright and pleased with herself as she comes into the consulting room; but it soon becomes apparent that she is also troubled by something. There is a mixture of excitement and fear, as she proceeds in a rather confused way to tell me about her weekend. She is in a state of hyperarousal as I immerse myself in our conversation, allowing her story to develop, just letting her know through short verbal and non-verbal responses that I am listening. She becomes distressed, yet wants to tell me about something that happened, as I speculate with her—she wants to tell me, but at the same time she does not want to delve into it, for fear that it will overtake her. This theme repeats itself in several different ways—her coherence diminishes as she begins to relate a recent experience that appears to have qualities of a past experience, but is "currently" happening. Staying with her and providing her the safety of our relationship, she begins to talk about the traumatic experience of the weekend as if in a dream, into which I feel myself entering. There is a confusion of time, persons, and places for her, and she worries that they might be false memories—"Did they really happen?" she asks. I feel myself dissociating. I struggle to be with her, as her childhood experiences become entangled with this most recent experience. There is no boundary between past and present—a state of fusion exists: Though she is telling me about this most recent experience, she is also reliving a past traumatic experience, which I struggle to stay with. However, I must not wrench myself away; neither should I become engulfed in her experience. I gradually disentangle myself and remain on the periphery of her experience. To withdraw abruptly would leave her bereft and alone. Attempting to take the patient off track will not help either, as some therapists are prone to do, because the patient would not be able to process the traumatic memories if left alone.

Two different phases are clearly experienced: While I attempt to reestablish a sense of equilibrium and containment, the experience of the patient becomes clearer. The therapist must enter the dissociative world of the patient. Being aware of her, being curious as to what has happened, being aware of my own feelings in response to hers, and connecting with words, sounds, shifts in posture, facial expressions, or movement shows willingness on my part to be there with her, allowing myself to be experienced more fully in relationship. It sometimes feels as if you are not there, but the patient is acutely aware of your presence. A relationship is required in the therapeutic space in order to be aware of the nuances of a dissociative episode.

A core feeling is a necessary part of every state of consciousness—and so is the relatedness that becomes disorganized whenever it is interrupted by a traumatic memory. Paradoxically, by entering at her level of consciousness, one can move it to an emergent, coherent state of relatedness (Graham & van Biene, 2007). The patient's state of mind dictates what the therapist says.

Describing her early life, Jennifer says, "Every day was like walking through a minefield." This presence of a "minefield" maintained her in a state of wariness: "It was funny afterwards, I hated the punishment, but punishment brought me peace."

Her state of mind conveys uncertainty, a fear of repetition: "I feel like, in a bit of a bind, because something happened on Sunday, in fact, I am not wanting to delve into things." This statement calls for understanding on my part, as I speculate with her that something happened on Sunday, but there is a fear of delving into the experience that confuses her. This is followed by an opposite feeling: "I don't want to delve into things, but then I am afraid of separating myself from them as well—I am afraid of blocking it out, of pushing it away— living like a false—a false life." She feels that, if she becomes happy, "It's just going to come back again."

Jennifer sees herself in a bind, wanting to work through things, but fearing the difficulty she would experience; at the same time she is afraid of blocking out those things and living like nothing has happened, which is just as difficult for her. She is also afraid that when she is relaxed, she is lulled into a false sense of security, from which she could suddenly be aroused. She is unable to "trust feeling better." For example, she reported:

"Then it came again, just when everything was relaxed. I think, is it me or is there a connection? Is it something that it is real you just remember or see that is what was happening in my teenage years? I would see something and I would keep having, um . . . I would hear voices . . . that I . . . eh, and it wasn't me, but I was watching a woman doing stuff . . . sort of, um . . . and they were taking photos." A brief response from me, "It's confusing, the present and the past?", results in her saying "I don't know. I just want to see him again, and it makes me feel dirty that it makes me feel, um—why am I thinking?"

She seems to wander into and out of several levels of consciousness. Her voice changes when "every time I think about it, you know, it is just there, you know what I mean, I just looked and looked . . . and then I turn away and it is like a rock that hits like a thump and you hear things and I turned the other way and started to walk—it's just —it feels so real, and there is a connection with it and it feels so distant as well." Then she was once more in the present, with me, telling me about the events of the weekend, as she started to place the events of her childhood in the past.

As the session moved on, Jennifer dissociated less frequently and was gradually able to maintain a narrative: "I had to punish myself, every time I saw myself in a mirror, even in a window. I could not look at myself. I could not think of anything sexual—it was difficult, because the thoughts came even if I did not want them to. Afterwards, I hated the punishment, but punishment brought me peace. Scratching, punching, hitting myself became the way to punish myself, then starving—I was bad, so I could not eat."

Jennifer proceeded to talk about the development of her anorexia: "If I could have an apple or something like that for lunch—then you were allowed to have only half, and then I wasn't allowed any of it," she said, which led me to respond, "So by the time the half apple gets halved and halved, there's no apple left, and you are left starving." She said it was the norm —the punishment.

This session concluded with her telling me about a birthday party she went to when she was 13 years old, where she was introduced to masturbation and sexual intercourse, and when, in her words, she "freaked out." Notwithstanding this disclosure, Jennifer remained alert and together and was able to conclude the session with relatively little difficulty.

CONVERSATION AND THE UNCONSCIOUS

The linguistic approach to the therapeutic conversation resembles the psychoanalytic. It is based on the idea that the way in which a particular thought, memory, story, or other piece of information is expressed is not random. It treats as implausible assumptions that a particular semantic ensemble is merely a chance event. It is based, in short, on the notion of the unconscious. It suggests that the text of the conversation conveys more than either the speaker or the listener knows. The "meanings" of the discourse are unconscious in the sense that they (1) are realized by choices that few people could consciously report; (2) accumulate and ramify at a rate that cannot be monitored in real time, even by linguists; and (3) accumulate and ramify to complex quantities that require considerable reflective and statistical processing of implicit themes. Such themes might develop in parallel, creating a form of semantic "polyphony" (Halliday, 1975–2007).

The notion of the unconscious determinants of conversation includes the fact of the early development of the unconscious, which is prereflective, in the first and formative relationships with carers. Our taking on of personhood and the personalization of our brains are continuous with the meanings we take on and the meaning by which our relationships are sustained.

In essence, the linguistic approach depends upon the view that within a particular conversation, unconscious linguistic patterns can be discerned that arise on the basis of "motivated selection" (Tynjanov & Jacobson, 1928/1981). A nonrandom consistency in the choices of words is a textural realization of a state of mind.

Linguistic Method: Coherence versus Fragmentation

A straightforward means of tracking the connectedness between the words of a text is through the use of a cohesive chain. One form of a chain is based on the accumulation of words that "point" to an identical person or "thing." Such words are grammatical items like pronouns and demonstratives (e.g., *this, that, these, those*), which create threads of identity that are specific to the given text: hence, *identity chains*.

A second form of chain is built out of similarities. The similarities are based on relationships that are *not* specific to this text but that are carried over to any use of the word(s). These are chains of what are called *open system* items (i.e., *not* from a small set of grammatical choices such as pronouns, but drawn from the dictionary head words). These are interrelated by their various meanings, especially if they are standard logical relations of equivalence (synonymy), oppositeness (antonymy), class membership (hyponymy), or part to whole (meronymy).

A third kind of chain that figures in our analysis is built from explicit declarations of equivalence in the wording of a specific text: for example, "the birds, the birds were soldiers. . . ." In the semantics of this instance of text ("Dry Loaf," a poem by the poet Wallace Stevens), it is necessary, after this declaration in the text, to construe birds and soldiers together because that equivalence has been legislated by the text itself. The equivalence is only for this instance of text (*birds* and *soldiers* will not carry this relation beyond the text). Consequently we can refer to these texts, following Hasan (1984), as "instantial." Such texts weave in links between terms that are specialized, technical versions of experience (often made explicit in appositions), and the instantial chain will also capture metaphorical relations that become significant to the logical skeleton of meanings within a text (as in the "birds ←→ soldiers" text).

When the tokens (words) in the chains are set against the numbers of the units of text (i.e., clauses/sentences) in which they occur, we can see the threads of identity, of similarity, and of metaphorical equivalences (or of technical formulations) laid out in a diagram of the connectedness of words and referential items (i.e., pronouns, definite articles) in that text. The chain diagram is "iconic" (as C. S. Peirce, 1932, used the term) in that the chains display a "resemblance relationship with the semantic threading," from word to word, throughout the text or text segment. Such chains offer certain restrictive quantitative perspectives on the text—only the number and density of these cohesive devices, clause by clause. Such simple quantities will not discriminate sense from nonsense—or from fragmentation and other grades of incoherence. Yet such "bunchings" of items, when regarded from the point of view of speakers' motives, provide evidence of shifts or phases in the talk.

The issue of fragmentation demands that we introduce another quantitative principle, essentially an index of how the "threads" are interwoven. Hasan (1984) found that she could represent "chain interaction" by indicating where tokens in two different chains had the "same" relationship repeated, or "echoed." The *same relationship* means here that words in two chains serve in the same grammatical roles with respect to each other, at least twice (hence, their relationship is *echoed*). The crucial grammatical roles pertain to experiential roles (actor/acted upon, etc.). These interacting tokens (words) then take on a new analytical status: such "central tokens" do serve as a measurement of textual coherence (not merely cohesive stitching). In fact, a number of quantitative relations, based on central tokens, can be brought to bear on the question of textual coherence.

These relations are the number of central tokens (interacting tokens) as a proportion of:

1. The total tokens in the text
2. The total relevant tokens in a text (i.e., those that enter into chains)
3. The number of peripheral tokens (i.e., those that do *not* enter into any chain)

A further iconic sign of textuality might be thought of as the bridging or "step" function of the chain interactions: Does the diagram show any chain, or grouping of chains, without a bridge of interaction to other chains? Such "islands" of cohesive chaining suggest a failure of connectedness, or (depending on the genre) a segment that stands alone from the texture of the discourse, as in the case of an analogy or parable.

Transcript of the Dissociative Episode

The following is a transcript of what the therapist judged to be an overt dissociative episode occurring during a therapeutic session. Such episodes are frequent during the conversations between a therapist and someone suffering the borderline condition. They range from mild disturbance to catastrophic. Apart from those occasions when the patient clearly manifests an alteration in consciousness, these episodes are often unrecognized since the patient may seem little different from someone who is not dissociated. Inquiry, however, may reveal severe disturbance, even hallucinosis, going on as a background to a somewhat automatic form of conversational responsiveness.

The judgment that the patient is dissociated can only be presumptive because, of course, standard measures of dissociation cannot be taken from moment to moment in a session. The therapist's presumption is based on a number of factors, including, most importantly, the conversational structure and style and the therapist's own experience. The patient's expressions tend to become vaguer, nonspecific, and general, and at, the same time, constricted in range. The therapist's own experience may be a sense of confusion, of being caught up in something that is not one's own and that is unclear.

This transcript is taken from the point in the session when the therapist judged that the dissociation began. It clears quite suddenly. The shift is evident in the linguistic analysis that is briefly summarized in a section following the transcript. The emphasis is upon the fusion aspect of the dissociative experience.

79 Jennifer: Like on Sunday we, I, went to my sister's place on the weekend.

80 Therapist: Mmm-hmm.

81 Jennifer: (decrease volume) They have a few acres and they've got horses. /mm/ A few of us went out to see the horses. Everything was fine, and we were heading back—

seeing the horses, it's like, it's really disgusting. Everything was fine and we go to start heading back.

82 Therapist: Mmmm-hmmm.

83 Jennifer: Then it came again, everything was relaxed . . . (inaudible). That's when I think is it me or is there a connection? Is it something that is real you just remember, I just keep seeing what was happening in my teenage years. I would see something and I would keep having, um, I would hear voices . . . that I . . . And it wasn't me, but I was watching the woman doing stuff to the horse (silence) sort of, um (silence), and they were taking photos. It's always taking photos.

84 Therapist: It is very confusing. The present and the past, kind of mixed up?

85 Jennifer: I don't know. It's just what I see in my head and it makes me feel dirty that it makes me feel um . . . /yeh/ why am I thinking like that, it is not like I saw it and, um, started to think about it you know. It's just there, you know what I mean, and I looked and then I turned away and it is like a thump it hits you like a thump . . . and you see things and you hear things and I turned the other way and started to walk it's just . . .

86 Therapist: Yes.

87 Jennifer: And, um . . .

88 Therapist: Yeah.

89 Jennifer: I just want to know if I am making it up or if . . . ?

90 Therapist: Making it up?

91 Jennifer: Umm. (silence) I just saw it and thought maybe that happened too, you know what I mean, but it wasn't like that.

92 Therapist: Maybe that happened too.

93 Jennifer: (*silence*) It feels so real and it's like there is a connection with it and it feels so distant as well.

94 Therapist: Yes, yes.

95 Jennifer: It is so far away, it so . . .

96 Therapist: Yeah, yeah.

97 Jennifer: Umm.

98 Therapist: It seems like it is seeing the horse's penis, or the pony's penis, you immediately felt bad, like associated it with something sexual? Like you were bad for seeing the horse's, the pony's, penis?

99 Jennifer: No.

100 Therapist: No (*laughs*).

101 Jennifer: It is just the thoughts associated.

102 Therapist: The present and the past. The thoughts associated with it.

103 Jennifer: He thinks it is a part of his body, that it's just because human perverse of that, um.

104 Therapist: Mmmm.

105 Jennifer: That is what makes me feel crazy in the head . . . the thoughts.

106 Therapist: Mmmm. You mentioned the thoughts associated with it, Jennifer. The thoughts now or the thoughts in the past?

107 Jennifer: It is the images now. I don't know if it is the past or if it is something I am making up or is just my humanness doing that or . . .

108 Therapist: It is very confusing, but then from the past there were always images associated with anything sexual. Mmmm.

109 Jennifer: (*silence*)

110 Therapist: It seems to me like you are associating with the sexual images, the sexual connotations, with just something of what image is what you see now. You see the pony's penis—well, for that matter, one can see, you know, pictures, and one can see naked bodies in reality. Mmmm.

111 Jennifer: Yes.

112 Therapist: But does that mean something sexual? But it seems like the association . . .

113 Jennifer: It doesn't, it shouldn't, but with me it does.

114 Therapist: Yes.

The Fabric of Dissociative Conversation

The fabric of conversation can be displayed by means of lexical chains of identity and "similarity," developing during the conversation, which are stitched together by grammatical relations, manifesting the warp and weft of the verbal interplay. This mapping of the vertical and horizontal axes of the illustrative transcript is shown in Figure 8.1. Detailed consideration of these results is given in Butt et al. (2010). The brief discussion in this chapter is concerned with the more salient aspects of the analysis.

Certain of the vertical chains are unresolvable or equivocal, so that they do not provide an "anchor" to established states of affairs. With this failure of tokens to hold together, mutual coherence cannot grow; fragmentation is the result. The therapist finds herself caught in a semantic vertigo. The most prominent of these chains concerns "it." The last few turns in the transcript show some resolution of analogous items—*seeing, penis, sexual, images*—which are now more distinct. At the same time, the number of chains is reduced, the "it" now interacting with the key "similarity" chain (real vs. made-up; note, in the figure, the reduced horizontal spread of blue shading).

The more striking finding in the diagram is the great reduction in the horizontal lilac bands after turn 100. These bands show an exaggerated connection or fusion between contexts that are normally kept apart. The most obvious evidence in the transcript concerns time. Present and past are conflated as the dissociative episode beings (e.g., turn 83). At this stage, the therapist herself feels something of the dissociation. The state is hard to describe, resembling the head-spinning effect of being mildly stunned. The therapist does not back away from the experience, nor does she attempt to clarify what is going on. She "stays with it," representing their shared experience. "It is very confusing. The present and past, kind of mixed up?" (turn 84).

The therapist's demeanor and way of responding allow the dissociation to rapidly clear, so that by turn 98 she is aware that she herself is free of its effect. She makes a different kind of remark that is more reflective, to which the patient replies "No." The therapist laughs. They are now two people connected, but no longer a fused dyad.

FRAGMENTATION AND RELATEDNESS

This brief episode of dissociation is relatively mild. The partners in the conversation do not lose contact with each other or experience the alienation that is characteristic of dissociation. In this section, an illustration is given of a more obvious dissociation occurring in the context of a deteriorating relationship that precipitates a fragmentation, the discernment of which is clear, needing no linguistic help.

The relationship is a crucial aspect of the dissociation and cannot be separated from it. The co-occurrence of relationship and state of mind can be understood in terms of conception of a mental state. All states of mind, such as dissociation, necessarily arise from a certain way in which the brain is working. A brain, however, considered as an isolated machine, spinning away in its cranial box, is an abstraction. A brain is always in an interplay, though the sensory apparatus, with the world around—which, most importantly, is the world of others. The form of the interplay determines the brain state, and vice versa. In the terms of the relationship with others, the interplay is conducted by means of conversation.

Particular forms of conversation are associated with particular states of mind. These different kinds of conversation manifest and constitute not only a state of mind but also a form of relationship. In the preceding illustrative session, the therapist's ability to establish a different form of relatedness to that which is part of the dissociative experience, at the same time staying

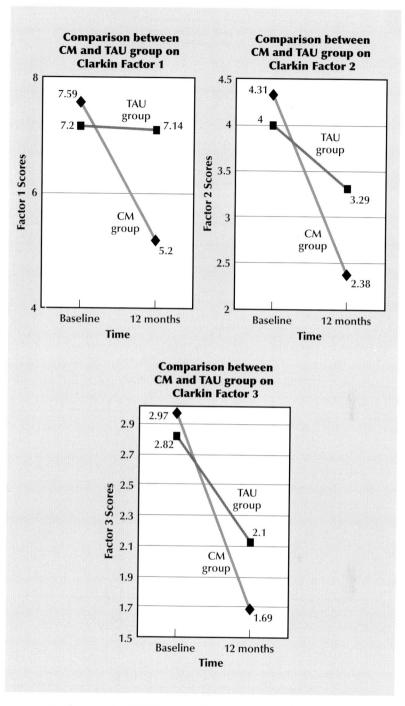

FIGURE 3.1 Changes in BPD factors of 1. Self, 2. Emotional dysregulaton, 3. Impulsivity over one year's treatment by two different forms of treatment, Conversational Model (CM) and Treatment as Usual (TAU)

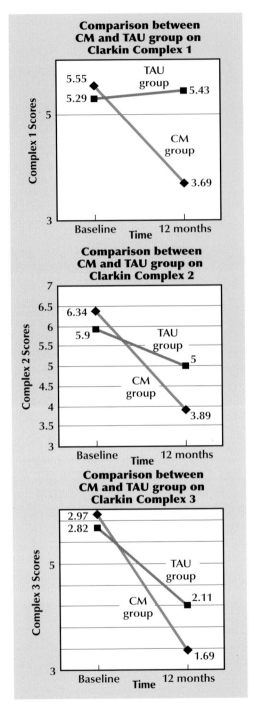

FIGURE 3.2 Changes in BPD complexes of DSM-IV criteria 1. Self, 2. Emotional dysregulation, 3. Impulsivity over one year's treatment by two different forms of treatment, Conversational Model (CM) and Treatment as Usual (TAU)

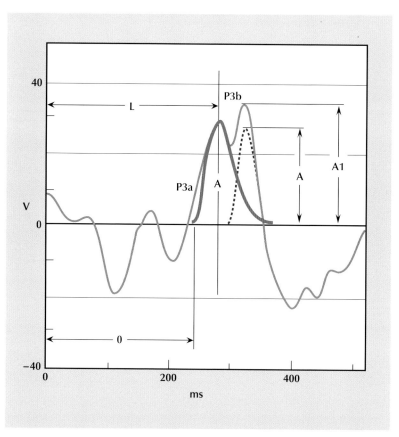

FIGURE 5.1 The solid line exemplifies single trial event-related potential record with identified P3a and P3b. Ordinate scale is for voltage (V, µV). Bold solid and dotted curves show models of P3a (A=28. µV, O=244 ms, L=280 ms) and P3b (26.9, 300, 324), respectively. Resolution of the temporal overlap-corrected estimate of P3a and P3b provides an overlap-corrected estimate of P3b peak amplitude, A. A1 is the peak amplitude of the P3b peak in the single-trial record.

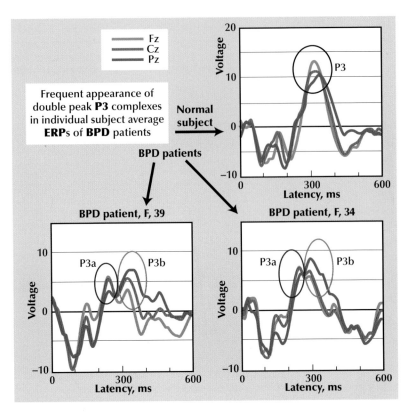

FIGURE 5.2 Disconnection between P3a and P3b produces in BPD a P3 with two peaks.

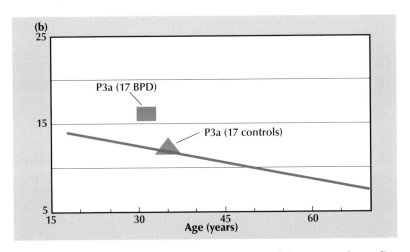

FIGURE 5.3 (Cz recording site) (a) Dependencies of the P3a peak amplitude on the number of target stimuli. (b) The bold solid line shows P3a normative age dependency between the ages of 18 and 70 years (normative group). The square and triangle show P3a peak amplitudes for patients with borderline personality disorder and the control group, respectively. Ordinate scales (a) and (b) are for peak amplitude (μV).

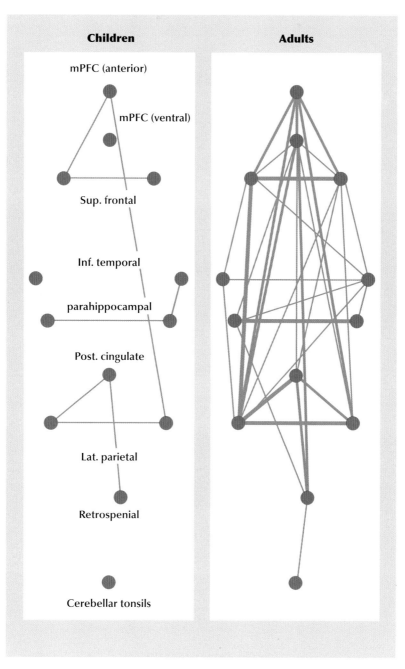

FIGURE 6.1 Different connectivity of DMN in children and adults.

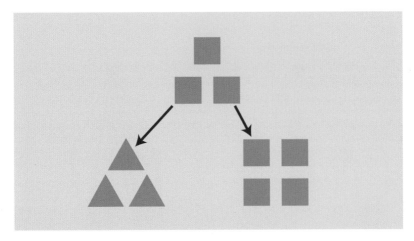

FIGURE 7.1 Choosing best match between two options below with figure above.

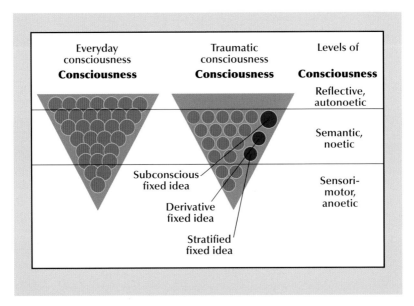

FIGURE 7.2 Schematic representations of traumatic and non-traumatic consciousness.

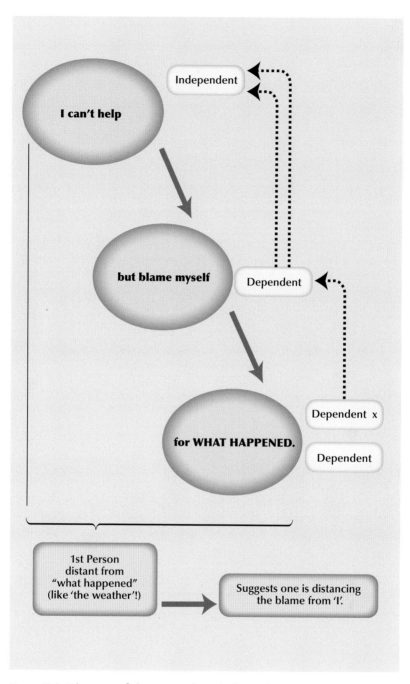

FIGURE 8.1 Diagram of the semantic "stitching" between words—the lexical chains—is presented in this figure. It is an iconic version of the identity between certain items ("identity chains") and the relatedness of meaning (relations of similarity, oppositeness, class membership, part-to-whole, etc: hence "similarity chains") (see text).

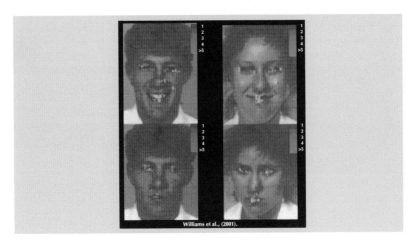

Williams et al., (2001).

Figure 9.1 Facial Expressions of Different Emotions. Top images depict sample scan paths for happy faces; bottom images depict scan paths for neutral expression. Squares (marked in black) indicate Duchenne crows feet regions, and dots indicates number of fixations to each facial region.

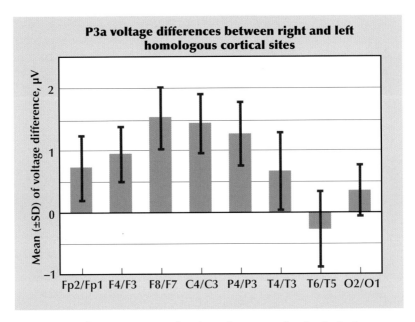

Figure 15.1 Illustrates Lateralization of P3a Amplitudes in Patients with BPD. The bars (± standard errors) show the mean differences, 7A, in P3a amplitudes between eight homologous electrode sites in the right and left hemispheres: Fp1 vs. Fp2, F4 vs. F3, F8 vs. F7, C4 vs. C3, P4 vs. P3, T4 vs. T3, T3 vs. T5, and O2 vs. O1. With exception of nonsignificant differences at T6 vs. T5 and O2 vs. O1, the 7A for remaining pairs of cortical sites are statistically significant ($p < .05$). The positiveness of the differences indicates larger P3a amplitudes in the right hemisphere.

within it, so that connection is not lost, enabled her to shift her patient's state of mind to one that was more integrated and that showed greater differentiation between things that are normally differentiated. If she had failed to establish the different form of relatedness, it is likely that the patient's state would have deteriorated, perhaps manifesting the severe and florid dissociative experience that had kept Jennifer in a psychiatric hospital for 3 months before her referral. An opposite situation is illustrated in the following short transcript, in which a therapist, not trained in working with those suffering from BPD, meets a new patient. Commentary appears in brackets and indented.

The patient is a 37-year-old man working as a copywriter at an advertising firm. He is seeking treatment because he feels himself to be unproductive and uncreative. The patient and therapist exchange a few pleasantries as they walk from the waiting room.

Patient: Why am I seeing the world like I am? I have been to therapy before—it made no difference. I'm unattractive, unaccomplished, mundane, immature—to every human being in my orbit. I know that people don't care, but they don't wish me ill. I'm disinterested—I don't care much about them either. I don't need them. I don't like anything I achieve, because I did it—I created it. Even if I made money, I would hate it.

Therapist: It's hard to enjoy anything? Anything that you are involved in?

[Disconnection immediately occurs. The therapist tries to imagine what the patient's experience is like. What she says, however, does not use anything that he has told her. She does not "stay with" what she has been given. This may be an effect of an "expectational field," to be discussed in the next chapter. He seems to take no notice of the disjunctive response.]

Patient: I'm lazy. I'm on my own quite a lot. I just sit there and stare into space. I can't just sit there and do nothing. The ultimate inertia!

[Following a disjunction, the actual words of the patient frequently tell what has happened. "I'm on my own quite a lot" betrays his feeling of disconnection and the isolation that follows the therapist's remark.]

Therapist: It's pretty difficult!

[Again, there is no connection with the expression and immediate experience of the patient.]

Patient: I will be better off dead—there's nothing here for me.

[His reply can be understood both as a general one and as one related to the present situation, in which he might have sensed that "there's nothing here for me."]

Therapist: Nothing here for you?

Patient: You tell me. What is the point? I am unlikeable. This is my life. It can't be removed or exorcised. No one can do anything—I would not want it anyway.

[The therapist is now frustrated, challenged, and indeed, quite rattled.]

Therapist: We will have to see if you need medication.

Patient: What do you mean, *medication*? I've had heaps of it—no help whatsoever.

[At this point, the therapist tries to regain her footing and to gather herself together.]

Therapist: I am hearing you say that medication has not been of any use. I also hear you say that no one has been helpful, nothing has helped. I wonder . . . I wonder if you're feeling that coming to see me would also be of no help?

Patient: Never expect anything . . . never get disappointed, don't deserve anything anyway.

(*There is a period of silence.*)

Therapist: It's about not having expectations, and therefore not being disappointed, but at the same time, "don't deserve anything anyway"? . . . It must be hard . . . very hard.

["It must be hard" is apparently heard by the patient as sympathy, not empathy, as can be seen in his reply.]

Patient: The world is full of do-gooders—do things for others, not their own, think they can change the word —(*moves his chair further back*)—damn it—it's terrible—worst piece of work—don't think you'll be up to any good.

The patient's speech exhibits severe disintegration—a remarkable shift from the lucidity of his opening remarks, which include words such as *orbit* and *mundane*, indicative of a relatively higher-order consciousness. It seems the therapist's failure to connect with him has triggered an aspect of an unconscious memory system, with the words "don't think you'll be up to any good" presumably echoing the words of an abusive parent.

The therapist is now thoroughly caught up in the experience, disconnected from him, confused, and also afraid, aware of the anger in his movement and face.

SUMMARY

The two transcripts in this chapter illustrate certain main aspects of the dissociative experience. First, the experience of dissociation involves not only a loss of connectedness between those aspects of existence that are usually connected, but also a connection between those that are usually separate. Secondly, this experience cannot be conceived as distinct from the context, particularly the human context, in which the dissociation occurs. The form of relatedness between the subject and other people mirrors the subject's state of mind. Relationships arise in which there is, paradoxically, both fusion and disconnection.

The second transcript illustrates how quickly a situation can arise with someone suffering from the borderline condition that is difficult, highly emotionally charged in a negative way, and even frightening. The transcript also illustrates that the situation is the outcome of the way in which the other has responded to the subject's expressions. In many cases, particularly in hospital wards, staff may be unaware of the effect of their way of responding, considering the patient's behavior to be simply a manifestation of his or her psychiatric condition.

The first transcript, on the other hand, shows the opposite state of affairs in which a dissociative episode is corrected by skillful but apparently simple responsiveness on the part of the therapist. The two transcripts together show (1) that a dissociative state of mind potentiates the emergence of a particular form of relatedness, characterized by disconnection between the partners; and (2) that different forms of relatedness either rectify or precipitate dissociation. BPD, then, is not a condition to be understood as equivalent to a medical condition, held within the confines of the body. In the case of psychiatric illnesses, and most particularly BPD, the individual is not an isolated system but part of a larger organism that includes the social world.

Chapter 9

THE EXPECTATIONAL FIELD, REVERSALS, AND OTHER ASPECTS OF DISINTEGRATED RELATEDNESS

A FORM OF CONSCIOUSNESS, to recapitulate, is not to be conceived as an isolated entity, standing alone, but as a part of a larger system that includes a relationship with the world, whether extrinsic or intrinsic. This connection with the world is what consciousness is for: Its purpose, in its most primitive form, is to enable the organism to respond adaptively to the environment. In lower forms of consciousness, the relationship is unidirectional, a response to stimulus, of which the fright–flight response is a complex example.

Seen in this way, a form of life that comprises the organism and its environment is, as French philosopher Henri Bergson put it in a letter to William James (as cited in Richardson, 2007, p. 430), a "phenomenon of attention."

UNSTABLE RELATIONS: SELF AS "A PHENOMENON OF ATTENTION"

A more evolved organism has an enhanced attentional capacity and is able to respond, not only to exogenous but also to increasingly complex endogenous stimuli. In the higher-order consciousness of the human primate, the endogenous stimuli to which attention has access include visualization of past events and, as importantly, of events that have never occurred. Such internally generated stimuli can serve as the origins of activity that is new and free of environmental stimuli. As Frederic Bartlett (1932) put it in his great book on *Remembering*, we have developed "constructive imagination and constructive thought wherein at length we find the most complete release from the narrowness of time and place" (p. 314).

As a consequence of our enhanced attentional capacity we are able to cope with an environment of greater complexity, created by the evolution of the social world. The relationship with the environment in this setting takes a new form. It becomes bidirectional, or more exactly, a continuing interplay, in which internally generated material can, as it were, be "traded" in ordinary converse (*trading* is an essentially human capacity, illustrated in the thesis of Marcel Mauss, 1969). Such a relationship is potentially "intimate," this term being used in the quasi-technical sense of "inmost, most inward" (Oxford English Dictionary, 1971). This new form of relatedness is one of many patterns of relatedness we have available to us in our daily exchanges with those around us.

Our increased attentional capacity, which gives us the experience of self, allows us to respond appropriately to the expressions of those in our social environment, which are shifting from moment to moment. These circumstances demand a flexibility of response that is made possible by the nonlinear, associative, and constantly evolving background of subject consciousness—which might be seen, in a figurative way, as analogous to the current conceptions of consciousness arising from the ceaseless patterning and repatterning of neural networks. We are able to maintain coherence through changes in relatedness, each one manifested and giving rise to slightly different states of self–identity. The integrity of the self–identity complex is dependent upon an attentional system that allows each of us, in varying degrees, to achieve a stable but flexible standpoint in relation to others in our social world.

In those who suffer from BPD, attentional function is impaired. The coherence of the self–identity complex is deficient, leading to unstable relations in which forms of relatedness are distinct, shifting, and disconnected from each other. The situation resembles adolescence in which, for example, a boy keeps his relationships with his friends separate from his family because he relates to them in different ways and feels unable to be two different "selves" at the same time.

The forms of relatedness characteristic of those with BPD differ from the type of relationship dependent upon highly evolved awareness of inner events. A reduced capacity for such awareness leads to a state of mind in which, in subtle ways, the scope of imagination and memory is reduced. Relationships tend to be more reactive, more unidirectional, and somewhat inflexible. The sense of reciprocity is also impaired. Diminished attentional range seems to restrict the ability to create and tolerate models of reality that are not one's own. Put another way, "perspective taking," an aspect of theory of mind, is limited.

ATTACHMENT VERSUS INTIMACY

A cardinal feature of these forms of relatedness in people with BPD is an absence of intimacy, this term being used in the technical sense referred to previously. Intimacy is sometimes confused with attachment. The two terms, however, are not synonymous. Bowlby (1969, 1973) was quite clear in his description of attachment as a distinct form of relatedness. It has the apparent evolutionary purpose of protecting the animal from predators. It is first manifest, as is well known, in the separation anxiety shown by the child in the second half of the first year. An early analogue of it is displayed by a baby 3 months old, in a similar kind of distress when the mother is present but behaves as if she were absent (Milgrom-Friedman, Penman, & Meares, 1980).

The behavior of attachment is maintained by anxiety. Intimacy depends upon no such fuel. Moreover, it can be gained in a meeting with a stranger, as exemplified by Bertrand Russell's remarkable description of his first encounter with Joseph Conrad:

> At our very first meeting, we talked with increasing intimacy. We seemed to sink through layer after layer of what was superficial, till gradually both reached the central fire. It was an experience unlike any other I have known. We looked into each other's eyes, half appalled and half intoxicated to find ourselves together in such a region. (Russell, 1971, p. 203)

Whereas anxiety is a spur to attachment, an anxiety is an impediment to intimacy. There is fear that those experiences found in "the central fire" will, in some way, be devalued or harmed, inflicting damage on the individual equivalent to a physical hurt (Meares, 1976). In most cases, those who suffer from BPD have had such wounds inflicted upon them. As a consequence of such a past, many of those with BPD avoid intimacy. Rather than having frequently disrupted relationships, they live alone; a considerable number of our patients with BPD have had no intimate relationships. Although it can be argued that a failure to gain a sense of self deprives those with BPD of the opportunity for intimacy, it can equally be argued that harm inflicted on the proto-intimate expressions of the developing person stifled the emergence of self.

A third kind of relatedness is affiliation (Murray, 1938), which, like attachment, is akin to a drive, in this case toward companionship and toward belonging to a group, a tribe, a gang. It emerges before intimacy and after the onset of attachment. In maturity, the three forms of relatedness can be "compounded" into a single relationship, a marital one, for example. According to a neo-Jacksonian approach to the development of human relations, a failure to develop the most recently evolved form will result in an exaggerated expression of earlier forms. As a consequence, attachment needs are a salient aspect of the BPD picture, as reflected in DSM-IV's first diagnostic criterion.

THE EXPECTATIONAL FIELD

The disintegrated forms of relatedness seen in those with BPD are essentially traumatic. The nature of this kind of relationship, in which the higher-order systems controlling and modulating limbic activity may be hypofunctional, create a peculiar interpersonal effect that I call *the expectational field* (Meares, 2005, pp.114–125). This field is produced by what Bowlby (1973) would have called an internal working model (IWM). This term refers to the representation in memory of a particular relationship, which necessarily includes the attributes given to both partners in the relationship and their roles in relation to each other. When a particular IWM is triggered, the individual feels him- or herself to be in relation to the other in accordance with the "script" of the IWM (Meares, 1998). If, for example, the person has been the victim of relentless criticism and devaluation, he or she will expect, unconsciously, the other to behave in this way. With this expectation comes his or her assumption of the role of one devalued. This person is rarely aware of either the expectation or the role he or she plays in it.

The other person in the dyad, when this traumatic memory system is activated, tends to become influenced by the expectation of the subject. The other, without being aware of the influence of this expectation, comes to play out, or at least tends to play out, the role the subject has cast for him or her. The therapist, for example, may make remarks which are implicitly critical of the individual in a way which is uncharacteristic of him or her.

Although an effect of expectation upon the other partner is

present, to some degree, in all relationships, one is not generally aware of it. In the traumatic relationship, however, there may be sensed a subtle coercion to behave, or not to behave, in a particular way, in accordance with the expectation. This feeling and tendency are the clinical bases of the conception of projection identification (Ogden, 1982), which Kernberg, in a series of publications (e.g., 1967, 1984), has described as a principal feature of BPD. Segal summarized Melanie Klein's formulation of this concept as follows: "Parts of the self and internal objects . . . then become possessed by, controlled and identified with the projected parts" (Segal, 1973, p. 27). The theoretical assumptions underlying this definition are no longer generally agreed upon. A more empirically based term for this important clinical phenomenon is preferred.

Three studies from Lea Williams's laboratory suggest how the expectational field is formed and how the force of this field is magnified when one enters a traumatic relationship, as compared with entering a nontraumatic relationship. The first study showed that the other, the therapist in this relationship, is likely to register signs in the voice, facial expression, and posture of the patient so small that he or she is not consciously aware of them. Williams's observations depended upon a machine that charts with great accuracy the movements and gaze fixations as a subject looks at a face on a television screen. The usual scan path, evident when the face has a neutral expression, is triangular, moving from eye to eye, to the mouth, and then back again. In expressions conveying affect, the scanning becomes more complex and includes, in the case of a smile, fixations on the wrinkles at the corners of the eyes. These fixations are so fast that the subject would not have been aware that he or she was making such a check (Williams, Senior, et al., 2001). (See Figure 9.1.) Nevertheless, subliminally they create an impression. In the case of absent wrinkles in a smiling face, for example, one becomes wary without knowing why.

In another set of experiments, Williams and her group showed that these unconsciously registered signs are likely to be more potent than the same signs of which there is a conscious awareness. These experiments involved the study of brain responses to images of fearful and neutral faces that were exhibited for either a long duration (500 ms) or briefly (16.7 ms and masked). In the latter case the individual was not conscious of the visual perception (Williams, Liddell, et al., 2006). Although the fearful face was presented subliminally, the amygdala was activated: The face had evoked a flicker of fear in the subject. The imaging data were correlated with skin conductance recordings showing that subliminal fear perception evoked arousal. An earlier study (Liddell et al., 2005) suggested that the subliminal response may involve superior colliculus and pulvinar activity, regions believed to be associated with blindsight (Morris et al., 2001), which is the capacity of an individual blinded by damage to the occipital cortex to locate objects in space.

The brain response to conscious perception was different and seemed likely to involve a different neural pathway that included the medial prefrontal cortex. Activity in this region modified amygdaloid excitation. These findings supported those of an earlier study from the laboratory, showing enhanced amygdaloid responses to unconsciously perceived stimuli using ERPs as the measure of responses (Liddell et al., 2004).

These data suggest the workings of a strange dynamic in the intersubjective field during the conversation with a patient who has BPD, particularly during a period when an unconscious traumatic memory system has been triggered. Since it is unconscious, the modifying prefrontal effect upon it is lacking, and the subject is in the state of amygdaloid activation that is manifest in the body via the autonomic system. The small signs of this activation are picked up by the therapist, albeit unconsciously, so that their effect is magnified. A further study, described in an earlier chapter, showed that amygdaloid responses to unconsciously perceived stimuli in traumatized people are greater than in those who are not traumatized (Felmingham et al., 2008).

REVERSALS

The studies coming from Lea Williams's lab offer a means of understanding the faint sense of coercion to behave, or not to behave, in a particular way that the therapist might feel in a conversation with a patient with BPD, and which might lead to an uncharacteristic response on the part of the therapist. The studies do not, however, explain another phenomenon that may occur in the same conversation, which term a *reversal* (Meares, 1993a, pp. 87–100; 1993b; 2005, pp. 104–113).

In the case of a disintegrated self, in which there are multiple and shifting states of personal existing, each one correlates with a particular form of relatedness. These forms of relatedness both constitute and manifest a state of personal existing, a certain kind of mental state.

The change in the manifestations of these IWMs might be figuratively conceived as occurring, at any moment, in three dimensions. First there is a range of people, occurring in the present, who are good, bad, likeable, incompetent, and so on, and who, as it were, are confronting and linking to a range of experiences of the other. *Who one is*, here, occurs along a horizontal plane. A second category of experiences is vertical, fluctuating up and down a chronological axis. The individual's states range between those of a young person and those of someone who is more nearly mature. The third dimension is also in the horizontal plane, orthogonal to the first. It involves a back-and-forth change in which the subject *becomes* the other. The poles of relatedness in a particular IWM are transposed. The subject takes on the role of the abuser as if inhabited by the original other.

Although originally remarked upon by Freud (1915c), this oscillation between the poles of a traumatic IWM has been the subject of very little discussion since that time. The rapid switching between poles that Freud (1924) characterized as active–passive and sadistic–masochistic is a disconcerting feature of the relationship with those suffering from BPD. Peter Hobson and his colleagues (1998) give an account of the rapid switches in attitude those with BPD exhibit in their exchanges with others. They might shift, for example, from seductive to contemptuous. These investigators suggested that such shifts reflect the malign experiences those with BPD have had with others.

The appearance of a reversal often signals a sharp deterioration in the frail connectedness established between patient and therapist. It can be understood as a reflection of an increased state of fragmentation.

The behavior of reversal and the experience of the expectational field are the bases of the psychoanalytic concept of projective identification (Meares, 2000b), as previously remarked. In my view they should be considered as separate but related phenomena, not to be understood as having a defensive purpose.

DISINTEGRATED RELATEDNESS

Fragmentation of self–other representations can be conceived as a reflection of a failure of maturation. Seen in this way, the "splitting" between the manifestations of IWMs, characteristic of BPD, is not primarily defensive, although in certain circumstances it may become so.

That integration comes with maturation is supported by child developmental studies. Perhaps the best known studies come from Tom Bower (1971). One of his experiments involved a clever system of mirrors in which an image of the same person could appear simultaneously in two or three cubicles at the same time. Infants were presented with two situations. In the first, the mother was in one cubicle while strange women occupied the others. In the second, the mother seemed to be in each cubicle.

Infants younger than 20 weeks responded to the first situation by smiling at mother and in various ways interacting with her while ignoring the other women. In the multiple-mother situation created by the mirrors, the baby happily cooed and waved to each mother in turn. Older infants responded to the first situation similarly, but when confronted by multiple images of the mother, they showed distress as if their concept of mother as a single person had been upset.

Numerous other studies, beyond the scope of this chapter, support the notion that the perceptual and conceptual world of the child is as if in pieces relative to the adult. Although integration of small fragments of personal reality into larger wholes comes with maturation, it is not inevitable, at least in terms of higher-order functions and systems. This integration depends upon suitable responses from the social environment. Such was the thesis of Vygotsky & Luria (1994) whose concept of sociogenesis was influenced by the ideas of Janet: "Janet was arguing that all higher, typically human conducts have a social origin. They exist first between people, as social acts, and only afterward as intraindividual, private acts. These private acts, however, retain their social character" (van der Veer & Valsiner, 1988, p. 58). Janet had speculated that the process he called "*personal synthesis*" involves a coherence in the responses of the caregivers that fosters unification. He wrote: "The child creates his individuality because one always mentions him in the same way and because one's behaviour towards him has a certain unity" (Janet, 1929, p. 268). Failure of sociogenesis not only results in disturbance of the coherence of "individuality" but also of that individual's stability in the way of relating to others.

The basis of fragmentation of IWMs has been conceived in terms of attachment. Bowlby (1973) suggested that unsatisfactory relationships between the developing child and the primary caregivers may lead to a disturbance of attachment in which, instead of a relatively unified system of IWMs, representations of particular forms of relatedness develop that are multiple and disconnected. This idea has gained support through the work of Mary Main and her colleagues. These studies led to the description of a disorganized form of attachment (Main & Solomon, 1990), a fourth category added to the trio identified by Ainsworth and her collaborators (1978; i.e. secure, insecure-avoidant, insecure-resistant). Disorganized attachment was found to be related to unresolved traumata in the lives of the caregivers. Main and Hesse (1990) suggested that traumatized caregivers may behave in a way that is frightening to the child and, worse, offers no resolution to the fright. These data led Main (1991) to argue that disorganized attachment results in multiple, incoherent, disaggregated representations of self and other.

Liotti has reviewed this background to his own work as a prologue to putting forward a model of dissociation and BPD that depends upon the implicit view that dissociation as a *state of mind* cannot be separated from dissociation as a *form of relatedness*. In a series of papers, Liotti (1992, 1994, 1995, 1999) proposed that disorganized attachment is the first step in a developmental pathway that might culminate in the clinical expression of dissociation in adult life. The caregiver who relates to the child in a way that is associated with the development of disorganized attachment in the child, behaves in a manner that is not only frightening at times but also unpredictable and contradictory. The mother might, for example, be frightened of the child. The child is now placed in a situation in which simultaneous but incompatible perceptions of the caregiver are received. The child's need to respond appropriately is overwhelming, since the bond to the caregiver is felt as necessary to existence. The discordant and incongruent signals, however, do not indicate how to behave. The child might be immobilized, as if stunned, or in an apparent trance state analogous to the adult state of dissociation.

Liotti (1992) suggested that disorganized attachment has three possible main outcomes: (1) satisfactory adaption, in response to the integration of disaggregated IWMs though later secure attachments; (2) the development of a propensity for dissociation in later life; or (3) dissociative disorders due to later traumata amplifying the earlier vulnerability associated with disorganized attachment. In later papers Liotti (1995, 1999, 2000, 2004) proposed that the disorders that are the outcome of the third pathway include BPD and complex posttraumatic stress disorder.

In essence, Liotti's work suggests that a relationship dominated by an individual whose behavior is determined by multiple and disconnected IWMs creates in the partner a state of mind that mirrors the relatedness; that is, it produces a disaggregated form of consciousness. In circumstances where the maturational process of integration in psychic life is facilitated by a suitable interplay with the caregiving environment, the original difficulty may be overcome. If not, dissociative pathology may emerge in more florid forms.

Liotti's theories are given evidential support not only by his own studies (Liotti & Pasquini, 2000; Pasquini et al., 2002) but also by the observations of other groups. The Minnesota Longitudinal Study (Carlson, 1998; Ogawa et al., 1997) reported the outcome of 168 young adults whose attachment patterns had been observed in their second year of life. Those who had displayed disorganized attachment in childhood had higher dissociation scores in adult life than those with other forms of attachment. In addition, those who had suffered subsequent traumata had higher scores than those who had not (Ogawa et al., 1997). Three subjects in the study had developed clinically diagnosable dissociative disorders. All had exhibited disorganized attachments as infants (Carlson, 1998).

A later study from Dutra and Lyons-Ruth (2005) confirmed and extended the findings of Ogawa and colleagues. They followed 56 infants at social risk from birth to the age of 19. At the age of 19, they found that five measures of infant, childhood, and adolescent maltreatment failed to predict dissociation at age

19. In contrast, infant disorganization, maternal lack of involvement with the infant at home at 12 months, and disrupted maternal affective communication in the laboratory at 18 months contributed to the prediction of dissociative symptoms at 19. In addition, concurrent dissociative symptoms in the mother, but not PTSD, depression, or anxiety, were related to those of the adolescents' dissociation scores.

The findings of this study suggested that the measures of maternal care are better predictors of a dissociative outcome than infant disorganization itself. They found, surprisingly, that hostile, frightening, and intrusive behaviours on the part of the mother were weak predictors. Less salient behaviors were more pathogenic: for example, "withdrawing from emotional contact, being unresponsive to the child's overtures, displaying contradictory, role-reversal, or disoriented responses when the infant's attachment needs are heightened" (Dutra & Lyons-Ruth, 2005, p. 69).

REVERSALS IN THE CHILD'S BEHAVIORS

Reversals, as noted previously, characterize the relatedness of those with BPD. This kind of behavior was strikingly evident in schoolchildren who had shown disorganized attachment during infancy as they seemingly mirrored the contradictory, role-reversed behavior of their mothers. Lyons-Ruth and Jacobvitz (1999) reviewed two longitudinal studies of infants who had exhibited disorganized attachment. At this stage in development they were hesitant and apprehensive in their behaviors. Their school-age behavior was typically discontinuous with such demeanors. Over 80% of the children displayed either punitive-dominant or caregiving behavior toward the attachment figure. Both those behaviors can be conceived as "controlling."

Liotti (2006) points out, using the evidence of Hesse et al. (2003), that these reversals may be conceived as defenses that are helpful to the child in maintaining some kind of integration. When, however, anxiety is activated, the defensive strategy collapses and the original disorganized IWM again becomes manifest. In the Hesse study, 6-year-old controlling children were shown pictures from a separation anxiety test. These children, who initially presented as well oriented and organized in their thinking, gave incoherent, unrealistic, and catastrophic narrative responses to the pictures. Such observations may have significant implications for our understanding of reversals in the behavior of those with BPD.

MENTALIZATION, THEORY OF MIND, AND TRAUMATIC ATTACHMENT

The foregoing observations have focused on "relational traumata" (Schore, 2003a & 2003b) in those with BPD that impede a particular aspect of the maturation of self, namely, its coherence. Fonagy and his colleagues (2003 report on deficiencies in BPD of another cardinal aspect of self. They suggest that traumatic early attachment experiences hinder the emergence of "mentalization." *Mentalization* is a term coined by Uta Frith and her colleagues (1991) to refer to the ability that underlies the mental accomplishments in having a "theory of mind" (Premack & Woodruff, 1978). Fonagy and Bateman (2008) define mentalization as "the capacity to make sense of each other and ourselves, implicitly and explicitly, in terms of subjective states and mental processes" (p. 5). They further note: "It is not the fact of maltreatment but more the family environment that discourages coherent discourse concerning mental states and it is this that is likely to predispose the child to BPD" (p. 13).

Fonagy and his colleagues (2003) used measures of reflective function and theory of mind to evaluate the two main features of mentalization in BPD. Recent evidence, however, does not support the supposition that those with BPD perform poorly on theory of mind tests (Fertuck et al., 2009; Arntz et al., 2009). In the Fertuck study, those with BDP showed an enhanced ability to judge mental state as indicated by the "reading the mind in the eyes" test (Baron-Cohen et al., 2001). This is consistent with clinical observations that many of those with BPD are acutely aware of facial expression and have the capacity to make very sensitive discernments, enabling them to respond in a way that they believe is expected or necessary.

The study of Arntz and colleagues (2009) depended upon a more advanced theory of mind capacity devised to test those with subtle deficiencies (Happé, 1994). The subject is asked questions about double bluff, mistakes, persuasion, and white lies. It is not surprising that those with BPD did not perform poorly on these tests, since strategies involving deception are familiar to those with BPD. The capacity for pretense develops at 2–3 years, earlier in human life than the conception of self. Moreover, sympathy may be well developed, enabling the patient with BPD to have, at times, startlingly accurate intuitions about the mental life of others that are based on their own experience. Sympathy, however, is not empathy. These same patients may make assumptions about the other that are grossly inaccurate since they derive from an understanding of their own desires, beliefs, and so forth, rather than from the capacity to imagine a personal reality that differs from their own.

Theory of mind may not adequately identify the specific deficit in attributing mental states to others that those with BPD often display. Those with BPD, it should be remembered, include politicians and highly successful entrepreneurs whose success has depended, in part, on very efficient "mind reading." On the other hand, they can be remarkably obtuse in dealing with others. Their specific deficit is in the capacity for what may be called empathy, which, contrary to the assertion of Arntz and colleagues (2009), is not exemplified by appropriate responses to someone bereaved, a behavior dependent upon sympathy. In my view, the capacity to empathize with others is related to, and arises from, the development of self, identified by a reflective awareness of mental states sensed as one's own. The realization that one has a unique and personal world that differs from others gives rise to another realization: that others also have their own unique, personal and private worlds.

Episodic memory, involving the recall of events from one's life, is a cardinal indicator of self. Theory of mind tests, however, can be performed normally by a person without episodic memory, as demonstrated in two rare cases of people who, through injury to the brain, were unable to recollect personal happenings in their own lives (Rosenbaum et al., 2007). Thus, although episodic memory and theory of mind performance depend upon similar areas of brain function (Buckner & Carroll, 2007) they appear to be independent. On the other hand, linguistic analyses of a patient who was studied early in treatment and again 6 months later suggested that the emergence of reflectiveness on inner events, evident in the second analysis, was related to a capacity for empathy (Meares, Butt, et al., 2005).

HOSTILE/HELPLESS, ANACLITIC, AND OTHER FORMS OF IWM IN BPD

That those suffering from BPD relate to others according to a disintegrated system of IWMs is implicit in the DSM catalogue of criteria for BPD. The interpersonal style is "unstable," vacillating, for example, between polar extremes of idealization and devaluation. Attempts to categorize these IWMs follow the early studies from which emerged the notion of disorganized attachment. Two kinds of Adult Attachment Interview (AAI) transcripts related to disorganized attachment have been designated "unresolved" (U) and "cannot classify" (CC; Hesse, 1996). The unresolved classification can be made only if there is a history of trauma or loss. This raises a methodological difficulty since a transcript characteristic of the U code cannot be given that code in the absence of trauma. U transcripts reveal a lack of coherence in the discussions of trauma and suggest deficient integration of the trauma event into conscious life. The integration may be impaired by contradictory maternal behaviors, particularly of being frightening to and frightened of the infant.

The CC classification is co-called because the transcript suggests different and shifting forms of attachment, reflecting a disintegration of IWMs. In the first part of the interview the subject displays a "dismissing" attitude to attachment and then shifts, without apparent awareness of the contradiction, to a "preoccupied" state in which is given a jumbled, confusing, often angry, and prolonged account of early childhood. Fonagy and his colleagues (1996) found that those with BPD are particularly likely to be associated with "unresolved" and "preoccupied" types of attachment. Choi-Kain and her colleagues (2009) report that preoccupied and fearful attachment styles differentiated individuals with BPD from depressed people and from another comparison group of nonborderline subjects. Furthermore, being rated as having both styles of attachment confers a greater risk for being diagnosed with BPD than either style alone.

In his review of this subject, Liotti (2006) points out that U and CC attachment classifications are particularly common in dissociative and borderline groups. This observation is consistent with the main thesis of this chapter, that dissociation and a particular form of interpersonal style are interrelated.

In more recent studies Lyons-Ruth and her colleagues (2005) have developed a new coding that develops the U category but is not contingent upon a history of trauma or loss. They call this coding *hostile/helpless* (H), and it is given when the subject, now an adult, gives contradictory and unintegrated emotional descriptions of the main original caregiver. Lyons-Ruth has stressed how H/H relations between a mother and infant predispose to the formation of disorganized attachment. H/H coding is particularly common in patients with BPD (Lyons-Ruth, Menick, et al., 2007).

Another main category of IWM in BPD is related to the fear of abandonment and of being alone, a prominent feature of the disorder noted by pioneers of the syndrome (Stern, 1938; Adler & Buie, 1979; Gunderson, 1996). Bornstein and colleagues have thoroughly reviewed the evidence concerning "dependency" and BPD (Bornstein et al., 2010). Levy et al. (2007) suggest that dependency in BPD is of a particular kind. They used Blatt's methods in their investigation. Using Rorschach methods, Blatt and Auerbach (1988) described two kinds of BPD pathology associated with depression, which they called anaclitic/dependent and self-critical introjective. Following this, Blatt and his coworkers (1976) developed a 66-item scale covering a wide range of depressive feelings, beliefs, forms of relating, and so forth. Factor analysis revealed three factors composing the scale, entitled the Depressive Experiences Questionnaire (DEQ). The factors were Dependency, Self-Criticism, and Efficacy. The Dependency factor was subjected to a further analysis, from which emerged two scales: Anaclitic Neediness and Interpersonal Depression (Blatt et al., 1995). The former covers separation fears and the latter, loneliness and loss. This investigation was conducted with attachment theory in mind, suggesting that it is not inappropriate to call these factors and subfactors IWMs. Levy and colleagues (2007) conclude that Anaclitic Neediness and Self-Criticism are characteristic of BPD pathology. On the other hand, the over-arching Dependency factor did not distinguish BPD and non-BPD groups.

TRANSGENERATIONAL TRANSMISSION OF BPD

The evidence presented so far regarding the developmental background of individuals with BPD gives support to ideas that were put forward a century earlier. William James, building on the observations of Pierre Janet, wrote: "Children are not born with a sense of unified identity—it develops from many sources and experiences. In overwhelmed children, its development is obstructed, and many parts of what should have been blended into a relatively unified identity remain separate" (1983, p. 264). It might be expected that those who have been "overwhelmed" by inappropriate responsiveness of the caregiving environment and who develop BPD in later life will be likely to create a similar caregiving environment for their children. Their disconnected and unpredictable interpersonal style, derived from "enmeshed," "unresolved" (Patrick, 1994; Crandell et al., 2003), and other attachment patterns, might result in the transgenerational transmission of BPD.

This possibility is being investigated by Peter Hobson and his group at the Developmental Psychopathology Unit at the Tavistock Clinic, London. In a study of mothers with BPD and their 2-month-old babies, Crandell et al. (2003) videotaped the dyad at play; during a period when the mother maintained a still face; and during the recovery period from the unresponsive still maternal face. During the baseline period the mother with BPD and her baby were indistinguishable from the control dyads. The differences in the still face period were not marked, but babies of mothers with BPD showed increasing looking away and dazed expressions. The dazed expressions continued in the recovery period when the mother's behavior seemed relatively ineffective in facilitating the baby's regrouping. These mothers were judged "intrusively insensitive" compared with controls. It seems important that evidence of disturbance in the mother–child relationship did not properly emerge until stress was introduced.

A second study concerned ten 12-month-old babies and their mothers who suffered BPD (Hobson et al., 2005). The investigation involved three different situations: (1) A still-faced stranger subsequently attempted to engage the infants in a game; (2) the babies were confronted by the Strange Situation of Ainsworth and Wittig; and (3) the mothers were asked to teach their infants to play with a toy train and miniature figures. Compared with 22 controls, (1) the infants of mothers with BPD were less organized and allowed less opportunity for positive engagement; (2) a higher proportion (8 out of 10) rated as showing disorganized attachment; and (3) the mothers were more "intrusively insensitive."

In a second study of mothers with BPD and their year-old infants, the dyads were compared with dyads in which the mothers were depressed mother and in dyads with mothers who had no psychiatric disorder (Hobson et al., 2009). As expected, a higher proportion (85%) of women with BPD showed disrupted communication with their infants. They also displayed frightened/disoriented behavior.

These data provide compelling evidence that children of mothers diagnosed with BPD are at risk. Treatment of mothers with BPD might therefore confer a double benefit, not only helping the mothers but also, hopefully, diminishing the chances that their children will suffer the same disorder. The phenomenon of reversal repeatedly displayed by the parent might be particularly pathogenic. Our own studies have shown that treatment of patients with BPD is associated with beneficial changes in their family relationships (Gerull, Meares, Stevenson, Korner, & Newman, 2008).

SUMMARY

This chapter has concerned the disintegration of representations in memory of traumatic forms of relatedness. These different "scripts" record the role of the subject and his or her relatedness with the other in the traumatic scene. The disintegration causes the individual to shift, typically quite sharply, from one way of relating to another. Each shift is associated with a different expectation of the other. The expectation is that the other will behave as the original traumatizing other. Certain neuro-physiological data are presented in order to show how this expectation is heightened where traumatic memory is activated and has a subliminal effect upon the other which is perceived unconsciously. Another aspect of the disintegrated form of relatedness arises when the poles of the traumatic "script" become as if reversed, and the subject takes on the role of the traumatizer.

Developmental aspects of the disintegration are discussed. These data suggest that the disintegration may arise in early life through the child living in a parental atmosphere, which leads to disorganized attachment. The disorganized behavior of the child mirrors the later disintegration of psychic life, which is referred to as dissociation.

Chapter 10

THE POLYSYMPTOMATIC NATURE OF BORDERLINE PERSONALITY

THIS CHAPTER IS SPECULATIVE. The view is put forward that the disorders that are so frequently found to be comorbid or in the life history of someone who is eventually given the diagnosis of BPD are not separate and distinct illnesses, occurring as if in a random manner, but are part of the same systematic disturbance, manifest to its greatest degree as BPD. Furthermore, it is suggested that what is common to BPD and the disorders with which it is apparently comorbid is a history of trauma. Such traumata are likely to be of different kinds, predisposing the individual to develop a particular comorbid condition.

KERNBERG'S OBSERVATIONS

In the classic description of *Borderline Personality Organization* given by Kernberg (1967, pp. 647–648), he included, as part of this syndrome, the following features:

1. "Chronic diffuse, free-floating anxiety"
2. "Multiple phobias," including social phobia, specific phobias, and particularly those phobias "which impose severe restriction on the patient's daily life"
3. "Obsessive–compulsive symptoms"

4. "Multiple elaborate, or bizarre conversion symptoms," including those "bordering on bodily hallucinations or involving complex sensations or sequences of movements of bizarre quality"
5. "Dissociative reactions" including fugues and amnesias
6. "Hypochondriasis"
7. Paranoid trends which develop into delusions under certain circumstances; for example, "when classical analytic approaches are attempted in these patients"

The important implication of this description is that patterns of symptomatology now called Axis I disorders are not merely comorbid with BPD but *part of it*.

The implications of Kernberg's observations are often overlooked, presumably because they are inconvenient. They upset the apparent tidiness of the DSM compartments. Kernberg's account, however, is supported by a study using the Symptom Checklist–90–Revised (SCL-90-R; Derogatis & Cleary, 1977). The SCL-90-R reflects most Axis I disorders. It is a 90-item checklist widely used as a measure of general clinical distress. The checklist, completed by the patient, consists of nine subscales measuring somatization, obsessive compulsion, interpersonal sensitivity, depression, anxiety, hostility, phobic anxiety, paranoid ideation, and psychoticism. Hull et al. (1993), in charting change in BPD, found that the changes in each subscale were very similar, as if there were a coherence among them—as if they were all part of a single measure. This finding suggested that the measure might indicate change in an aspect of BPD not encompassed by the DSM catalogue of diagnostic criteria.

THE EXTENT OF COMORBIDITY

The comorbidity of BPD with Axis I disorders has been considered by Zanarini, Frankenberg, Dubo, and her colleagues (1998) in an interesting way. The co-occurrences of Axis I disorders in

379 subjects was compared with another group of 125 people who had other personality disorders. A whole range of Axis I disorders could be diagnosed significantly more frequently in those with BPD than in the other group. The illnesses included depressions, panic disorders, agoraphobia, social phobia, simple phobia, obsessive–compulsive disorder, PTSD, somatoform disorders, and eating disorders. The investigators concluded that a "lifetime pattern of Axis I is characteristic of borderline patients" and "a particularly good marker for borderline personality disorder" (p. 1733). This important inference from their data implies that Axis I disorders, when appearing in conjunction with BPD, are not to be explained as random co-occurrences. Rather, these disorders are related to BPD. A later study from Zanarini, Frankenberg, Hennen, and her colleagues (2004) seemed to give further support to the possibility that Axis I disorders are linked to the BPD diagnosis. In a 6-year follow-up of 290 patients, they found that in those whose BPD remitted, there was a decline in the number of associated Axis I disorders, whereas "those whose borderline personality did not remit over time reported stable rates of co-morbid disorders" (p. 2108).

The so-called comorbidity of Axis II disorders with BPD is also considerable. There is an overlapping with other Cluster B personality disorders—that is, BPD, narcissistic, histrionic, and antisocial personality disorders (Fossati et al., 2000; Grilo & Mc-Glashan, 2000; Moldin et al., 1994; Zimmerman & Coryell, 1989, 1990; Zimmerman et al., 2005). Cluster A group, on the other hand, comprised of schizotypal, schizoid, and paranoid personality disorders, overlaps very little with Cluster B (McGlashan et al., 2000). The case is less clear for Cluster C personality disorders, which is disparate. It is composed of avoidant, dependent, obsessive–compulsive, and personality disorder "not otherwise specified." Dependent personality disorder overlaps with BPD (McGlashan et al., 2000), as does avoidant, though to a lesser extent (Zanarini et al., 1987; Zanarini, Frankenburg, Vujanovic et al., 2004).

Such observations are consistent with the idea that the comorbidity of Axis I and Axis II disorders with BPD is not a random co-occurrence, which is one of the several meanings of *comorbidity*. It is more in line with the second of the two main meanings proposed by writers on the subject of comorbidities, which is that the conditions are found together because they have a common etiology or pathophysiology, or at least some type of causal relationship between them (Caron & Rutter, 1991; Kendall & Clarkin, 1992; Widiger et al., 1991).

DEPRESSION AND THE EFFECT
OF TRAUMATIC SYSTEMS IN BPD

The most common focus in evaluating the nature of the comorbidity of BPD and Axis I disorders has been the relationship between depression and BPD. Summarizing the outcome of their own work, Levy and his coworkers (2007) conclude that a depression having peculiar qualities is not to be explained as the co-occurrence of two discrete disorders. Rather, "those feelings seem central to the pathology" of BPD. In support of their conclusion, they cite the evidence of Gunderson and Elliott (1985), Westen et al. (1992), and Zanarini, Frankenberg & DeLuca et al. (1998).

Structural equation modeling techniques have been used by Klein and Schwartz (2002) to examine the relationship between BPD and atypical depression, as exemplified by dysthymic disorder (DD). By means of assessing 84 outpatients with DD over 5 years, the researchers tested four competing models of the relationship between DD and BPD symptoms over time. The models were (1) no association; (2) contemporaneous direct effects in which BPD and DD symptoms influence one another over a rela-

tively short time period; (3) lagged effects of a similar kind operating over a longer period; and (4) a fixed common factor
underlies both DD and BPD, along with influences that are
unique to each condition. The *fixed common factor* was the best fit-
ting of these models, providing an excellent fit to the data.

A main aspect of the study by Levy and his colleagues (2007)
involved the relationship between what can be seen as two IWMs
(Bowlby, 1973), or traumatic memory systems, and different aspects of the BPD syndrome. The IWMs were dependent/anaclitic
and self-critical/introjective, both of which Blatt and Auerbach
(1988) had proposed as central to BPD pathology. In order to
consider which elements of the BPD syndrome might be linked
to these forms of relatedness, Levy et al. (2007) used the three
factors isolated by Clarkin and his colleagues (1993). They found
that anaclitic/neediness correlated with all three factors. The self-
critical/introjective score correlated only with Factor 1, the self
factor, comprised of emptiness, identity problems, fear of abandonment, and unstable relationships. These findings suggest that
the phenomenon of BPD might be created by two relatively independent traumatic memory systems, each of which is related
to a particular grouping of phenomena.

It is often said that those with BPD might suffer not one, but
two or more, kinds of depression, each having a characteristic affective state or mood. The first of these is related to the anaclitic/
neediness form of vulnerability, which might result in depression
arising from abandonment or fears of abandonment. The second
arises from a different vulnerability, and has a different quality.
Whether or not it is the same as the ongoing state of "psychic
pain" is yet to be determined.

The self-criticism measure is regarded as a reflection of introjective processes in which the critical caregiver or "object" is internalized, so that the subject takes over the role of the object,
inflicting the harm that had once come from another. Its most
famous formulation came from Freud. The notion of the "critical

agency" has been seen as the origin of object relations theory (Ogden, 2002).

Freud's (1915a) "Mourning and Melancholia" is considered by some authorities to be his most significant work. It was one of the first fruits of Freud's shift in thinking, the so-called "turning point of the 1920's" (Laplanche & Pontalis, 1973). It must have been an extremely difficult work to write, since it is unlike his previous theory based on the consequences of unacceptable drives. To read this paper written in 1915 and "Introductory Lectures," written about the same time, is to enter into two different intellectual universes.

The tone of "Mourning and Melancholia" is uncharacteristically humble, as if Freud were making his way toward a formulation of which he is not yet clear. Freud makes no claim for the universality of his argument. He warns "against any overestimation of the value of our conclusions" (1915a, p. 243). He finds it unlikely that his proposal will be relevant to all forms of depression so that "we shall, therefore, from the outset drop all claim to general validity for our conclusions" (p. 243). A key passage in "Mourning and Melancholia" is the following:

> Let us dwell for a moment on the view which the melancholic's disorder affords of the constitution of the human ego. We see how in him one part of the ego sets itself over the other, judges it critically, and, as it were, takes it as its object. Our suspicion that the critical agency which is here split off from the ego might also show its independence in other circumstances will be confirmed by every further observation. (p. 247)

This observation concerning "the critical agency" is central to my argument. In this passage, "ego" can be seen as a general word for self or psyche. It was not until the 1930s that Freud eventually distinguished between ego and self (Strachey, 1961). The part of the psychic system that is split off, acting as if independent of the main stream of consciousness, is equivalent to the notion of the unconscious traumatic memory system. This "critical agency" repetitively acts upon the system of self, inflicting the same devaluation, derogation, derision, humiliation—the same wounds—as the original traumatic situation. The association, in the Levy et al. study (2007), between the self factor of Clarkin et al. (1993) and the self-critical/introjective scores in those with BPD is in line with the story of the "critical agency," since the original source of the criticism is internalized, or introjected, in the BPD sufferer, sometimes experienced as a voice.

HUMILIATION: ATTACKS UPON VALUE

According to the theory of introjection, the self-criticism variable reflects traumatic criticism. It is not, however, simple criticism that is traumatic. A particular form of personal damage is becoming increasingly recognized as pathogenic. Its essence is harm inflicted on the positive feeling at the heart of selfhood that gives rise to the sense of worth (Meares, 1999b). These positive feelings have not been scientifically designated. They are, however, often referred to as the tender or intimate emotions. James spoke of "warmth and intimacy" as the feeling at the core of self. This feeling is an essential aspect of the nuclear experiences of personal existence. James sensed this region as a "sanctuary within the citadel" of self (James, 1890, p. 297), which is not to be defiled, devalued, or in other ways violated. Damage to this "self of all the other selves" (James, p. 297) may come through mockery, shaming, or apparently innocuous behavior such as disinterest or lack of response when the child reveals a need for tenderness (see Dutra & Lyons-Ruth 2005, Chapter 9).

The most serious of the various kinds of attacks upon value is sexual abuse, in which the violation of tender feelings is, in the usual case, of greater consequence than the anatomical and behavioral facts of the abuse. A body of evidence now suggests that sexual abuse is the most pathogenic of the various traumata that can be inflicted upon the child, apart from extreme neglect. The harm that comes through physical abuse may come not through pain and terror but most particularly through the humiliation associated with the abuse. Psychical traumata are themselves felt as blows. Derogation, belittling, derision, or whatever it is, is felt like a hit. There is a sharp and instantaneous feeling of distress, and this instant is not connected to the rest of life. It is an interruption in the ongoing sense of personal being. A frequently cited report suggests that the pain of humiliation evokes a pattern of brain response in the anterior cingulate region that is similar to the response induced by pain due to a physical cause (Eisenberger et al., 2003).

Recent findings point to the significance of humiliation in the pathogenesis of atypical depression—that is, a form of depression associated with BPD. In one study, 20 treatment-resistant patients with depression were compared with 20 people who were responsive to treatment (Kaplan & Klinetob, 2000). The treatment-resistant individuals "reported significantly greater levels of childhood emotional abuse, and experienced current day-to-day sequelae of childhood emotional abuse" (p. 597).

Another study concerned 489 subjects who were interviewed and then followed up in order to examine associations between the findings of this interview with subsequent depression (Murphy et al., 2002). "Feeling worthless" at first interview was highly predictive of subsequent depression. In this article reference was made to two other studies with the same findings. In a third study Kendler and colleagues (2003) also found that loss, humiliation, entrapment, and danger predict onsets of major depression and generalized anxiety. In their study 7,322 adult twins were blindly rated on dimensions of humiliation, entrapment, loss, and danger. The authors remarked that "humiliating events that directly devalue an individual in a core role" were strongly linked to risk for depressive episodes (p. 789). Loss and humiliation, when combined, were the most pathogenic events. An example of such a situation is other-initiated separation. These findings replicated earlier studies from London reporting experiences of loss, humiliation, and entrapment among women developing depression (Brown, Harris, & Hepworth, 1995). Another study supported the hypothesis that loss and humiliation are particularly relevant in the provocation of depression onset (Farmer & McGuffin, 2003). It might be supposed that a significant proportion of these findings can be explained in terms of traumatic memory systems concerning devaluation. These symptoms can be triggered by the circumstances of current existence and lead to the onset of clinical depression.

Humiliation and similar attacks upon value are essentially attacks upon self, as previously remarked. The self-criticism variable used by Levy and his colleagues (2007) represents the introjective consequence of such traumata. They showed that a particular kind of depression, measured by the SCl-90-R depression subscale, correlates with self-disturbance in BPD, where self is reflected in scores for identity problems and emptiness.

Another series of reports, although not directly concerned with humiliation and devaluation, showed that an atypical depression, relatively resistant to antidepressant medication, is associated with the background characteristic of BPD: that is, traumata. The depression in these reports is characteristically persisting and resistant to antidepressant medication. Levitan and coworkers (1998), using a community-based sample of 653 individuals with major depression, demonstrated a significant association between early childhood physical and/or sexual abuse and atypical depression but not the endogenous symptoms of depression (i.e., the neurovegetative features). Nemeroff and his fellow investigators (2003) studied 681 patients with chronic forms of depression. They found that those suffering early childhood trauma (loss of parents at an early age, physical or sexual abuse, or neglect) did not respond well to antidepressant medication and in this way were atypical. Psychotherapy achieved a better outcome.

A Finnish study of 1,405 depressed subjects who were followed up by means of a self-rating inventory 2 years after the baseline screening found that those who remained depressed ($n = 217$) were more likely to have a history of multiple traumatic experiences than those who recovered (Tanskanen, 2004). Parker's group found that those women who suffered from childhood abuse developed certain symptoms that are characteristic of BPD. Sexual abuse was associated with deliberate self-harm, whereas physical abuse was related to adult interpersonal violence (Gladstone et al., 2004).

IS TRAUMA THE COMMON FACTOR LINKING AXIS I DISORDERS IN BPD?

The works of Kernberg, Zanarini, and others suggest that the co-occurrence of BPD and Axis I disorders is not comorbidity in the strict sense of the term when it refers to conditions that are unrelated. It is possible that these illnesses and disorders that co-exist share some common etiology or pathophysiology. A hypothesis concerning the common factor can be inferred from a case such as that of Jennifer, briefly described in Chapter 8. She had received multiple diagnoses during her life, in addition to BPD, including anorexia nervosa, obsessive–compulsive disorder (OCD), depression, panic attacks, dissociative identity disorder, and schizophrenia. Her successful treatment by Joan Haliburn, in each of these illnesses, revealed their basis in several forms of interpersonal traumata. The basis of her panic attacks, for example, could be understood in terms of separation–abandonment fears, whereas the OCD was related to an intrusive and controlling traumatic parental background which may provide a specific vulnerability to OCD (Meares, 2001a).

Whether trauma or, more particularly, traumata of different

kinds provide the link between BPD and Axis I disorders is a question to which the answer is largely speculative since adequate data are not available. Nevertheless, it is not unreasonable to suppose that within the typically traumatic background of those with BPD, it may be possible to identify subcategories of trauma beyond those coarsely distinguished forms of sexual, physical, and emotional abuse reported in retrospective studies. A more detailed account of these subcategories of trauma appears to be arising from studies of childhood development. Each of these subcategories may contribute to the etiology of a certain proportion of the Axis I disorders. This idea has implications for treatment: It suggests that in those circumstances when a "comorbid" Axis I disorder arises in a patient suffering BPD, the principal focus of treatment should be upon the basic illness— that is, BPD. However, a multimodal treatment regime, specifically constructed for a particular Axis I disorder, is a useful additive measure.

Depression is an example of the polysymptomatic nature of BPD, which is not a single condition but comprises several different mood states that are distinguishable and that presumably have different bases. It is not suggested that all forms of depression that coexist with BPD can be considered aspects of the syndrome. Melancholic forms of depression might be more truly comorbid, suggesting that two kinds of depression can coexist in a person suffering from BPD. In the same way, it is also *not* suggested that all subcategories of the Axis I disorders can be understood as particular manifestations of the systematic disturbance that produces the patterning of symptoms diagnosed as BPD.

Finally, the multiple patterns of symptoms that may manifest in the life course of someone with BPD may be a further illustration of a basic disconnectedness at the core of BPD. The bases of these symptoms may be conceived as an effect of different systems of unconscious traumatic memory, which are not organized in a single coherent traumatic complex but are largely, though not wholly, disconnected from each other and therefore have different consequences in terms of symptomatology. The polysymptomatic character of BPD, then, mirrors on a much larger scale the broken-up quality of some sessions with the patient who suffers from BPD, in which the effects of various IWMs fleetingly emerge, shifting from one to the other.

Chapter 11

EMOTIONAL DYSREGULATION

EMOTIONAL DYSREGULATION is considered by a number of authorities (e.g., Corrigan et al., 2000; Herpertz et al., 1999; Linehan, 1993; Silk, 2000; Stiglmayr et al., 2001) to be the core characteristic of BPD. Indeed, there has been some support for the proposal that, in the forthcoming DSM-V, the diagnostic term *borderline* be abandoned in favor of "emotional dysregulation disorder." Emotional dysregulation is seen as one of the two principal phenotypes of BPD (Siever et al., 2002), the other being impulsivity. These two phenotypes have different natural histories and may therefore have somewhat different bases. In this chapter, however, they are considered together.

Emotional dysregulation is a principal means of identifying BPD, since the DSM focuses particularly on behavioral phenomena. The more subjective elements of BPD represented in the triad of criteria composing the "self factor," considered in Chapter 3, are only sketchily described. This triad—identity problems, emptiness, and abandonment fears—is often confused with depression (Silk, 2011) and is seen in this book as the core of BPD, with emotion dysregulation related to it and secondary to fluctuations in the self system. Some indirect support for this proposal came from our outcome studies (Korner et al., 2006;

Meares et al., 1999b; Stevenson & Meares, 1992). The focus of the twice-weekly treatment was upon self generation and regeneration. No attempt was made to train or to instruct the patients in self-regulation, yet significant change occurred in its indices.

The notion that emotional dysregulation in BPD is related to self-disturbance is consistent with a study by Koenigsberg et al. (2001), in which they showed that this trait of dysregulation is correlated with the DSM criteria of identity problems and emptiness; that is, with the self factor. It also correlated with inappropriate anger and suicidality.

REACTIVITY AND DISINTEGRATION

Emotional dysregulation in BPD is authoritatively considered to be reactive to psychosocial stresses, as Koenigsberg (2010) points out, using the evidence of Gunderson and Lyons-Ruth (2008) and Stiglmayr et al. (2005). In this way it is distinguished from the emotional instability of bipolar disorder (Henry et al., 2001; Paris, Gunderson, & Weinberg, 2007). The reactive nature of emotional dysregulation in BPD is enshrined in DSM-IV.

The reactions of people with BPD are most frequently precipitated by those close to them (Gunderson & Phillips, 1991; Tolpin et al., 2004). Glaser et al. (2008), however, in a study using a structured diary technique accessing current context and mood in daily life, found that the small disturbances that continually happen in the natural flow of daily life, outside the home, are also likely to trigger emotional reactions in those with BPD. This research showed that these people have more such reactions than patients suffering from psychosis or healthy controls. This study confirms a number of other investigations of a similar kind reviewed by Nica and Links (2009).

The experience of devaluation, through belittling, shaming, criticism, and other forms of invalidation, is a particularly powerful trigger of affective shift. Linehan and her colleagues have highlighted the significance of shame in self-inflicted injury (Brown et al., 2009). An experimental study from Gratz et al. (2010) supported this clinical observation. They compared subjects with BPD to outpatients without personality disorder in their responses to two laboratory stressors, one general, and the other involving negative evaluation. They found that, compared with non-BPD individuals, the subjects with BPD showed heightened reactivity to the negative evaluation but not to the general stressor. Furthermore, their results provided support for shame-specific reactivity in BPD.

Devaluation, however, is not the only trigger to a reactive shift in affect in people with BPD. Rejection, or at least the perception of rejection or possible abandonment, and also frustration, may trip the sufferer from BPD into a negative state. These states are typically somewhat different from those produced by devaluation. In the first case, anxiety is likely to form a significant component of the emotional response, whereas anger is the usual outcome in the second case. Anger, anxiety, and a sense of personal devaluation (i.e., of chronic low self-esteem) are characteristic affects of those with BPD (Reisch et al., 2008). Therapeutic behaviors that amplify and regularly precipitate such affects are unlikely to be beneficial and indeed may be harmful (Meares & Hobson, 1977).

The article from Gratz et al. (2010) also offered evidence about two other characteristics of affective dysregulation in BPD. The first of these is the intensity of response. The subjects with BPD reported higher levels of shame in response to negative evaluation. This observation supported earlier reports indicating intense negative emotions following social interactions in those with BPD (Russell et al., 2007).

The second characteristic of BPD reactivity is its prolongation. In the Gratz et al. (2010) study, the levels of shame remained elevated as if the subjects had no suitable way of "turning off" the unpleasant affective state. This finding again corroborates earlier work. Stiglmayr et al. (2005) found that subjects with BPD experienced longer periods of distress than healthy controls. Domes et al. (2006) found deficiencies in inhibitory functioning in those with BPD, which might reflect impairments in the capacity to reduce both intensity of emotional experience and its duration. These researchers compared a group of women with BPD ($n = 28$) to age-matched healthy controls ($n = 30$) in their performances on neuropsychological tasks that involved both neutral and emotional material. Their data suggested that individuals with BPD have difficulties in actively suppressing irrelevant information when it is of aversive nature.

A third characteristic of BPD reactivity was not addressed in the Gratz et al. (2010) study. It is the extremely rapid rise time of the response, which comes so sharply that it seems as if automatic, with inadequate cortical involvement, the nervous impulse apparently traversing LeDoux's "quick and dirty" low road through the brain (2003, pp. 122–123).

The clinical observation that those with BPD are emotionally hyperactive is not always supported by experimental data. Linehan, for example, who had described emotional reactivity in BPD (Linehan, 1993), could not replicate this kind of responsiveness in a laboratory investigation (Kuo & Linehan, 2009). Jacob et al. (2009) were also unable to demonstrate unusual emotional reactivity in BPD in an experimental study. They reviewed current evidence on the matter and found that some of it supported what they called "the hypothesis of emotional reactivity," but other reports were contradictory. Herpertz and her colleagues, for example, found no exaggerated startle responses in those with BPD (Herpertz & Koetting, 2005; Herpertz et al., 2000) and, strangely, psychophysiological evidence of low arousal (Herpertz et al., 1999).

Findings from so eminent a researcher as Sabine Herpertz cannot be ignored. Equally, however, the clinician cannot ignore what his or her senses have revealed when working with patients who have BPD: namely, sudden shifts into negative states often produced by apparently trivial interpersonal events. How are there these contradictory findings explained? At least two explanations come to mind. The first, touched upon in more detail in the following chapter, depends upon a propensity for those suffering from BPD to enter a state of secondary dissociation that involves the activation of coarse, or lower-order, inhibitory mechanisms leading to lowered arousal. A laboratory situation may be sufficiently unnerving to trigger such a response. The second explanation is that watching pictures or listening to stories in a laboratory does not replicate an interpersonal situation, particularly one in which attachment might play a part.

The phenomenon of reactivity in BPD can be conceived in terms of the neo-Jacksonian hypothesis, in the following way. The incident that triggers the affective shift (e.g., a gesture, word, or tone of voice that suggests devaluation) activates the unconscious traumatic memory system. An ill-developed system of higher-order consciousness relating to self-awareness is overturned by the intruding traumatic complex, which is underpinned by a neural patterning in which activity is reduced in the prefrontal orbitofrontal cortex (Schmahl, Vermetten et al., 2004) and amygdala activity is enhanced (Donegan et al., 2003; Herpertz et al., 2001). Minzenberg et al. (2007) also showed a disconnection between frontal areas of the amygdala in subjects with BPD who viewed facial expression of fear. They showed an exaggerated amygdala response and impaired emotional modulation of the anterior cingulate cortex (ACC). A different kind of consciousness now prevails, in which reflection is lost and the person is unaware that he or she is in the grip of memory. The "facts" of an original series of traumata now dominate the subject's experience, albeit unconsciously, so that the subject feels once again in the role of victim and in a form of relatedness in which the other is sensed as devaluing, critical, controlling, contemptuous, or whatever part the original other played in the traumatizing events.

This state of mind—its structure, its accompanying affect, and the form of relatedness in which it is experienced—is sharply discontinuous from that which preceded it. Other social triggers characteristically produce a somewhat different complex of changes, also discontinuous from a previous state of mind. The quality of the affect alters. The form of relatedness in which it arises is also changed. There are discontinuities, then, not only in emotional expression and its style, but also in forms of relationship. Both are necessarily aspects of a particular form of consciousness in which the lineaments of self are lacking.

Koenigsberg et al. (2009) have put forward a similar approach to an understanding of emotional dysregulation in BPD. They distinguish between two main forms of brain–mind function. The first of these, termed "reflective," refers to the system of higher-order consciousness, or self. The second, "reflexive," refers to lower-order brain functions, which resemble simple reflexes. Each depends on a different network of neurocircuitry. The phylogenetically older system underpinning the reflexive mode "provides an automatic, fast operating emotional response, while the latter, incorporating the lateral and medial prefrontal areas, the medial temporal lobe and the rostral anterior cingulate (rACC), provides a more nuanced, experience-based, but slower responding emotional appraisal. We hypothesize that the increased emotional reactivity characteristic of BPD patients may be a consequence of their inability to adequately engage the reflective system" (p. 193). Consistent with this hypothesis, patients with BPD showed greater amygdala activity than healthy controls when viewing pictures of social interaction likely to trigger negative affective states. These data were consistent with those of Herpertz et al. (2001) and Donegan et al. (2003). The overactivity of the amygdala is seen as a consequence of disconnection from the modulating effects of the higher-order system.

Disconnection is a main component of the theme of hyperreactivity in BPD. The findings reported in the foregoing paragraphs are resonant with the disconnection reflected in the failure of coordination between P3a and P3b in BPD, which is discussed in Chapter 5.

DETECTION OF FACIAL EMOTION

The emotional dysregulation in those with BPD, which is related to disconnections among particular areas of brain activity, is compounded by a heightened sensitivity to social signals, particularly those that may have negative valence. Herpertz and her colleagues (2001) performed a study whose findings led them to suggest that "borderline subjects' perceptual cortex may be modulated through the amygdala leading to increased attention to emotionally relevant environmental stimuli" (p. 292). Domes et al. (2009) reviewed a number of such observations. In summary they revealed a pattern of alterations in discernment of facial emotion in people with BPD: subtle impairments in basic emotion recognition, negativity or anger bias, and a heightened sensitivity to detection of negative emotions. The overall picture was one in which those with BPD showed subtle impairments in accurately labelling emotions, with a tendency to interpret ambiguous faces in a more negative way. The researchers suggested that a bias toward the perception of anger shown in their work (Domes et al., 2008) might reflect the anticipation of rejection or threat.

A heightened sensitivity to the implications of facial expression in those with BPD has been observed by clinicians, who sense, at times, the patient scanning their face. This is usually understood, in the manner of Domes and his colleagues (2008), as a manifestation of the fear that the traumatic relationship of the past may be played out once again. There is, however, a second explanation put forward by Brandchaft (2010) that concerns a hypersensitivity to all facial and tonal expression, not merely the negative aspects. It is driven by anxiety that arises out of a disturbance of attachment, characteristic of those suffering from BPD. Their drive to maintain the bond with the other, however difficult, may cause them to respond in a way that they believe the other wishes, even to the point where their behavior is false. It is dictated by what they detect of the emotional life of the other rather than their own feelings. They "accommodate" to the other, developing systems of pathological attachment. This need might determine hyperacuity in the judgment of relatively neutral emotional expressions that could be sensed as ambiguous. A recent study of discrimination of emotion, conducted by Fertuck and his colleagues (2009) using a methodology that differed from previous studies of this kind, supported the notion that although those with BPD have a generally enhanced capacity to discern the nature of others' emotional expressions, this enhancement is particularly marked in the case of neutral stimuli.

Fertuck et al. (2009) used the reading-the-mind-in-the-eyes test, one of the so-called theory of mind evaluations, in their investigation. This test assesses the subject's ability to discriminate the mental state of others using only the eye region of the face. The subject was asked to make a choice from four words (three distractor words and one correct word) to describe the mental state portrayed in their eyes. The investigators found that for both neutral and positive emotions, patients with BPD performed better than healthy controls. There was also a nonsignificant trend toward better discrimination of negative emotional expression.

Although not all reports on this issue show that participants with BPD discriminate the emotional impact of facial expressions better than healthy controls, the consensus supports this conclusion. However, an interesting finding from Minzenberg et al.

(2006) suggests a modification to this conclusion. These researchers showed that subtle impairments in recognizing emotional expression may occur when these expressions of emotion are made in more than one sensory modality. They found that their patients with BPD had a normal ability to recognize isolated facial or prosodic expressions of emotion but had impaired recognition when the stimuli were presented together. A possibility implied by such findings is that although those with BPD may be hypercompetent in recognizing simple emotional expression, identified by a single word, this competence is diminished when confronted by complexity, when higher-order functions of integration are required.

Much of the data in this area must be considered preliminary. Most of the reports concern comparisons only between those with BPD and healthy controls. A third cell, comprised of patients suffering another psychiatric disorder, is usually lacking. Studies of patients with depression, however, suggest that, in contrast to those with BPD, they are impaired in the recognition of emotional facial expressions (Gur et al., 1992; Persad & Polivy, 1993; Rubinow & Post, 1992). Nevertheless, the possibility cannot be discounted that the differences between those with BPD and healthy controls in discrimination of emotional signaling of the face may not be specific to BPD. Further study is required. Research attention also needs to be paid to the integrative aspects involved in judging the emotional lives of others. As Livesley (2008) points out in considering the way forward in personality disorder research, "it is important not to lose sight of the importance of studying these integrative aspects of personality and the way they are impaired in personality disorder" (p. 557).

Despite the limitations in current data, they are consistent with the view, expressed by Sadikaj et al. (2010), that emotional dysregulation in BPD should not be considered a matter of disturbed regulatory mechanisms alone but also as a process involving interpersonal perceptions. The view was based on findings of an investigation that hypothesized that affective dysregulation in people with BPD would involve greater persistence of negative affect involving interpersonal events and also a heightened reactivity to stimuli indicating risk of rejection or disapproval, specifically perceptions of others' communal (agreeable–quarrelsome) behaviors. A total of 38 participants with BPD and 31 controls collected information about affect and perceptions of their interaction partner's behavior during interpersonal events for a 20-day period. Negative and positive affect persisted more across interpersonal events for individuals with BPD than for controls. In addition, individuals with BPD reported a greater increase in negative affect when they perceived less communal behavior and a smaller increase in positive affect when they perceived more communal behavior in others.

FAILURE OF NORMAL REGULATORY MEASURES

A further factor in the disturbance of affective regulation in BPD may be a diminished ability to mobilize normal methods of coping in the face of unpleasant or threatening interpersonal stimuli. This subject has not received a great deal of research attention. Koenigsberg and his colleagues (2009), however, tested a group of people with BPD ($n = 18$) and compared them with healthy controls ($n = 16$) in their effective use of the strategy of "distancing"—that is, a way of viewing stimuli as if from the standpoint of a detached and objective observer.

All subjects were trained in this technique. They were told that during the test they were not to look away from the images to be presented nor to close their eyes. After mastering the technique to the satisfaction of their instructor, they practiced on a laptop on 20 occasions. During the actual test the subjects were shown pictures of social situations, some neutral and others designed to evoke negative emotions. As these pictures were shown, the subjects were asked, at each presentation, to "suppress" (i.e., to distance) or to "maintain" their gaze while not attempting to diminish their emotional reaction. Brain activity was imaged by fMRI during these procedures.

The imaging showed that during the distancing task, when pictures arousing negative emotion were shown, both groups showed decreased negative affect ratings and increased activation of the dorsolateral prefrontal cortex, areas near and along the intraparietal sulcus (IPS), the ventrolateral prefrontal cortex, and the posterior cingulate/precuneus regions. However, there were also differences, suggesting that those with BPD did not engage the neural control systems to the extent of the healthy controls. They showed less activation in the dorsal anterior cingulate cortex and IPS, less deactivation in the amygdala, and greater activation in the superior temporal sulcus and superior frontal gyrus.

The procedure of distancing is only one of many measures the individual might use, usually unconsciously, to modulate the intensity of affect. The process begins at birth. Brazelton has shown that infants are able to soothe themselves when distressed, suggesting that the capacity is innate, presumably genetically determined (Als et al., 1977). It is not, however, fixed. A propensity evident soon after birth may be potentiated or diminished through interplay with the social environment. Regulation, then, is partially inbuilt but early in life is strongly influenced by the interaction with the mothering figure. It is a widely accepted view, as Manian and Bornstein (2009) point out, that regulation in infancy depends, in part, on two people. The mother or other caregiver has a role in regulation which is eventually taken over by the child.

Emotional regulation, in essence, is the child's management of arousal levels so that they do not exceed a certain optimum. In the beginning of life, a very large part of this management comes from the mother. From time to time she enters a state that Winnicott (1958) called "primary maternal pre-occupation." In this state she builds a kind of attentional cocoon around the pair of them. We studied this state in a series of newborns with their mothers (Meares & Horvath, 1974). We gauged the capacity to screen out irrelevant stimuli during feeding by comparing the mother's rate of her habituation to a meaningless stimulus during feeding with her habituation on another occasion. Habituation was much faster during feeding. We also monitored the baby's heart rate during feeding; it significantly increased. The mothers who displayed very effective screening capacities had babies with higher heart rates than those of mothers with less effective methods. This difference seemed to be independent of the babies' weight gain (i.e., milk intake during feeding). The findings suggest the possibility that arousal, as indicated by the babies' heart rate, may be necessary to the initial stages of the attachment process and that it occurs in a paradoxical context of calm, created by the mother's attentional "cocoon."

The baby soon begins to manage his or her own arousal, albeit in a behavioral way since internal methods such as distancing are not yet available. Gaze aversion is typically used by the baby to regulate arousal, and its effectiveness is shown by a reduction in autonomic arousal (Field, 1981). This tactic, however, is one that develops in concert with the mother's congruent behavior. We studied this aspect of what Brazelton called "behavioral synchrony" (Brazelton, 1979; Brazelton, 1975). The babies were assessed by the Neonatal Behavioral Assessment Scale (Als et al., 1977) 2 or 3 days after birth. This scale measures four dimensions of neonatal behavior: (1) interactive ability, which rates responsiveness to social stimuli such as voices and faces, and social responsiveness; (2) motor maturity, which rates, in particular, coordination; (3) state control, which rates the neonate's ability to remain calm despite increased stimulation; and (4) physiological response to stress, which rates the baby's response to unpleasant stimuli.

On another occasion the mother's response to stimulation was also assessed. Her screening capacity was measured in terms of her rate of habituation to a meaningless stimulus.

When the infants were 3 months old, they and their mothers were videotaped for 15 minutes while they sat opposite each other, the mothers being instructed to play with their babies as they might normally do. We analyzed the tape according to a method proposed by Tronick et al. (1977). The data showed the complexity of what seems, to the ordinary observer, a very simple engagement. The outstanding finding, however, was that infants who were more socially responsive had mothers with greater capacity for "screening out" redundant stimuli. These dyads had a characteristic cycling pattern that differed from the other dyads. They spent a lot of time gazing at each other before one or other, usually the infant, averted gaze. It could not be said that this was the "normal" pattern, since the rapid cycling of the other dyads was also "normal" and adaptive for these pairs. In both cases, the mothers seemed to be "attuned" to what their babies required, in shifting in and out of engagement. It has been claimed that the better attuned the mother is to the arousal level of her baby, the more she allows him or her to recover quickly during periods of disengagement. Stern (1977) has argued that the development of such synchronized interactions is fundamental to healthy affective development.

The mother–baby pairs behaved in a way that suggested a "fit" between them which may have been influenced by common neurophysiological capacities. We postulated that in some cases a mismatch of these capacities might occur, in which mother and baby cannot establish a suitable to-and-fro engagement. In a subtle way the mother feels that she and her baby are out of sync. She may blame herself, think she is a bad mother, or feel that the baby does not like her. On the other hand, she may harbor a negativity toward this infant, who may feel different to her than her other babies. The stage is set for disturbance of normal regulation (Penman et al., 1983).

The child who cannot regulate him- or herself is labeled "difficult." Thomas et al. (1978) identified a particular constellation of temperament traits in "the difficult child." They include disturbances of regulation in biological functions, such as sleeping and eating, slow adaptability to change, and intense and negative mood expressions. As far as I know, there has been no longitudinal follow-up sufficient to provide evidence about the vulnerability of such children to the later development of BPD.

In our study of some origins of the difficult child, 32 mothers of newborn babies were interviewed by a woman who herself was a mother within 48 hours of birth (Meares et al., 1982). The interview was semistructured. It concerned the mother's preparation for the birth; her feelings about pregnancy, labor, and her baby; and her assessment of herself regarding her flexibility, general coping ability, and confidence capacity/tolerance. The mother's expectation of her infant's "difficulty" was rated by the Neonatal Perception Inventory (Broussard & Hartner, 1971). The babies were rated on the Brazelton Neonatal Behavioral Assessment Scale (Als et al., 1977).

The study showed that, within 48 hours of their babies' births, mothers could make a decision about the expected difficulty of their newborns. This judgment came from two main sources: (1) the mothers' own characteristics, and (2) the mothers' finely made observations of their infant's behavior. Three months later some of these babies were indeed "difficult," and the only prediction of their dysregulation was the mothers' expectation. The Brazelton scores were not predictive.

We could not distinguish between the two main influences on the mothers' expectations of their newborn infants in terms of which was the more powerful. Presumably however, with a larger sample it may have been possible to differentiate between those mothers who predicted the child's difficulty on the basis of a fairly accurate perception of the baby's innate disposition and those who foresaw the development of the child in terms of their own characteristics.

THE "DIFFICULT CHILD" AND DISORGANIZED ATTACHMENT

Although they did not directly study the origins of the "difficult child," Spangler, Fremmer-Bombik, and Grossman (1996) produced data suggesting that for at least some children, innate disposition is an important determinant in being given this label. They found, in a "low-risk" sample of mother–baby pairs, that disorganized infants (i.e., those showing poor self-regulation) displayed poor self-regulation as newborns. They could detect no differences in maternal sensitivity between mothers of organized and those of disorganized infants. Their findings were consistent with earlier reports that ratings of poor regulation in the baby and reduced orientation to social stimuli predicted the formation of insecure attachment (Crockenberg, 1981; Grossman et al., 1985; Waters, Vaughn, & Egeland, 1980).

The data from "high-risk" samples of mother–baby pairs contrasts with those from "low-risk" groups. About 15% of 1-year-old infants from low-risk pairs and over 80% from a high-risk group showed disorganized attachment behavior in the Strange Situation (Barnett, Ganiban, & Cicchetti, 1999; Main & Solomon, 1990; van IJzendoorn, Schuengel, & Bakermans-Kranenburg, 1999). Studies of high-risk samples show high levels of unsuitable and insensitive maternal responsiveness among mothers of infants showing disorganized attachment. They behave, for example, in a hostile-intrusive way, making communication errors (Lyons-Ruth et al., 1991; Lyons-Ruth, Bronfman, & Parsons, 1999; Madigan, Moran, & Pederson, 2006).

It seems likely, at least to me, that children now given the attachment status of disorganized are those who would once have been called "difficult" children. "Difficulty" was conceived in terms of temperament. The child, in short, was born "bad." In contrast, disorganization is seen by current researchers and therapists as a relational problem. Nevertheless, the epithet of the "difficult child" persists as a lay expression and is not infrequently the precursor of the borderline condition. Yesterday, for example, I saw two patients with BPD for the first time, both of whom had been labeled in this way. The labeling appeared to be a self-fulfilling prophecy.

The first of these patients was the child of a feckless father and a mother who died young. The child was parceled out to a grandmother, who found that she was not a "good girl" and a burden. She was bundled off to the boarding school at the age of 8, where her status as a "difficult child" was confirmed. She was expelled and returned to the grandmother, eventually running away at 13 to live on the streets. She endured a life of deprivation, depravation, and horror that included prostitution, drugs, and abuse. Amazingly, she survived, now living alone and working in a refuge for runaway adolescents. The second patient's story was similar. Although, as remarked previously, there is no evidence available about the relationship between the parental designation of the "difficult child" and the adult diagnosis of BPD, it may well resemble that between disorganized attachment and BPD.

Psychopathology of the infant's principal caregiver, leading to deficient responsiveness to the child's emotional expressions, is associated with a disturbance of normal methods of emotional regulation. A simple example is the baby's use of gaze aversion to control arousal. In a study of depressed mothers ($n = 48$) compared with a group of nondepressed mothers, Manian and Bornstein (2009) found that there were differences in gaze behavior when babies tried to adjust themselves during a 2-minute period. The mothers were asked during this period to act as if tired and unable to play with their babies properly, to speak in a flat dull monotone, to keep their faces expressionless, and to minimize body movement and contact with the baby. The babies of nondepressed mothers used the strategy of gaze aversion and attention to objects significantly more than the babies of the depressed mothers, as if the latter were relatively unable to use this simple method of coping with negative arousal.

Certain evidence suggests that the child's ability to use external or behavioral means of emotional control tends to be internalized if adequate attachment develops. One of these pieces of evidence comes from Kochanska, Philibert, and Barry (2009), who studied children who, at 15 months of age, were judged to be insecurely attached. The researchers found that these insecurely attached children failed to develop a form of internally generated self-regulation. They had difficulty in the effortful control of a dominant response toward a desired goal. The capacity to control a dominant response in favor of another begins to emerge in the second year of life.

A well-known test of the capacity for effortful control and response inhibition is a go/no go task. In a study of subjects ranging from 8 to 20 years, the capacity to inhibit responses increased with age, and aging was associated with increased orbitofrontal activity (Tamm et al., 2002). Damage to this region results in emotional liability, and decreased impulse control (Knight et al., 1995).

A GENETIC CONTRIBUTION TO DYSREGULATION

Livesley (2008) proposed a two-component conception of BPD comprising (1) a disintegrated self system and (2) emotional dysregulation. He considers, as others do, that the second component has a significant heritable, or genetic, basis. The dysregulation characteristic of BPD also includes behavioral regulation (i.e., impulsivity). The two forms of dysregulation are considered the two major endophenotypes of BPD. They presumably contribute to the formulation of the two subgroups of BPD identified by Shedler and Westen (1998) and Westen and Shedler (1999). The first is labeled "emotionally dysregulated"; the second, called *histrionic*, was characterized by an exaggerated manner and impulsive behavior.

Much of the research on impulsivity focuses on *impulsive aggression*, as distinguished from *instrumental aggression*. The former is reactive and likely to involve deficient orbitofrontal cortex function, leading to a failure to sufficiently "inhibit" inappropriate behavior. Instrumental aggression, on the other hand, is calculated and a feature of psychopathy. It is associated with amygdala dysfunction (Blair, 2004).

The two forms of dysregulation, affective and impulsive, must be related since the motor discharge of impulse is necessarily driven by affect. Nevertheless, their genetic backgrounds are believed to differ. Research evidence suggests that impulsive aggression involves a deficit in serotonin activity, whereas the cholinergic system has been implicated in affective instability (New & Siever, 2002). Since serotonin is an inhibitory transmitter, deficits in its function provide the basis for a plausible hypothesis for origins of behaviors that can be seen as the consequence of failed inhibition. A disturbance of serotonergic activity has been postulated for a range of dysfunctional behaviors (Lucki, 1998). Depue and Lenzenweger (2001, 2005) point out, however, that it is premature to conceive behavioral disorder in terms of a single neurotransmitter, and that behavior is the outcome of complex interactions among multiple systems.

The degree to which genetic and/or environmental factors influence the emergence of BPD is not yet known. Torgerson and his colleagues (2008) provide a reasonable estimate. They assessed 1,386 Norwegian twin pairs between the ages of 19 and 35 using the Structured Interview for DSM-IV Personality. Their statistical analysis provided heritability estimates for Cluster B personality disorder traits as follows: 38% for histrionic personality disorder, 24% for narcisstic personality disorder, and 35% for BPD traits. The authors of this report point out that the estimates of genetic influence on the emergence of BPD were far lower than in their previous study (Torgerson et al., 2000). This report concerned 221 twin pairs (92 of the twins were monozygotic and 129 dizygotic) involving BPD, either "definite," meaning all criteria were fulfilled, or "broad," meaning one or two criteria were present. The concordance for definite BPD was 35% in monozygotic pairs and 7% in dizygotic pairs. The authors calculated an additive genetic effect of .69, which is quite high, probably too high. This study had certain limitations. Distel et al. (2008) point out that "this heritability estimate must be considered approximate due to the small number of twins, the ascertainment method (sampling those who were treated for mental disorder) and the fact that the zygosity and diagnostic status of co-twins was not hidden from the interviewers" (p. 1220). Drawing on a sample of 5,496 twins between the ages of 18 and 86 from the Netherlands, Belgium, and Australia, the researchers calculated that additive genetic influences explain 42% of the variation in BPD features in both men and women. This heritability was similar across the three countries. Unique environmental influences explained the remaining 58% of the variance. Another recent study produced a somewhat similar heritability estimate of BPD (Kendler et al., 2008).

Investigations into the specific nature of the heritable contribution to the origin of BPD are at a very early stage. Research thus far has focused on the relationship between genes and the dysregulation aspects of BPD. The main studies in this area to date have been summarized by Goodman et al. (2010) and Reichborn-Kjennerud (2008). The principal evidence concerns an association between impulsive aggression and reduced central serotoninergic activity. This evidence is reviewed by Perez-Rodriguez et al. (2010), who conclude that "the link between decreased serotoninergic function and impulsive aggression across psychiatric diagnoses is one of the most robust findings in biologic psychiatry" (p. 2). Their own study concerned the tryptophan-hydroxylase 2 (*TPH2*) gene, which codes for first enzyme in serotonin synthesis in the brain. Using the approach of Zhou et al. (2005), who identified a *TPH2* "risk" halotype associated with anxiety, depression, and suicidal behavior, they found that those with this halotype, among 251 people with various personality disorders, had higher aggression and affect lability and more suicial/parasuicidal behaviors than those without it. There was an association with BPD. Their findings gave support to an earlier study by Ni et al. (2009).

Other studies have focused on polymorphisms in the serotonin transporter gene (*5-HTTLPR*). *5-HTTLPR* S (short) allele carriers are more likely than noncarriers to develop PTSD (Lee et al., 2005), and they also have greater amygdala response to threatening stimuli (Munafo, Brown, & Hariri, 2008), suggesting that they might also be associated with BPD. This hypothesis was supported by the findings of Steiger et al. (2007), who found that the presence of the S allele significantly predicted a diagnosis of BPD in patients with bulimia. Lyons-Ruth, Holmes, et al. (2007) found that the numbers of short *5-HTTLR* alleles were significantly related to the incidence of BPD and antisocial traits in a group of low-income young adults. Other studies, however, did not find the S allele overrepresented in BPD patients (Pascual et al., 2008; Tadic et al., 2009). Finally, Distel and colleagues (2008) reported on the outcome of a major study involving 711 sibling pairs with phenotype and genotype data, and 561 additional parents with genotype data. BPD features were assessed on a quantitative scale. The researchers believed this investigation to be the first linkage study on BPD features. It showed that chromosome

9 is the richest candidate for genes influencing BPD. They note, in addition, that association studies in this region are required to detect the actual genes.

Gene-Environment Interaction

In the year following their report, Distel and colleagues (2009) produced their estimate that 42% of those influences culminating in the diagnosis of BPD were genetic. In commenting on the considerable environmental component in the development of BPD, they concluded their article by noting that the interaction between gene and environment had not been studied in BPD. In the presence of such interaction, "individuals with a 'sensitive' genotype will be at greater risk of developing BPD if an undesirable environment is present, than individuals with an 'insensitive' genotype" (Distel et al., 2009, p. 8). This is an idea developed in some detail by Gunderson and Lyons-Ruth (2008). Their argument began with a consideration of the likelihood that those who develop BPD have a constitutional diathesis for relational reactivity; that is, for hypersensitivity to interpersonal stressors. Their next consideration concerned the possibility that such a diathesis might predispose the developing individual to the formation of disorganized-types of attachment. This attachment style, as noted earlier in the book, may be an important precursor to the eventual diagnosis of BPD.

Perez-Rodriguez (2010) and colleagues attempted to investigate a gene–environment interaction. They put forward the hypothesis that not only would the presence of the "risk" halotype increase the likelihood of the development of BPD, so also would a history of trauma. They also supposed that the difference between aggression scores among the "risk" halotype would be amplified by trauma compared with those who were not carrying it. Since such data would have provided indirect support to the proposals of Gunderson and Lyons-Ruth (2008), it was unfortunate that there were not sufficient subjects without a history of trauma to make a statistical comparison. Nevertheless, such a study provides a model for future research in this area.

This model has been followed in a number of child studies that have focused on the expression of the *5-HTTLPR* gene and the influence upon it of the type of attachment the child forms. For example, Zimmerman, Mohr, and Spangler (2009) studied 92 twelve-year-old adolescents and found that the short-allele serotonin transporter gene was associated with a higher overall rate of autonomy behaviors in relation to their mothers. The form of attachment displayed by these children influenced the style of their autonomy. When the autonomy was threatened, a genetically based higher negative reactivity was moderated by a secure attachment. The subjects were less hostile than those insecurely attached.

Another study from the same group (Spangler et al., 2009) was much in line with the Gunderson and Lyons-Ruth (2008) proposals. These researchers studied children who were 12 months old and found that there were significant associations between attachment disorganization and the short polymorphism of the serotonin transporter gene, attesting to a genetic predisposition to the development of attachment disorganization. When considering a gene–environment interaction, they found that the genetic association was valid only for infants of mothers exhibiting low responsiveness.

This kind of maternal behavior does not, at first sight, seem sufficient to create disorganization. When, however, the consequences of a failure of the mothering figure to respond to the child are considered, a disorganized outcome is explicable. A baby depends on the mother's facial and tonal expression to understand the meaning of a particular situation. An example is provided by a well-known visual cliff experiment (Sorce et al., 1985). A baby crawls along a glass floor, then stops, realizing that there is a space below it. He looks up towards his mother, who is at the "deep" end of the space below the glass. His emotional state is presumably one of undifferentiated arousal, involving both apprehension and interest. The mother now represents this state, as she understands it. Her understanding gives it a "shape" and meaning. If she smiles and shows pleasure, he knows that this endeavor is interesting and perhaps even fun. He scuttles towards her. If, on the other hand, she shows fear, he turns back, perhaps in some distress. The meaning she conveys through her nonverbal expression leads to an action. What, however, would the baby do when no meaning is supplied, when the mother's face is still? What action should the child take? Go back or forward? The child is presumably bewildered and confused, perhaps frozen to the spot, without sufficient information, on his own, to determine danger versus safety.

Another recent study also gives support to the gene–environment interaction hypothesis. Kochanska et al. (2009) assessed 89 children for secure or insecure attachment at 15 months and followed them up at 25, 38, and 52 months in order to make judgments about their capacity for self-regulation. In addition, genotyping at the *5-HTTLPR* was determined on each child. At the follow-up points, the children were tested on their ability to suppress a dominant response and instead to make a nondominant response. The tasks became more difficult at each assessment point. Early tasks included waiting to unwrap a present and to take turns while building a block tower. Such tests gave an indication of the child's ability to suppress or inhibit impulses, a principal aspect of self-regulation. Among the children who carried a short *5-HTTLPR* allele, those who were insecurely attached developed poor regulatory capacities. Of these 40 children, 12 displayed disorganized attachment. The remaining 48 children developed good regulatory capacities regardless of their genetic status.

The investigators suggested that their findings supported the "maternal buffering" hypotheses of Suomi (2006). He noted that he and his colleagues have repeatedly demonstrated that monkeys with ss [short-short] or sl [short-long] genotype show a range of significant self-regulatory problems (impulsivity, inappropriate aggression, orienting problems, risk taking) but only if they had been separated from their mothers and raised in a peer nursery. For monkeys raised in natural, supportive mother–infant relationships, there was no effect of genotype. These findings led Suomi to state that "secure attachment relationships somehow confer resiliency to individuals who carry alleles that may otherwise increase their risk for adverse developmental outcomes" (Suomi, 2006, p. 52).

CONCLUDING REMARKS

Although the data on self-regulation in children does not directly contribute to our understanding of BPD, they suggest an ecological view of the etiology of this disorder—that is, one in which the individual is conceived as a system that is necessarily part of a larger system, which includes the environment. No single factor, whether it be trauma, the circumstances of early life, genetics, or a characteristic neurophysiology, is likely to be the sole cause. Nevertheless, the theme of disconnectedness is an important one, the most salient being that between prefrontal systems and the amygdala. Further, subtler reflections of disconnectedness are evident in the bodily markers of emotion in autonomic activity. Disconnections in the autonomic system in those with BPD are discussed in Chapter 13.

Chapter 12

SOMATIZATION AND STIMULUS ENTRAPMENT

SOMATIZATION IS COMMON in BPD, as it was for hysteria. It comes in three main forms: (1) the conversion disorders, better called "somatoform dissociation"; (2) symptoms that are bodily representations of trauma, discussed in the following chapter; and (3) symptoms that can be understood as amplifications of sensations that, under usual circumstances, cause discomfort but not distress. The third kind of somatization is the topic of this chapter. A "vicious circle" hypothesis is put forward for this kind of somatization. Two compounding mechanisms are seen to be operative: (1) a failure of higher-order inhibitory systems involved in the "medial pain system," and (2) amplification of stimulus intensity produced by the effect of attention. Attention is enhanced by the salience of stimuli, which is consequent upon the failure of sensory intensity modulation, resulting from deficient inhibitory mechanisms. Attention is also enhanced by psychosocial factors.

THE BACKGROUND OF HYSTERIA

Although somatization does not appear in the standard lists of criteria for identifying BPD, the ancestry of the borderline syndrome suggests that it should be, as noted earlier. Authoritative descriptions of hysteria, such as those of Pierre Janet and others at Salpêtrière, make clear that somatization, including pain, is central to the condition.

When the DSM abandoned the term *hysteria* in 1980 and the syndrome was "split asunder" (Hyler & Spitzer, 1978) into its component parts, as if they were unrelated to each other, somatization disorders became a separate clinical entity. However, in subsequent editions, as it became apparent that the 1980 categorizations did not fit the clinical facts, there has been a trend toward reconstitution of the original syndrome. The DSM-IV version of somatization disorder must now include conversion or dissociative symptoms in order to be diagnosed; dissociative phenomena are also among the criteria for BPD.

In this chapter the definition of the term *somatization* is derived from Lipowski (1988), who described somatizing patients as "those who frequently complain of physical symptoms that either lack demonstratable organic bases or are judged to be grossly in excess of what one would expect on the grounds of objective medical findings" (p. 1358). The additional criterion of seeking medical help for these symptoms is not included in my definition.

The main theme of the chapter is an attempt to understand the basis of such complaints. It is consistent, in a broad way, with Janet's view that a disturbance of attentional mechanisms is central to the disorder. His view is supported by the finding of a remarkable failure of habituation to meaningless stimuli in such patients (Horvath et al., 1980; Meares & Horvath, 1972). These studies, as noted in previous chapters, prompted the hypothesis that the basis of hysteria involves a relative weakness of higher-order inhibitory mechanisms.

ATTENTION AND PAIN

The hypothesis advanced here about somatization and pain has two aspects, which are both opposite and related. The first involves *amplification* or *augmentation* of the intensity of sensation through attention paid to it. The second involves a failure of systems usually effective in modulating the intensity of sensation. They are likely to involve neural circuitry with prefrontal connections.

Early studies of vulnerability to the experience of pain explored the first aspect, drawing on the concepts of Petrie (1967), who identified subjects as either "augmenters" or "reducers." The former group had a low threshold for pain. Buchsbaum and his colleagues (Buchsbaum & Pfefferbaum, 1971; Buchsbaum & Silverman, 1968) translated the Petrie paradigm into one based on EEG. They showed that in certain individuals, as stimulus intensity rose, so also did the amplitude of the event-related potential (ERP) evoked at the cerebral cortex. On the other hand, some people showed a tendency to reduce the amplitude of the ERP as the stimulus intensity arose. These people, "reducers," showed a relatively good tolerance of pain compared with those who augmented.

In a series of studies Buchsbaum and his colleagues investigated individuals with depression for whom complaints of pain are particularly common. Consistent with such clinical evidence, they found that an augmenting response was unusually common in depression (Buchsbaum et al., 1971, 1973). Backed by evidence that augmentation may have a genetic basis (Buchsbaum, 1974), Buchsbaum and colleagues inferred that augmentation was a biological marker of depressive illness (Gershon & Buchsbaum, 1977). Our studies, however, suggested something else. Whereas Buchsbaum's studies involved individuals when they were ill with depression, we investigated our subjects not only during their illness but also during recovery. When the patient had recovered from depression the amplitude of the ERP fell (Friedman & Meares, 1979c). The increase in the size of the ERP during the depressed episode correlated, in a broad way, with the severity of the illness (Friedman & Meares, 1979b).

Our findings in depression led us to surmise that the augment-ing pattern found during a depressive illness is a consequence of the illness, and that a change in neurophysiological function during the depression might be a contributing factor to the pain experienced by those with depression. This possibility leads to the related possibility that a similar disturbance underlies com-plaints of pain in people with borderline personality disorder. Such a possibility is supported by the finding that amplitudes of the ERP in somatization disorder are enlarged (James et al., 1989, 1990). Furthermore, a "pain-prone" personality style, namely extraversion (Bass & Wade, 1984), is associated with increased amplitude of ERPs (Friedman & Meares, 1979a). Extraversion has long been associated with the diagnosis of hysteria (Eysenck, 1967).

As might be expected from the Buchsbaum studies, the ampli-tude of the ERP is related, in a rough way, to the intensity of the stimulus. Pain evokes high-amplitude waveforms. Moreover, at-tention paid to the stimulus greatly influences the amplitude. The P200 (i.e., that positive component of the ERP occurring about 200 ms after the stimulus) evoked by stimuli to which the subject was asked to attend was shown by Miltner et al. (1989) to be three times the size induced by those stimuli which the subject had been told to ignore. The facts that powerful stimuli evoke high-amplitude ERPs and that attention can augment these amplitudes suggest the possibility that attention itself might produce pain even in the absence of a painful stimulus. Bayer et al. (1991) conducted a study that seemed to demonstrate this very effect. Normal subjects were connected to a sham stimulator and were told that a headache could occur as a result of the elec-trical current they received. Half of the subjects reported pain fol-lowing the sham stimulation. More recent studies involving the use of neuroimaging expand the implications of such a finding, showing that expectation of pain shapes the neural processes that underlie the sensed experience (Koyama et al., 2005).

The concept of augmentation has been transposed into the field of somatization by Barsky, who used the term *amplification* instead. This theory supposes that the somatizing patient experiences his or her normal bodily sensations as more intense than other people do (Barsky & Klerman, 1983). Barsky and Klerman argued that attention is one of the most important factors in altering the perceived intensity of, and distress caused by, bodily sensation.

The concepts of augmentation and amplification continue to direct inquiry into psychological pain. Additional terms such as *hypervigilance* and *catastrophizing* (i.e., hyperbolic descriptions of pain) have now been introduced into the argument. For example, a study by Crombez et al. (2004) of 64 patients with fibromyalgia, in which psychogenesis is presumed to play a part, found that vigilance to pain was correlated significantly with the pain intensity, negative affectivity, and catastrophic thinking about the pain. These patients differed in these respects from 46 patients with chronic low back pain. This study gave support to earlier studies, for example, by McDermid et al. (1996), whose findings on questionnaire responses by patients with fibromyalgia favored the generalized hypervigilance hypothesis and suggested that these patients have a perceptual style of amplification.

CEREBRAL PROCESSES UNDERLYING PAIN AND ATTENTION

Recent advances in neuroimaging are beginning to illuminate the cerebral processes underlying pain and attention. The affective experience of pain depends on the *medial pain system*. Its main structures include the midline and interlaminar thalamus nuclei (MITN), which projects to the limbic cortex, the periaqueductal grey, the amygdala, and the anterior cingulate cortex (ACC) (Vogt & Robert, 1993). The ACC has a main role in both of the two main forebrain networks underlying pain processing. They have opposite functions. The system that opposes the medial pain system, and which operates to modulate and diminish the intensity of unpleasantness, depends on the rostral part of the ACC (rACC) and also on the lateral orbitofrontal cortex. When pain is made to abate either by distraction or nonhypnotic suggestion (e.g., placebo), there is increased activity in the rACC (i.e., BA24) and the lateral orbitofrontal cortex (Bantick et al., 2002; Petrovic et al., 2005), suggesting that these are involved in inhibitory mechanisms. They operate so as to "turn off" the system underpinning the unpleasantness of the sensation by reducing activity in the amygdala (e.g., Petrovic et al., 2004).

The medial pain system is coordinated with a lateral one that has sensory and discriminative functions, whereas the medial system concerns affective and motivational factors. The processing of pain by these two subsystems is illustrated in a number of studies. For example, a PET study used laser to provide nociceptive (i.e. painful) stimuli without the contamination of touch. It was found that the lateral system is concerned with localization of pain, whereas in contrast, attention to unpleasantness increased responses in the medial system (Kulkarni et al., 2005). The dorsolateral prefrontal cortex is part of the lateral system underpinning "stimulus awareness" (Buchel et al., 2002).

The medial–lateral distinction, however, is not confined to pain but also concerns emotional processing. Emergent evidence suggests that the medial system is involved in the processing of "feeling" whereas the lateral is concerned with "facts" (Williams, Phillips, et al., 2001). Such data lead to the conclusion that the medial pain system is only one function of a more extensive processing system that evokes the emotional states that give a meaning to environmental stimuli, and, in the view of Damasio (1998), provides the meanings necessary to a system that is still larger— that of *self*.

INHIBITORY DISTURBANCE
AND STIMULUS ENTRAPMENT

A main background to this chapter is the view that patients with BPD suffer pain as a consequence of a deficiency in the sphere of self. The pathophysiology of pain in BPD is that of BPD itself. The deficit that is the prime basis of excessive pain in the patient with BPD is reflected in a large P3a, which is the outcome of a disturbance in prefrontally connected inhibitory neurocircuitry.

Enlarged P3a amplitudes and a failure of habituation are produced by damage to the orbitofrontal cortex (Rule et al., 2002). Rule and colleagues (2002) suggest that orbitofrontal damage might underlie a vulnerability to the experience of pain. They remark that "damage to the orbito-frontal cortex impairs the ability to modulate or inhibit neural responses to aversive stimuli" (p. 264).

Structural studies using MRI suggest that it is not the orbito-frontal cortex alone that is relatively dysfunctional in BPD. The circuitry disturbance is likely to include the ACC, particularly BA24 (Hazlett, et al., 2005; Tebartz van Elst et al., 2003). This structure is necessary to the system involved in the reduction of the intensity of pain (Bantick et al., 2002; Petrovic et al., 2005).

The attentional disturbance in BPD, reflected in P3a abnormalities, is correlated with a characteristic clinical picture. Since the individual is unduly alerted by stimuli, including those from the body, the contents of consciousness are constantly determined by external events. The individual's conversation consists of a "readout" of the impacts of these events on consciousness. The appearance of autobiographical memory and the emergence of imagination are relatively impeded by the effect of stimuli. The conversation manifests little evidence of the movements of inner life but instead takes the form of a "chronicle" (Meares, 1998). The individual, moreover, is as if entrapped by this situation, since removal of stimuli leaves him or her exposed to a painful state of emptiness, a state that must be avoided. This formulation leads to the proposal that a therapeutic approach to "stimulus entrapment" is likely to benefit those manifesting somatizing behavior.

TWO STUDIES OF SOMATIZATION IN PATIENTS WITH BPD

The foregoing remarks suggest that disturbed function of the medial pain system, which depends upon structures also involved in emotion, arousal, and attention, is likely to underlie the phenomenon of somatization in patients with BPD. In essence, the vulnerability to pain in those with BPD is seen to arise, in large part, from an attentional disturbance in which these individuals are unduly focused on external stimuli, including those from the body, and unable to modulate and inhibit these stimuli in the usual way. "External" is used here to refer to experience beyond that of psychic life, which is sensed as "inner." It might be supposed that a therapy that encourages a focus upon inner rather than outer events might diminish somatization in patients with BPD. This hypothesis was tested using two different data sets that are briefly presented here.

Study 1

The first study was part of a larger study evaluating the outcome of treating patients with BPD (Korner et al., 2006), which replicated the findings of our original study that concerned the effect of treating these patients by means of the conversational model (CM) with treatment as usual (TAU). Our unpublished data included results from the SCL-90-R, which is composed of nine primary symptom dimensions, one of which concerns somatization. The somatization dimension consists of five items (Derogatis, 1994). Estimates of internal consistency (coefficient) of this scale range from .86 to .88, and estimates of test–retest reliability after 10 weeks range from .68 to .86. Scores on the So-matization scale correlate well with the diagnostic index for the DSM category of somatization disorder (Hunter et al., 2005).

Data were analyzed by repeated measures ANOVA using the statistical software package SPSS for Windows (version 12). The group × time interaction provided the measure of the significance for the treatment effect. The significance level was set at 0.05. The 29 CM patients obtained a mean score of 1.49 (*SD* [standard deviation] = 0.18) at baseline, and the 31 TAU patients had a mean score of 1.54 (*SD* = 0.15). After 12 months of treatment the mean score for the CM patients had fallen to 1.08 (*SD* = 0.17) whereas the TAU cohort showed an increase in score to 1.75 (*SD* = 0.15). The group × time interaction was significant for the Somatization scale, which is evidence that the treatment effect had significantly altered the difference between the groups after 12 months: Wilks' lambda = 0.79, $F(1, 53) = 14.13$, $p < 0.001$.

These findings show that somatization is an extremely promi-nent feature in BPD. The somatization scores are much higher than a normative sample of 974 nonpatients (*M* [mean] = 0.36, *SD* = 0.42) and considerably higher than a group of 1,002 psychi-atric outpatients (*M* = 0. 87, SD = 0.75; Derogatis, 1994).

Study II

The second study concerned one patient in the CM cohort, as-pects of whose treatment have been touched upon elsewhere (Meares 2001b; Meares et al., 2005). The patient received 160 sessions of treatment, all of which were audiotaped. The patient's scores on the Somatization scale of the SCL-90-R were 0.70 at baseline; 0.70 at 1 year; and 0.30 at 2 years. Every eighth tape was analyzed. All somatization references (e.g., headache) in the first 5 minutes of the session were counted and the number com-pared with the number of somatization references emitted in an-other 5-minute period beginning 20 minutes into the session.

To test the hypothesis that the number of somatic references differs in the first 5 minutes of the session from another 5-minute period 20 minutes later in the session, the Wilcoxon signed ranks test was applied. Within the patient's conversation there were significantly fewer somatic references in the second 5-minute period (20 minutes into the session) than in the first 5 minutes of the session ($z = 3.256$, $p < 0.001$). The mean number of somatic references during the first 5 minutes was 2.8, whereas in the second period, the mean was only 0.2. Although no generalized conclusions can be drawn from a single case study, the finding is consistent with the proposal that somatizing behavior can be reduced by a therapy that engages a shift in focus from bodily and other external stimuli to inner events.

TREATMENT IMPLICATIONS

The kind of somatization that occurs in those with BPD discussed in this chapter is common. Headache is the most frequently presented symptom. Briquet (1859, p. 213), for example, interviewed 356 women who had been given the diagnosis of hysteria and found that 300 of them complained of headache constantly or were afflicted in this way very often and very easily. The main thesis of the chapter is that these patients suffer a form of attentional disturbance in which they are unduly focused on external stimuli. This idea has certain treatment implications that arise from the notion of amplification and its clinical consequence of stimulus entrapment.

Stimulus entrapment must be seen as dependent upon more than the physiological mechanism of deficient inhibitory activity. Such a mechanism implies that all sensation is likely to be amplified in those with BPD. The typical patient reports particular symptoms. A second mechanism is likely to be operative that determines the specific symptoms and involves social and cultural influences.

The focus of attention may be directed to a particular aspect of bodily function that is determined by social factors (Meares, 1997). For example, in certain families and societies, bodily distress may become the main means of expressing more personal distress. The individual, or child, may be driven by attachment needs, so that somatic complaints become a form of "care-eliciting behavior" (Henderson, 1974). Models of such behavior may come not only from personal experience but also from members of the individual's family who have physical illnesses (Hartvig & Sterner, 1985; Kriechman, 1987; Mechanic, 1980; Shapiro & Rosenfeld, 1986). The person chooses from a mass of sensations those that are more significant, as decreed by the familial or larger social environment. Psychodynamic influences may also determine the focus of attention. The symptom fixed upon may reflect some personal anxiety not explicable in terms of culture. For example, a woman complained of vertigo-like symptoms that were subjected to intensive medical investigation that proved fruitless. On being referred for psychiatric care, it emerged that she suffered from panic attacks. Out of the multiple sensations and emotions that compose this syndrome, she experienced as most salient the fear of falling, reflecting a fear of death related to abandonment fears.

The fact that the bodily state the person reports is likely to be a selection from a welter of sensory impressions dictates a therapeutic approach. The patient's preoccupation with the symptom has sometimes been seen as a resistance in the patient to talking about more "inner" matters. Instead of trying to avoid the subject, the therapist working in the CM approach takes an opposite and paradoxical stance. Rather than avoiding any discussion of somatic complaints for fear of reinforcing them, the therapist focuses on the somatizing behavior, listens to it intently, and attempts to have the patient outline the total experience as much as possible, beginning with the feeling. Put another way, the therapist works on the assumption that the somatizing behavior, although apparently impersonal, is personal in that it involves a selection. The therapist, having established a feeling associated with the symptom, then works imaginatively to attempt to discover a metaphor that might represent a larger and more central element of the patient's personal being.

SUMMARY

An important feature of BPD, not included in the DSM catalogue of diagnostic criteria, is a form of somatization in which complaints of pain and other symptoms of bodily distress are unduly salient aspects of the clinical picture. The origins of these symptoms may resemble those underlining emotional dysregulation. A common factor in determining these two categories of symptoms in BPD is a relative failure of those systems modulating the experienced intensity of sensation and emotion. Psychosocial and cultural factors influence attentional focus, which, in the case of pain, causes its amplification. An understanding of this focus helps to structure a therapeutic approach.

Chapter 13

A MALADY OF REPRESENTATIONS
Dysautonomic Aspects of BPD

THERE IS AN IMPORTANT CATEGORY of BPD phenomena that is very often overlooked but that may relate to the core of the disorder. It is overlooked, first, because the patient does not report it and, second, because, if reported, it seems incidental to the main clinical picture and also inexplicable. It appears as an almost literal imprint in the body, particularly the skin, of a fragment of traumatic experience. The symptoms of this phenomenon can be understood in terms of a disconnection theory of BPD. They seem to reflect autonomic nervous activity that is independent of, and uncoordinated with, higher systems, particularly the prefrontal cortex. Rule et al. (2002) have proposed that the orbitofrontal cortex is central to the top-down regulation of subcortical functioning of structures such as the autonomic system, the hypothalamus, and the amygdala, all involved in the induction, activation, encoding, and elicitation of emotion. The phenomenon considered in this chapter appears to reflect a loss of this regulation and to manifest a "dissociation" of the autonomic nervous system activity from prefrontal regulation, particularly as it controls the dermal vascular bed. Quite intricate patterns of skin sensation and even skin markings arise in some traumatized patients with BPD, like sensory "maps" of parts of the trauma. Here are some examples:

- A young woman who had been in therapy for about a year telephoned her therapist some time after a session, which was an unusual thing for her to do, and reported that as she was preparing for a shower, she noticed a number of bruises behind her knees, which bewildered her. The therapist saw her the next day and found several linear but incomplete lesions behind the patient's knees. This incident might perhaps have been anticipated since, several years before entering therapy, the patient had been investigated by a physician for large linear bruises that occurred intermittently on her arms and legs. The physician was baffled by these bruises and could find no cause for them. They became a focus of therapy. One day the patient recalled being made to face the wall and, while she was caned, to keep her legs perfectly straight. "Phew!" she said. "She used to be cruel. Nowadays you would call it child abuse." It was following this session that the bruises appeared spontaneously behind the patient's knees.

- A middle-aged woman had an intermittent sensation of a male hand under her chin, grasping it between thumb on one side of her chin and fingers on the other. It turned out that this symptom had its origin in her being forced to commit fellatio regularly with her father as a preadolescent.

- A woman in her 30s had the strange sensation, from time to time, of something like a silken cord moving obliquely across her face in a wavering line. This sensation occurred particularly when she was anxious. Eventually a link was discovered that related her facial sensation to a car accident some years before. In the moment before impact, she could see that the accident was about to happen and at that instant felt the terror of knowing she was about to die. She was not, however, seriously injured, but, as she lay on the roadside, blood from a scalp wound trickled obliquely across her face.

- A woman in her 40s who had been sexually attacked by two men would feel, intermittently, the skin of her forearms twisting laterally. This was a "body memory" of being held down by the arms by one man while the other raped her.

- The skin on the face and hands of a woman in her early 30s would, from time to time during a therapeutic session, become blue and mottled, as if from cold. When her therapist inquired about the skin changes, the patient had no explanation for them. It later emerged, however, that during childhood she was punished by being locked in a closet that was totally dark and in a part of the house that was freezing cold. This experience was frightening.

In each of these examples, the symptom represents an element of traumatic memory that was initially unconscious. Janet called hysteria an "ensemble of maladies of representation" (1901, p. 488). Breuer and Freud concurred, noting that "the hysteric suffers mostly from reminiscences" (1895, p. 4). Until recent years, there have been few reports of phenomena such as these. Presumably they were ignored as medically meaningless or discounted as mere fabrications. In the years before World War I, however, they formed part of the descriptive background of the complex condition then called *hysteria*. The possibility that at least some of these phenomena reflect changes in the blood supply to the skin is suggested by the observations of Janet. He found, for example, that anesthesia of the arm is associated with markedly reduced blood flow (Janet, 1901, p.11). He also described the remarkable case of a young woman, observed over a period of 10 years, who had a persistent pulse of 100 and a temperature about 2 degrees Fahrenheit above the normal, suggesting a disturbance of autonomic regulation of body temperature (Janet, 1925, pp. 1050–1051). Her symptoms could not be explained in terms of illnesses such as thyrotoxicosis. Her abnormal temperature did not inconvenience her. She complained, however, of fever when she had a slight attack of influenza. Janet noted that the "disorders of the peripheral circulation taking the form of passive dilation of the blood vessels or of vasomotor spasm" (1925, p. 1051) were not uncommon. "A great many of these patients are continually becoming affected with redness or pallor of the skin of various regions" (p. 1051). In several of his patients, "patches on the skin, at first red and hot, and then pale and very cold, [are] apt to become blue on the following day, and that for a long time in these areas a bruise is left" (p. 1052). In one case the bruising was associated with "actual ecchymoses" (p. 1051).

ARE THESE DERMAL REPRESENTATIONS DISSOCIATIVE?

The sensations and/or marks on the skin representing traumatic memory in some patients with BPD are like analogues of the PTSD flashback and nightmare. The dermal imprint might be conceived as another form of what Lenore Terr (1988) called a "burning in" of the trauma (p. 105). The visual representation, which "is often the repetition of the actual experience without transformation of any kind," as W. H. R. Rivers remarked (1922, as cited by McDougall, 1926, p. 138), is larger and more coherent than the dermal one. The latter is also qualitatively different from PTSD in that the individual is typically unaware of the origin of the skin phenomena. Are they, then, dissociative?

In terms of the hypothesis being put forward at the beginning of the chapter about the origins of this category of BPD phenomena, the imprints on the skin representing trauma are dissociative. They can be understood in terms of Rivers's use of the great neurologist Sir Henry Head's (1918) definition of dissociation. Head considered it a process "whereby one set of nervous functions are separated from others with which they are normally associated so that they become capable of independent study"

(Rivers, 1922, p. 71). Rivers considered "the word 'dissociation' [to be] peculiarly appropriate to the psychological process" (p. 72).

Janet's description of cases involving dermal representation and trauma suggest a dissociative basis. The famous case of Marie provides an example (Janet, 1901, pp. 282–285). Marie was a young girl from the country who had been hospitalized because she was judged insane and incurable. Janet discovered a number of traumatic incidents in her past. A principal one involved the onset of menstruation at the age of 13. For some reason, "she took it into her head that there was some shame connected with the affair, and sought some means whereby to stop the flow as soon as possible. In the course of some twenty hours she went out and secretly plunged into a big tub of cold water. She succeeded completely, the courses stopped suddenly, and notwithstanding the severe chill that followed, she was able to reach home" (pp. 283–284). This episode was followed by an illness in which she was delirious for several days.

Her periods stopped for 5 years but when they returned, she suffered a crisis at each menstruation. Twenty hours after the onset, the flow stopped suddenly and a severe chill shook her whole body. Then followed a dissociative delirium with florid symptomatology, including hallucinatory representations from other traumata. The episode, which lasted about 48 hours, "ended with several blood vomitings." She remembered nothing of the experience. Janet remarked that the scene of the cold bath "takes place below the surface of consciousness" (1901, p. 284).

Although accounts as exotic as that of Marie are rare, it is becoming evident that much lesser forms of the phenomenon are not uncommon. This evidence suggests that they may be an aspect of dissociation. For example, Madhulika and Adilya Gupta (Gupta & Gupta, 2006) asked 360 people—44 psychiatric outpatients and 314 nonclinical participants—to complete both the Dissociative Experiences Scale (DES) and an extensive checklist of cutaneous symptoms. They found that the symptom score correlated with the DES total score. They then considered those 17 people whose DES scores were considered pathological and found that their mean score on the cutaneous symptoms scale, 360, was much higher than the mean score of the remaining participants, which was 70. Pain, itching, and numbness were the best predictors of the DES score.

Although numbness, and to some extent pain, have long been associated with the phenomenon of dissociation, itching has not. Pruritic states, however, may represent "body memories" of traumatic memory. One of our own cases supported this possibility. The patient, a woman of late middle-age, presented to a physician with a 15-month history of recurrent episodes of formication and pruritus, particularly in the pubic area. This formication, described as a creepy feeling that bugs were crawling under her skin, was accompanied by feelings of being "unclean" and unfit to be around others. A provisional diagnosis was made of connective tissue disorder. She was intensively reviewed by an immunologist, who found no abnormalities. Since she was also depressed, she was referred to our clinic. It emerged that her symptoms had begun soon after an incident in which she felt as if she had been physically assaulted in the stairwell of the apartment house in which she lived. During this "assault," an obese male neighbor thrust his large abdomen into her abdomen in an intimidating way, as if he were trying to bump her out of the way. She was extremely distressed by this incident. Her symptoms remitted during therapy (Meares & Jones, 2009). A traumatic precursor to the bumping incident was not revealed, nor was it sought.

Two remarkable case histories from R. L. Moody, reported in *The Lancet* in 1946 and 1948, suggest an association between the state of dissociation and the representation of trauma by vascular changes in the skin.

In the first of these cases a man of 35 was admitted to a hospital in 1944 "because of somnambulism accompanied by aggressive behaviour" (Moody, 1946, p. 934). He was an Army man, but no account was given of his military service. In a previous hospital admission in 1935 for a minor septic condition, he had been "retained five months because of somnambulism" (p. 935). During this admission various restraints were imposed upon him to prevent his nocturnal wanderings. "On one such occasion his hands had been tied behind his back during sleep, as a precautionary measure. Waking in a dissociated state he had struggled unsuccessfully to free himself. He had then managed to evade his bodyguard and had escaped into the surrounding countryside from which he had returned a few hours later" (p. 935).

One night, during a later admission in 1944, "the patient was observed to be tossing and turning violently in his bed. He was holding his hands behind his back and appeared to be trying to free them from some imaginary constriction. After carrying on in this way for about an hour, he got up, and with his hands still in the same position, crept stealthily into the hospital grounds" (Moody, 1946, p. 935). He came back after 20 minutes in an apparently normal state of mind.

Two nights later Dr. Moody abreacted the patient by means of intravenous narcosis:

> He slept for a few minutes and then began reciting poetry (this was a common prelude to his somnambulism). Then minutes later he began to toss and turn on the couch, with his hands behind his back. As he appeared to be in a completely dissociated state, I turned the light full on him. I watched him writhing violently for at least three quarters of an hour. After a few minutes weals appeared on both forearms; gradually these became indented; and finally some fresh petechial haemorrhages appeared along their course. (Moody, 1946, p. 935)

A photograph of these indentations was included in Moody's *Lancet* paper.

In this article, Moody briefly mentioned three other cases of abreaction of traumata being followed by bodily "representations" of an aspect of the trauma. Swelling at points on a man's body recurred where he had been injured by a flying bomb; a seaman who had been immersed in very cold water for a long time showed localized ischemia of the extremities; a woman injured in a riding accident at the age of 10 showed petechial hemorrhages along the tenth rib, which had been fractured in the accident.

In each of these cases, the history given was insufficient to infer a BPD diagnosis. However, the background of the case presented in Moody's 1948 article was very like that told by a person who would now be given the borderline diagnosis. The patient was a married woman in her late 30s, who had had "an extremely unhappy childhood in which a sadistic father had played a prominent part" (p. 964). During Dr. Moody's abreactions of her traumata, "swelling, bruising and bleeding were observed on at least thirty occasions" (p. 964). They included the following: (1) "The morning after abreacting an incident in which she had been thrashed with a cutting whip at 8 years, three large bruises of appropriate shape appeared on her left buttock" (p. 964). (2) A few minutes after abreacting an incident in which she had cut herself rushing through a window, long red streaks appeared down each leg. The patient reported that these bled during the night. (3) Bruising after an abreaction had a "curious sharply defined pattern" resembling an elaborately carved stick her father had used to beat her.

None of the symptoms observed by Dr. Moody or by my colleagues and myself could have been explained by trickery or as factitious. Certain of the phenomena resembled the famous story of Padre Pio, whose body at times bore the signs of the stigmata, the wounds that Christ suffered on his hands, feet, and side at the crucifixion. In the 1920s the Vatican suspected that the oozing blood observed at the sites of the stigmata was factitious, and he was banned from celebrating Mass in public for over a decade. However, no evidence was ever found to suggest that the bleeding was self-inflicted and that he was a fraud. Padre Pio was extremely popular. Hundred of thousands of people converged on the Vatican for the occasion of his canonization by Pope John Paul II in 2002.

SHOCK AND DYSAUTONOMIA

The mechanisms underpinning the representations on the skin have not been investigated. They are likely to be complex. Nevertheless, the data suggest the hypothesis that shock to the central nervous system causes a disruption and destabilization of the autonomic system that is manifest particularly in the regulation of blood flow to the skin. In a mild way, the phenomena might resemble the syndrome of dysautonomia that may complicate severe head injury. The name of this specific syndrome may soon be changed, since it is often confused with a more general disturbance. Ian Baguley and his colleagues (2009) report that although dysautonomia can result from any form of acquired brain injury, it occurs most frequently after a moderate to severe traumatic brain injury. In most of these cases, there are episodes of accelerated heart rate, blood pressure, respiration rate, and body temperature, which, when they occur together, suggest a paroxysmal and widespread increase in sympathetic activation. Usually, these episodes pass; in about 10% of cases, however, they persist and are indicative of a poor prognosis.

Baguley and his colleagues regard dysautonomia as a spectrum disorder, ranging from mild to severe. It seems possible that just as a blow to the head might be followed by a period of dissociative-like amnesia, resembling psychogenic shock, such a shock may precipitate a minor form of dysautonomia, manifest particularly in the vascular system. Minor disturbances of blood supply to the skin, such as displayed in Raynaud's phenomenon, are now sometimes diagnosed as dysautonomia, although there is little research evidence to back up such a diagnosis.

It is of interest that Baguley and his colleagues (2009) suggest that, in dysautonomia, it is not the presence of overreactivity, per se, but rather a loss of the inhibitory processes for *control over* reactivity that contributes to dysautonomic "storming," in line with observations of emotion and pain dysregulation in BPD (see Chapters 11 and 12). In an earlier paper Baguley (2008) put forward the hypothesis that symptoms of dysautonomia, in common with a number of similar syndromes of autonomic dysregulation, display an increase in the ratio between excitatory and inhibitory influences. There is also a tendency of the individual to develop an overreaction to non-noxious stimuli (Baguley, 2008). These phenomena are not dissimilar to aspects of the pathophysiology of BPD.

THE POLYVAGAL THEORY

In the field of psychological science, Stephen Porges has been prominent in the investigation of autonomic regulation in mental illness. He has put forward a theory that is resonant with Jacksonian principles (Porges, 2009). The basis of his theory is derived from his experiences as a neonatal physician. Porges and his coworkers found that a disturbance of heart rate in neonatal distress could be explained as the outcome of a disconnection between the activities of two vagal systems, one of which evolved later than the other. During the distress period the more primitive system remained operative, whereas the later evolved form was no longer functioning (Reed et al., 1999).

Porges's (2009) polyvagal theory focuses on regulation of the heartbeat and an organization of parasympathetic activity that is determined by evolutionary history. The early, or reptilian, element of vagal regulation of the heart depends on an unmyelinated efferent pathway originating in the dorsal motor nucleus and terminating primarily below the diaphragm. The later evolved mammalian component is myelinated in the process of evolution. This new system is involved not only in the regulation of the heart but also of the muscles in the face and head subserving emotional expression via cranial nerves V, VII, IX, X, XI. These nerves together create an integrated social engagement system and provide the neural regulation of the muscles controlling eye gaze, facial expression, listening, and prosody (Porges, 2007). This mammalian myelinated system also links the rhythms of the heart to breathing, producing respiratory sinus arrhythmia (RSA).

In a study of patients with BPD, Porges and his colleagues (Austin et al., 2007) reported that at baseline there was little difference to be found between the BPD cohort and controls. However, when the two groups were stressed by means of film clips selected to elicit a strong emotional response, the patients with BPD showed diminishing RSA whereas the controls showed increasing RSA. In 1992, Porges had proposed that vagal tone, derived from an RSA measure, be used as an index of relative stress vulnerability.

In addition to the differences in RSA, the two groups showed another contrast during the stress condition. A correlation was found between the changes in RSA and heart beat period in the control group but not in the patients with BPD, suggesting that vagal mechanisms mediated the heart period responses only in the control group. These findings can be understood as a failure of connection between the vagal signals originating in the brainstem and the heart's response in those with BPD.

Porges and his colleagues saw the change in the patients with BPD as evidence of a stress-induced "dissolution," the term Hughlings Jackson (1958) gave to the reversal of the evolutionary trajectory of development of the human brain–mind. *Dissolution* implies a disconnection between neural systems that usually function together.

Porges describes a phylogenetically ordered and hierarchical sequence of autonomic response strategies to environmental challenges. The highest-order system operates in an atmosphere of safety. It depends upon an increase in the influence of the later evolved

> ... myelinated vagal motor pathways on the cardiac pacemaker that slows the heart, inhibits the fight–flight mechanism of the sympathetic nervous system, dampens the stress response system of the HPA axis (e.g., cortisol), and reduces inflammation by modulating immune reaction (e.g., cytokines). Second, through the process of evolution, the brainstem nuclei that regulate the myelinated vagus became integrated with the nuclei that regulate the muscles of the face and head. This link results in bi-directional coupling between spontaneous social engagement behaviors and bodily states. (Porges, 2009, p. 588)

The notion of "bi-directional coupling" is particularly important and intriguing. It implies that a particular state of vagal activity is likely to foster social engagement and that, conversely, certain kinds of social engagement have the capacity to promote activation of the later evolved vagal component. The latter possibility is supported by an interesting study from Schwerdtfeger and Friedrich-Mai (2009). Heart rate was recorded over 22 hours by means of ambulatory monitoring of subjects with depressive symptoms. The group was divided into those deemed high and low in depression. When those with high depression were alone, they had less heart rate variability (i.e., RSA) and a higher negative affect. However, when they were engaged with partners, family, or close friends, the heart rate variability increased, approaching that of subjects with low depression, and their mood improved. This effect was not achieved when the interactions occurred with strangers or colleagues.

When the sense of safety is lost, and when threat appears in the environment, an earlier evolved network of neural circuitry is triggered that leads to the fight–flight mode of experiencing and behaving. This system, which is necessary to immediate survival, overrides the calming, social engagement system. Porges proposes, in addition, a third and more primitive circuitry involving inhibition and manifest in freezing and immobilization. It is a response to extreme terror.

Data presented by Porges and his group (Austin et al., 2007) lead to two main inferences: (1) Patients with BPD are more easily tipped into physiological states of fight–flight than controls; and (2) this physiology shows a failure of coordination between neural systems that were previously connected.

A DISCONNECTION BETWEEN SYMPATHETIC AND PARASYMPATHETIC SYSTEMS?

The Porges data and related observations suggest a disturbance in autonomic function in BPD that can be conceived figuratively as "vertical" in the sense that later evolved higher-order systems become inactive and are thus disconnected from lower-order, more primitive systems. A second kind of disconnection may also occur in the autonomic function of those with BPD, which is metaphorically "horizontal": A failure of coordination between sympathetic and parasympathetic activity is suggested by findings from the research by my colleagues and myself, the data being collected prior to formal recognition of the borderline concept.

Four decades ago our patients were given the diagnosis of "chronic hysteria" (Meares & Horvath, 1972). Most of them would have fulfilled DSM criteria for BPD. The essential diagnostic criteria were evidence of a polysymptomatic personality disorder and a history of conversion, defined as loss of neural function. These patients showed a habituation failure of the electrodermal response to an intermittently sounded neutral tone. Such a deficit in selective inattention was shown in no other nonpsychotic group, but was characteristic of a nonparanoid form of schizophrenia (Horvath & Meares, 1979).

In a nonpsychotic population, a failure of habituation occurs only in the presence of extremely high levels of the arousal (e.g., Lader, 1967). Using spontaneous fluctuations of skin conductance, which Lader (1969) had shown to be a better measure of arousal than the level of skin conductance, we found that our group of patients had levels of arousal considerably lower than people with anxiety disorders. The anxiety group, however, did not show impairment of habituation to the extent of our group of patients who would now be diagnosed with BPD.

In this study, the two measures of habituation and spontaneous fluctuation of skin resistance reflect inhibitory activity, in the former case, and excitation, in the latter. Since the level of arousal could not explain habituation failure in "chronic hysteria," we put forward the hypothesis that a deficiency in higher-order processes of inhibition was a primary disturbance in this condition (Horvath et al., 1980). Seen in the light of data such as that of Porges, our findings give rise to a second hypothesis: They suggest a relative failure of coordination between inhibitory and excitatory neural systems. The normal reciprocal or inverse linear relationship between these systems was upset.

Against our inferences are the earlier findings of Lader and Sartorius (1968). They had shown, in a group of patients similar to our own, not only very deficient habituation but also very high arousal, higher than those with anxiety states. These patients, however, were different from ours in one crucial respect: They were still suffering from conversion symptoms, whereas the symptoms had remitted in our patients. Their remission status may have explained their low arousal, relative to the Lader and Sartorius cohort.

It is only in the last decade or so that some interest has been taken in the autonomic peculiarities of BPD. Herpertz et al.

(1999) and Schmahl, Elzinga, et al. (2004) measured skin conductance in patients with BPD and found no evidence of sympathetic overarousal relative to controls. On the other hand, Ebner-Priemer et al. (2007) found that those suffering from BPD do show evidence of increased heart responses to emotional stimuli, relative to controls, when ambulatory monitoring is used. Crucial observations of parasympathetic activity were lacking in the studies of Herpertz et al. (1999) and Schmahl, Elzinga et al. (2004). These measures were included in a study by Kuo and Linehan (2009). They found that when patients with BPD were shown film clips likely to excite a negative emotional response, they showed a reduced basal RSA. However, their skin conductance responses did not differ from controls. What Porges has called the "vagal brake" was not operative. These findings give support to the view that coordination between parasympathetic and sympathetic activity is impaired in BPD.

THE ANTERIOR CINGULATE CORTEX AND TOP-DOWN CONTROL

The developing evidence concerning abnormalities of autonomic nervous system activity in BPD must be considered in the context of the autonomic system's role in the larger functioning of the body's neurology. The autonomic system is part of the emotional processing system involving a complex coordination of functions ranging from higher-order capabilities, including evaluation of outer and inner events, to the most primitive, such as regulation of the heartbeat. The whole system must be seen as an ecology, with each part influencing the activity of all other parts. The determinants of this state, then, are not only top down but bottom up, a reciprocity understood by Darwin (1872/1934). He wrote: "When the heart is affected it reacts on the brain, and the state of the brain again reacts through the pneumo-gastric nerve in the heart, so that under any excitement there will be much mutual action and reaction between these two most important organs of the body" (p. 25).

Much investigation of the autonomic system has concerned the top-down influences. The anterior cingulate cortex (ACC) has been a particular focus of research, and findings show that it is composed of four main areas, distinguished histologically (Vogt, 2005). A "cognitive" role has been identified for the dorsal ACC, whereas the rostral and ventral ACC have an "affective function." The ventral ACC is particularly implicated in autonomic arousal (Critchley et al., 2005; Patterson et al., 2002; Williams, Gordon, et al., 2000). There is an interplay among ACC regions leading to coordinated output. Depending upon environmental requirements, dorsal, rostral, and ventral ACC activity is, at times, alternatively turned on and off, mirroring, at a higher level of the nervous system, Sherrington's reciprocal inhibition (Drevets & Raichle, 1998; Lane et al., 1998).

Diminished activity in the ACC is one of the better validated findings in BPD, as noted in previous chapters. Since the autonomic system is crucially involved in fundamental attentional processes such as orienting and habituation, it is unsurprising that the ACC is implicated in the focusing of attention, which involves autonomic activation, most prominently shown in skin and heart responses.

DAMASIO'S THEORY AND THE IOWA GAMBLING TASK

Damasio has put forward an influential theory that gives an explanation of poor decision making in people with damage to the orbitofrontal cortex (OFC). Central to the theory is what he calls "somatic markers," which, in short, are

> . . . *a special instance of feelings generated from secondary emotions. Those emotions and feelings have been connected, by learning, to predicted future outcomes of certain scenarios.* When a negative somatic marker is juxtaposed to a particular future outcome the

combination functions as an alarm bell. When a positive somatic marker is juxtaposed instead it becomes a beacon of in-
centive. This is the essence of the somatic-marker hypothesis
. . . on occasion somatic markers may operate covertly (without coming to consciousness) and may utilize an "as if" loop.
(Damasio, 1996, p. 174, italics in original)

Damasio and his colleagues devised a game that enables them
to study decision making. They call it the Iowa Gambling Task
(IGT; Bechara et al., 1994). In this game the participants are given
four decks of cards and a loan of $2,000 facsimile U.S. bills, and
asked to play so as to win the most money. Turning each card carries an immediate reward ($100 in decks A and B and $50 in
decks C and D). Unpredictably, however, the turning of some
cards also carries a penalty (which is large in decks A and B and
small in decks C and D). Playing mostly from decks A and B leads
to an overall loss; playing from decks C and D leads to an overall
gain. The players cannot predict when a penalty will occur, nor
calculate with precision the net gain or loss from each deck. They
also do not know how many cards must be turned before the end
of the game (the game in fact ends after 100 card selections).

As the participants play this game, their skin conductance responses are monitored. All participants show a skin response before and after making a decision. As the game goes on, normal
players begin to have a sense of the riskier choice. They start to
generate anticipatory skin responses in the 5 seconds before
choosing a card, leading to preferences for the good decks. The
anticipatory skin responses are not accompanied by any conscious apprehension, which generally, but not always, follows
later. The people with ventromedial prefrontal cortex damage do
sometimes become consciously aware that the high reward cards
are bad choices, but they fail to generate anticipatory skin conductance responses and continue to choose the cards disadvanta-
geously (Bechara et al., 2005).

Roberts and her colleagues, building on the work of Damasio

and his colleagues, showed that the representation of the aversive event (i.e. choosing the bad card) in those with OFC damage is not entirely cut off from interchange with the environment (Roberts et al., 2004). They studied the effect of unanticipated and anticipated responses to acoustic startles in patients with OFC damage. The patients showed intact physiology when the startle was not anticipated. Their faces showed more surprise than controls, and they reported more fear. On the other hand, when the startle was anticipated, they showed no anticipatory autonomic response, in this case, a decrease of heart rate.

These findings and those of the IGT are consistent with the idea that the representation in the brain of the event involves autonomically mediated somatic changes that are aspects of the emotional effect of that event that give it its meaning. This meaning, which determines a response, cannot be activated by conscious, higher-order cognitive processes in those with OFC damage, but it can be activated by relatively unconscious, automatic processing. This latter situation resembles that of patients with BPD in whom the primitive registration of the aversive event is activated by means other than those of normal consciousness.

A deficiency in orbitofrontal function has been proposed as a likely determinant of BPD symptomatology, as outlined in previous chapters. This proposal leads to the prediction that those with BPD will fare badly at the IGT. Haaland and Landrø (2007) tested this hypothesis, comparing the performance of 20 patients with BPD with 15 healthy controls. The patients with BPD made less advantageous choices than the controls. The difference could not be explained by indicators of general cognitive function or by symptoms of depression.

CONCLUDING REMARKS

The patterned skin sensations and marks that sometimes appear on the skin of those with BPD, as if "branded" by traumas, have no technical or medical name. They might appropriately be called *stigmata*, since the original meaning of the word *stigma* was "a mark upon the skin; . . . a brand" (*Oxford English Dictionary*, 1971). Charcot and Janet, however, used this term to designate a quite different group of symptoms that has no representational significance and that serves a defensive purpose. As noted previously, Janet gave the name of "accidents" to those clinical phenomena that are representations, on the body, of traumatic experience. His case of Marie was an example. "Accidents" include stereotyped patterns of movements that appear from time to time as repetitions of a fragment of traumatic memory.

A study of these phenomena may lead to a better understanding of the BPD syndrome itself. The phenomena may provide evidence, in miniature, of the essential forms of the larger disorder. Scientific data about the phenomena are few. Inferences are necessarily made from pathological states, which might mirror, in certain respects, the autonomic abnormalities that are involved in their production. Brain damage, particularly prefrontal and especially orbitofrontal, seems likely to provide evidence that could be the basis of hypotheses directing future research.

The skin changes representing trauma are an intriguing subject, given the common embryological origin of skin and brain. In the earliest stages of evolution, contact with the skin was the principal means of the organism's feeling and knowing. The feeling and knowing of any event is represented in the nervous system on multiple levels. Such representations, in the Damasio thesis, are encoded with "somatic markers" that provide the events with their meaning. This process depends upon the autonomic nervous system. The case vignettes of subjects with BPD given at the beginning of this chapter suggest that primitive representations of trauma, or more precisely, of fragments of the trauma, are activated by unconscious processes and that they are relatively inaccessible to higher-order conscious mental processing, which retrieves higher-order representations. In the case of severe trauma, it may be that these higher-order representations are not properly formed. This idea derives from the "dissolution model."

It is not known how common are the patterned skin sensations and marks that appear as if "branded" on the skin by trauma, analogous to the "burning in" of PTSD (Terr, 1988). They are only discovered by patient reports and not by the ordinary processes of psychiatric examination. If they are not particularly common, it may be because the situation that was their origin is also not particularly common. The incidents recounted earlier suggest that this is one of massive trauma inflicted on a highly vulnerable personality, someone young and lacking the "buffer" of resilience provided by a maturely developed sense of self. It might be supposed that in these circumstances, an event creating an emotional response of great severity and intensity, leading to terror, could cause a maximal disconnection between neural systems. At the same time, the more recently evolved functional "levels" would become deactivated, leading to a profound "dissolution" and a retreat down the hierarchy of consciousness. At this level the later evolved "distance receptors" of vision and hearing would lose their domination. The dominant experience would come from the more primitive receptors of touch and smell, and the trauma recorded in these terms. Registration of the event at higher levels would be impeded.

The data currently available (e.g., Kuo & Linehan, 2009) suggest that the disconnectedness of autonomic function in BPD is not only "vertical," that is, between higher-order systems of monitoring and control and lower-order systems, but also "horizontal," between excitatory and inhibitory mechanisms. This figuratively two-dimensional failure of coordination in neural functions that normally operate together may mirror the larger disconnectedness underlying the symptomatology of BPD.

Chapter 14

PARANOID IDEAS AND
DELUSION FORMULATION

PARANOID SYMPTOMS WERE a late inclusion in the DSM diagnostic criteria for BPD, appearing not in DSM-III but in DSM-IV, 14 years later. They are among those features of the syndrome that gave rise to the name *borderline* because they contribute to the picture of psychoticism that caused earlier clinicians to distinguish it from what were then called the "neuroses," while, at the same time, they were unable to fit it into the category of typical psychosis. Seen in this way, the paranoid criterion is central to the syndrome. Indeed, Skodol et al. (2002) point out that the "paranoid and dissociative features" criterion distinguishes BPD from other disorders better than any other criterion.

The DSM linkage between paranoid and dissociative features in a single criterion seems to suggest a functional association and that BPD paranoid features might arise in a dissociative context. Such a suggestion is consistent with the main gist of this chapter, in which the view is developed that the paranoid ideas and delusions that occur in BPD have an etiological basis in trauma/dissociation.

Paranoid ideas are more easily understood than delusion formation. They are explicable as an aspect of the "malignant internalization" (Meares, 1999b) of traumatic experience. In this chapter I first touch upon this experience and then follow with a consideration of delusion formation.

Delusional experience is fairly common in the general community. For example, a large population-based survey in Australia found that 11.7% of respondents endorsed one or more items designed to identify delusion-like experiences. The items consisted of questions such as "Do you ever feel as if other people can read your mind?" (Scott et al., 2006). Such experiences, then, are not confined to schizophrenia. Most research into the genesis of delusions, however, is based on studies of those who suffer this illness.

PARANOID IDEATION

It is traditional to conceive of paranoid ideas as arising through projective mechanisms. Freud (1915b) himself, however, contemplated, but did not pursue, a different viewpoint, presenting a case that seemed to overthrow his theory. He told a story of a young woman who had never sought any love affairs with men but who had lived quietly as her old mother's sole support. She had, however, become attracted to a man and had agreed to visit him at his apartment where some form of lovemaking took place. The following day he appeared at her workplace and had a whispered conversation with her supervisor, an elderly female. The young woman feared, and became concerned, that her secret had been revealed. At the first opportunity, she confronted her lover with his supposed treachery. He thought her accusation senseless.

The young woman's state of mind could be understood as having its basis in a fear of intimacy, the sense that within a relationship that induced positive feelings, some harm would come through their revelation, that some kind of damage would be inflicted upon her. This is a situation common to those who suffer from BPD and whose histories have taught them that self-revelation is a danger. They have come to know that damage will ensue through despoliation of tender feelings and through betrayal of trust by abandonment.

Harry Stack Sullivan (1953) gave an account of how a fear of intimacy might come about. His concept of "malevolent transformation" provides a powerful experiential view of how paranoid ideas may arise. The trauma upon which he focused is that arising from attacks on what Bowlby (1969,1973) called "affectional bonding," the tenderness which is at the heart of the mother–child relationship and which lies at the core of the satisfactorily developing self. This crucial feeling gives value to a sense of personal existence. Sullivan wrote: "A child may discover that manifesting the need for tenderness toward potent figures around him leads frequently to his being disadvantaged, being made anxious, being made fun of and so on, so that, according to the locution used, he is hurt" (p. 214). This hurt, involving shame and humiliation, is felt in an almost bodily way, as a psychic wound. The child comes to learn that he or she lives among enemies to whom no intimate emotions, such as the need for tenderness, can be shown. Powerful systems of avoidance come to be built around both the core of self and the collection of traumatic memory. Their purpose is to protect against further damage through a reexperience of the trauma.

In the Sullivanian system, personality development is skewed around trauma, distorted by systems of avoidance (Sullivan, 1953). Sullivan describes the high anxiety associated with the traumatic memory in terms of his concept of the uncanny. He cites awe, dread, horror, and loathing as the "uncanny emotions" that are the consequence of overwhelming anxiety. Such experiences can never be properly organized (p. 327) but are loosely held together in a "not-me" personification, which is almost beyond communication (p. 164). Words merely hint at this unthinkable anxiety. Aspects of the self system are devised "to keep one safe from any possibility of passing into that extremely unpleasant state of living which can be called the uncanny emotions; and these aspects of the self-system can be inferred except in the case of disaster" (p. 316). This conception describes a pathology of selfhood, analogous to C. S. Myers's (1940) "apparently normal personality (p.67)."

High avoidance as an aspect of BPD function is demonstrated in several personality questionnaires. For example, it is reflected in Cloniger's Harm Avoidance Scale, which is high in BPD (Korner et al., 2007). The Acceptance and Action Questionnaire (AAQ; Hayes et al., 2004), a nine-item, self-report measure of experiential avoidance, or the tendency to avoid unwanted internal experiences, is also higher in BPD than in other personality disorders (Gratz et al., 2008).

Such is the anxiety surrounding traumatic memory, particularly of a sexual kind, that the person may hide it even from those closest to him or her and from mental health professionals who are attempting to care for him or her. Subtle processes of secrecy and guardedness protect against revelation. Medical personnel may be unaware that they are operative. For example, one patient, Mrs. A., who was only apparently timid and submissive, offered no spontaneous conversation. She seemed to require that questions be asked of her in order "to get her going." A series of psychiatrists and other mental health professionals approached her in this way during the long period of her illness. They never discovered that, for years, she had been sexually abused by her father. A psychiatric nurse, however, established a different kind of relatedness with her, which eschewed the interrogative mode. Mrs. A. eventually admitted that she wanted her therapist to ask questions "because then you'll never get there."

A second system of avoidance guards against further damage to those aspects of selfhood that are sensed as most personal. They include, as both Sullivan and Bowlby pointed out, the "tender emotions," those feelings associated with intimacy. They are related to themes of thoughts, images, feelings, and memories that are given peculiar value and felt as the core of self. They are necessarily hidden in order to avoid harm. This leads to a dilemma. The individual has an overpowering need for attachment. Yet the ordinary means of developing an intimate relationship is denied him or her, since the risk involved in the exposure of what is secret is too great (Meares, 1976). A common outcome for a patient suffering from BPD is the development of nonintimate attachments (Meares & Anderson, 1993). The dilemma of many of those with BPD, who wish to be known but also fear it, is sometimes manifest in paradoxical behavior in which emotional incontinence is allied to expressions of rage following the experience of being known, when their hiddenness is breached.

Lord Byron and the Paranoid Stance

Paranoid ideas emerge when that which is precariously guarded as secret has been intruded upon. They are revealed in florid form when the traumatic memory system is reevoked and the attributes of self and other that are central to "malignant internalization" (Meares, 1999b) become overt. Those whose behavior precipitated the reemergence of traumatic memory are cast in the role of the original traumatizing other, liable to become the objects of violent abuse, usually verbal. This outcome is illustrated by an incident in the life of the great poet, Lord Byron (1788–1824).

Byron's early life was of the kind that induces "malevolent transformation" (Sullivan, 1953). His father, a profligate who may have killed himself, died when he was 3½. "I was not so young when my father died, but that I perfectly remember him; and had very early a horror of matrimony, from the sight of domestic broils. . . . He seemed born for his ruin" (Marchand, 1957, p. 32). His young widow was left impoverished, the mother of a crippled child. Byron's mother did not cope well with her situation. A domineering, unhappy woman, she blamed the child for his disability, even ridiculing him. His clubfoot became a source of shame and humiliation for Byron, making him feel an object of scorn. He said later that his mother's daily rages and explosions of verbal and physical abuse had "cankered a heart that I believe was naturally affectionate, and destroyed a temper always disposed to be violent" (MacCarthy, 2003, p. 7).

While at Cambridge, Byron feared vacations because of his "horror" of returning to his mother (Marchand, 1957, p. 106). His habitual demeanor also illustrated the paranoid stance characteristic of those who have been harmed and who expect to be harmed again.

At the ages of about 10 and 11, for a period of about two years, Byron was sexually abused by a nursemaid, to whose care his mother had entrusted him. This woman also "was perpetually beating him" (MacCarthy, 2003, pp. 22–23). The abuse was ended when Byron entreated the family solicitor, who had been friendly to him, to help him (MacCarthy, p. 23). Further abuse followed at the age of about 15 when he was almost certainly seduced by the young aristocratic tenant of Byron's Newstead property (MacCarthy, p. 36).

This story is similar to that of many who develop BPD. Indeed, as a small boy, the victim of his mother's rages, Byron seemed to be already a "borderline-child-to-be" (Pine, 1986). Stories were later told of his appalling misdemeanors, such as "wrecking the miller's wheel, striking Lady Abercromby in the face, getting out his little whip to chastise a kindly person sympathizing with his lameness," and, while in church with his mother, "entertaining himself at intervals by getting out a little pin and pricking her fat arms" (MacCarthy, 2003, p. 8).

Byron started at Harrow School when he was 13. He was particularly sensitive to insults, whether real or imagined (MacCarthy, 2003, p. 29), responding at times with rage. "He was a fighter and a terrorist, in perpetual motion of flailing arms and whamming fists" (p. 31). How is it that Byron emerged from this state? The headmaster, Joseph Drury, played an important part in the transformation that took place in the next few years. At their first meeting, he viewed the youth as "a wild mountain colt." His educational aim, Fiona MacCarthy tells us, was "to get inside the mind of the individual child" (p. 31). Unlike other schoolteachers of his time, Drury did not beat his charges. He found in Byron positive elements and promise, giving value to him. Byron wrote later that Dr. Drury "had a great notion that I should turn out an Orator from my fluency—my turbulence—my voice—my copiousness of declamation—and my action" (p. 44). This led to Byron's star appearances at school speech days.

Although Byron had, to a considerable extent, been rescued in terms of personality development through his school experience, the scars remained. At the age of 19, when his *Hours of Idleness* was published, the book received 17 reviews. Only one was negative. Byron massively overreacted, drinking three bottles of claret immediately after reading it and contemplating suicide (MacCarthy, 2003, p. 63). Enraged by this and other insults, which became magnified in his mind, Byron flung himself into the composition of a long and bitter satiric poem, entitled "English Bards and Scotch Reviewers," which, as MacCarthy says, was "bulging with animosities and prejudices" (p. 83). The tone was "one of unremitting ridicule, remarkable even in that remorseless age of personal vindictiveness" (p. 85). Byron's insults were scattered far and wide, not confined to the single reviewer. His targets included most of the revered writers of his time. Scott, Coleridge, and "vulgar Wordsworth" were objects of his scorn. He later regretted some of these attacks, particularly on Coleridge (p. 249). Byron's massive outpouring of invective, provoked by a single review, was presumably a consequence of the traumatic system created by his mother's verbal abuse and devaluing criticism.

As life went on, Byron developed various modes of defense against reactivation of this system. One of these was a posture suggesting that his poems did not mean much to him, that they were mere trifles that he could flick off with little effort. For example, he refused payment for "The Corsair," airily telling his publisher that "rhyming came so easily he deserved no remuneration" (p. 215). This posture is characteristic of the dilemma of both wanting and fearing to be known. Damage is avoided by the implication that such casual expressions are not the "real me" (Meares, 1976).

Byron knew what he was doing and he also knew, with remarkable insight, what was wrong with him. The dark and brooding hero of his poem "Lara" is essentially himself. The poem's narrator tells us that Lara's "madness was not of the head, but heart" (stanza XVIII). This is a beautifully succinct definition of the borderline condition. The narrator describes the course of Byron's own life:

> With more capacity for love than earth
> Bestows on most of mortal mould and birth
> His early dreams of good outstripp'd the truth
> And troubled mankind follow'd baffled youth (XVIII)

Lara is a portrait of the outcome of the "malevolent transformation." He lives as if among enemies, an alien:

> He stood a stranger in this breathing world,
> An erring spirit from another hurl'd;
> A thing of dark imaginings. . . . (XVIII)

And yet he plays the social part: "With them he would seem gay amidst the gay" (XVII). But those who observe him can detect the inauthentic smile, which

> waned in its mirth, and wither'd to a sneer;
> That smile might reach his lip, but pass'd not by,
> None e'er could trace its laughter to his eye (XVII)

Behind the mask of sociability Byron remained hidden, developing a "chilling mystery of mien" (XIX). He "rarely wander'd

in his speech, or drew his thoughts so forth to offend the view"
(XVIII). His silence was not evidence of a natural steeliness and
coldness, for

> there was softness too in his regard,
> At times a nature as not by nature hard (XVII)

Rather, it was to hide "his mind's disease" (XVI). The narrator
asks:

> did that silence prove his memory fix'd
> Too deep for words, indelible, unmix'd
> In that corroding secrecy which gnaws
> The heart to show the effect, but not the cause? (XVI)

Byron was an extraordinary man who knew the despair of the
borderline condition, as his poem "Darkness" suggests. It speaks
of a world void, dead, and silent. Despite this, he was able to live
an extremely productive, although tempestuous, life. He sensed
that poetry and imagination had saved him. He wrote, "Poetry is
the lava of the imagination whose eruption prevents an earth-
quake" (Marchand, 1957).

DELUSION FORMATION

Although there is a developing literature on the subject, there
is, as yet, no general view of the way in which delusions are
formed. The main proposals currently being put forward are discussed briefly later in the chapter.

A notable deficit in a number of recent investigations of delusion formation is the absence of any reference to clinical accounts
or to the subjective experience that might underpin paranoid
thinking. Although modern techniques of neuroimaging allow
us to explore psychiatric phenomena in a way that should eventually lead to a larger understanding of these phenomena, the
hypotheses that direct these explorations must begin with clini-

cal observation that is, as far as possible, free from preconception. The pioneers of psychodynamic thought, lacking the advantages of modern technology, necessarily based their formulations on what their patients told them. Freud, of course, was one of these pioneers. Freud's first essay on the paranoid process, in which he introduced the term *projection*, became the starting point of all subsequent theoretical explorations of the subject within the psychoanalytic tradition. It also foreshadows the present argument, since the most prominent feature of the case he presented suffered from a failure in "the act of secrecy," that is, a breach of hiddenness. The 32-year-old Frau P. had slowly grown more suspicious and distrustful, until "one afternoon she suddenly got the idea that people watched her undressing at night. From that time onwards she employed the most complicated precaution when undressing, slipping into the bed in the dark and undressing under the bedclothes" (Freud, 1896, p. 171).

The notion that certain forms of paranoid experience arise through a failure in "the act of secrecy," an idea first put forward by Janet (see Ellenberger, 1970, p. 390), was the basis for a proposal concerning the origin of paranoid delusions in BPD derived from clinical observation (Meares, 1988) and further elaborated here. It involves the notion of boundary. A fundamental aspect of the emergence of self is a growing sense of demarcation between one's own personal system and that of the world. The development of the distinction between me and not-me is presumably, at first, perceptual—that is, dependent upon sensory experience. Out of such experience develops the concept of one's separation from the world, while, at the same time, the world is inseparable from the subject. This separation is marked by the child's achieving the concept of "innerness" at about 4 years of age (Meares & Orlay, 1988). This is a momentous event in the child's life, heralding the birth of "self" as defined by Jackson and James.

Freud's Frau P., it seems, had lost the most basic experience of ordinary existing, the sense that one's own personal and private world is distinct and separable from the world of others. Put another way, she lost the boundary between self and other. In what follows, I suggest that this deficit is an essential element in delusion formation in BPD.

The formation of a self-boundary must involve systems that maintain a discrimination between external and internal models of the world. Knight et al. (1995) produced evidence suggesting that such discrimination is one aspect of attentional control, which depends upon prefrontal cortical activity (Knight et al., 1995). These observations suggest that when prefrontal cortical activity is diminished, so also will the inner–outer distinction fail. In those with BPD, whose prefrontal functioning can be upset in the interchanges with those in the social environment, it might be predicted that the boundary of self will also fail at times. This was the case for Mrs. A. When her illness was at its worst, she would believe that others could read her mind. At the same time, she perceived others' heads as shrouded in a kind of cowl. She was, then, in a state of dissociation in which personal disintegration was associated with loss of the inner distinction, a circumstance discussed in Chapter 8.

The notion that a sense of personal disintegration may be at the bottom of paranoid states was discovered intuitively by Winnicott. Acknowledging the background of Freud and Klein, he remarked that "there can be a deeper origin to paranoia, which may be associated with integration and the establishment of a unit self: I AM" (1963, p. 225). The emergence of the paranoid delusion out of such disintegration is illustrated through a reconsideration of the strange experience recounted by Rebecca West, some of which was retold earlier in this book.

In a dissociated state following a severe infection, she was afflicted by a sense of strangeness. One night, at the nursing home to which she had been taken, she had a vivid and ominous dream of events in the facility involving two uniformed and sinister men of terrifying appearance, who entered the building and abducted a person in a calico bag. She woke and remembered an incident in childhood, involving the death of an old lady. She was overcome by fear and thoughts of death and burst into "the exhausted weeping that follows prolonged pain, and lay crying till it was broad daylight" (West, 1971, p. 55).

The following day two men came to take away in a coffin someone who had died at the nursing home that night. Rebecca West, when she saw the men, "knew with absolute certainty that I was watching the incident of which my dream had been the fantastic rehearsal" (1971, p. 55). Although skeptical of such ideas, she could not shake the belief that supernatural forces were at work.

The power of this experience affected her afterward so that, as she said, she was more subject to terror than she had been before. Nevertheless, she realized that her belief was incorrect: "The special weakness that had made me liable to this revelation made me link it up with childish fears and clothe it in symbolism inspired by an infantile conception of death that I knew to be untrue" (West, 1971, p. 56).

This account of a transient delusional state provides experiential evidence from which a two-stage theory of delusion formation in BPD can be inferred. In the first stage, in which the inner–outer distinction is impaired, dreams and reality are not entirely separate. The failure of differentiation between zones of experiencing extends beyond the external and internal worlds. The past and present are also imperfectly distinguished, as exemplified in the case history in Chapter 8.

This peculiar state provides the background to the second stage of the delusion formation. The individual searches for a meaning that will give the experience coherence. The formulation of meaning is influenced by the prevailing and profound emotional tone, which is likely to be one of derealization, estrangement, and high arousal. As Jaspers (1997) put it: "Delusion draws its content from the world which it shapes" (p. 196).

The judgment of meaning is made on the basis of ineffective and faulty monitoring systems, which, once again, depend upon the prefrontal cortex. As a consequence, the judgment remains uncorrected.

The delusion formation is, to some extent, adaptive. The order produced by delusion formation allows sensory input to be accommodated and to take its place among the conceptual categories stored in memory, against which events in the outer world are matched. Once again, a "fit" is achieved with the sensory environment, and arousal decreases (Meares, 1977, pp. 52–54).

Reality is narrowed through the construction made of it by the delusional belief. The events and behavior of others, which make up this reality, are interpreted in terms of the delusion and provide evidence that seems to confirm it. Some of this evidence is objectively "correct" since the behavior of the subject provokes behaviors in others in relation to the subject's demeanor. Thus, a reverberating system is established that helps to maintain this delusion.

The delusion is also, in part, maintained by the powerful effect of the anxiety that underlies it. To give up the delusional belief is to face, once again, meaninglessness and high arousal. Nevertheless, for those suffering from BPD, the delusion is usually transient, although it may last for weeks. Some forms of delusion formation in BPD, however, are prolonged. A particular example is that form of incorrigible, incorrect belief once called *erotomania*, which may arise in a number of conditions, including personality disorder. It is manifest in the therapeutic situation as a form of erotic transference. Beth Kotze and I report on such a case that could be understood as a disturbance of the self-boundary concept brought about through particular developmental circumstances. The mother's nurturing behavior impeded her child's progress toward the experience and conception of "otherness" and self-boundary by usurping the role of transitional object, a role which she herself assumed (Kotze & Meares, 1996).

Current Theories of Delusion Formation

How do the foregoing ideas relate to other contemporary theories of delusion formation? Garety and Freeman (1999) have contributed a review of three current theories that provides a means of comparison. The theories include one formulated by Frith and colleagues (1992; "theory of mind" deficits); a second from Bentall and colleagues (1994; attributional style and self-discrepancies); and a third proposed by Garety and colleagues (1991; multifactorial but involving probabilistic reasoning bases). In a later publication (Freeman et al., 2000), Gerety's group rejected the Bentall formulation on the grounds that it is not supported by evidence (Freeman et al., 1998). In essence, Bentall and his coresearchers conceive persecutory delusions as a defense against thoughts of low self-esteem reaching consciousness. However, there seems to be no relationship between delusional intensity and levels of self-esteem. Nevertheless, the Bentall formulation, although not sufficient to explain delusion, seems resonant with a view of paranoid ideation based on traumatic devaluation.

The Garety proposals have a number of features that also resonate with the model put forward in this chapter. Importantly, they see the delusion being formed in an atmosphere of arousal that initiates inner–outer confusion (Fowler, 2000) in an individual vulnerable to such a state. Sensory overload may overpower the mechanisms regulating sensory input, so that inner reality barely exists. In the midst of new experience, the individual searches for meaning (Maher, 1988). Garety and her colleagues believe that the creation of delusional meaning involves a deficiency in evaluating, and making a response to, significant stimuli. They call such a response style "jumping to conclusions." Although they base their proposals on studies of patients suffering from schizophrenia and those at risk for schizophrenia, such a deficit may also be present in BPD, as suggested by two kinds of evidence, one concerning evaluation of facial expression and the other, ERP data.

The possibility that borderline patients "jump to conclusions" when viewing faces is suggested by the fact that they make judgments about the affective meaning of facial expressions more quickly than controls do. For example, Lynch et al. (2006) compared 20 patients with BPD with 20 controls in their ability to detect emotional expression when pictures of facial expression morphed from neutral to maximum. Those with BPD made correct identifications faster than controls, regardless of the valence of the emotion expressed. Moreover, those with BPD were as accurate as the controls.

Other studies, however, find that patients with BPD tend to see fear or anger in neutral expressions, consistent with previous reports of a negative bias in interpreting facial expression (Bland et al., 2004; Levine et al., 1997). Judgments, then, are influenced by the prevailing mental state.

The possibility that patients with BPD may respond to stimuli more rapidly than controls is supported by studies of ERPs, evoked using the oddball paradigm, in which the subject is required to respond to a tone that is uncommon and different from a background series of tones. The latency for the onset of P3a is shorter in patients with BPD than it is for controls (see Chapter 5).

THEORY OF MIND AND DELUSION FORMATION

The differences between the details of the formulation of Garety and Freeman from my own are, in the main, not contradictions. They largely relate to differences in clinical focus, theirs being schizophrenia. The proposals of Frith can be seen as complementary to those of Garety, Freeman, and their colleagues. They are also broadly consistent with my proposal, although this concordance depends upon what is meant by a *theory of mind*. It is therefore necessary to consider this subject briefly.

The term *theory of mind* was introduced by Premack and Woodruff (1978), who were studying chimpanzees. They concluded that these animals have the capacity to make inferences regarding the mental states of others, a capacity they called a *theory of mind*. This term is now widely used. It is also generally agreed that the capacity first appears in human life at about 4 years of age (Baron-Cohen, 2001). This popular conception involves two main oversimplifications. First, it implies that so-called mind reading does not occur before the age of about 4, which is untrue. The infant is able to tell what mother thinks–feels well before this, and able to discern meaning in very slight changes of facial expression. Second, the developmental change that occurs at about 4 years of age is complex and not limited to mind reading.

The human experiments upon which the concept of theory of mind was based concerned "false belief" (Wimmer & Perner, 1983). For example, a child is asked to watch a playlet. A little girl comes into a room with a box of chocolates. She places them in a drawer in a desk, then leaves the room. A wicked witch enters. She discovers the chocolates and hides them in a wardrobe. She leaves, and the little girl comes back. The child who is watching is then asked where the little girl will look for her chocolates. A child of 3 typically chooses the wardrobe, whereas children of 4 and 5 usually say the desk. They understand that the little girl will be acting on the basis of a "false belief." Later theorists call this realization a theory of mind.

The 4-year-old's grasp of the false-belief situation can be understood in at least two related ways apart from mind reading. First, it reflects the child's ability to hold in mind, at the same time, two models of reality, one's own and that of the other. The 3-year-old, using Winnicott's term, has a single reality that is "personal."

A second explanation concerns the notion of psychic privacy that emerges at about the age of 4. It is indicated by the child of this age understanding the concept of secrecy (Meares & Orlay, 1988) and also by having access to remote episodic or autobiographical memory (Nelson, 1992; Perner & Ruffman, 1995). An outcome of the emergence of this kind of memory is the knowledge that one has a world of personal and private experience that is sensed as inner and that is not the same as public reality. The child of 4 or 5, watching the experimental playlet, knows that what he or she knows is different from what the little girl knows.

The sense that one has a world of private experience, which is unique and one's own, brings with it the realization that others also possess such an experience that differs from one's own. This realization leads to the capacity for empathy. Empathy requires imagination because it depends on the ability to conceive a reality that is not one's own. Its emergence is demonstrated by a little experiment reported by Flavell (1968), which compares gift giving in young children compared with older children. For example, a little boy of 3, asked to choose a present for his mother from among a bundle of objects, selects a toy truck. Another boy of 5 or 6 chooses something he feels she would like, which is not what he himself would prefer (Flavell, 1968).

Mind reading is not equivalent to empathy. Forms of the former appear developmentally before the latter. They depend upon an understanding of facial expression and gesture. The activity of mirror neurons has been suggested as an explanation of this kind of mind reading (Gallese & Goldman, 1998). Such an explanation is plausible for sympathy, but not for empathy, which is a more complex behavior requiring capacities additional to those supplied by mirror neurons.

The term *theory of mind* is, in my view, an unsatisfactory one since it bundles together a wide range of capacities that reflect the activities of different, although presumably related, systems of neurocircuitry. Following the initial false-belief experiments, a plethora of theory-of-mind tests have been devised, not only for "first-order" and "second-order" false belief, but also for various other measures, including the detection of sarcasm, faux pas, and deception. Using several of these measures, Frith and his co-workers found that the medial prefrontal cortex activation was common to them (Gallagher et al., 2000). Shamay-Tsoory and Aharon-Peretz (2007), in a study of patients with localized brain lesions that included an extensive review of neuroimaging studies, found that affective theory-of-mind competence is associated with ventromedial cortical function.

The evidence in favor of Frith's theory-of-mind hypothesis concerning the basis of delusion (Corcoran et al., 1995; Frith, 1992) is equivocal. Although this group of researchers found that paranoid patients and those experiencing passivity feelings performed more poorly than normal controls on theory-of-mind tests, so also did depressed/anxious control patients (Corcoran et al., 1997). Other investigators did not find a specific theory-of-mind deficit in paranoid patients (Langdon et al., 1997; Sarfati et al., 1997).

If theory of mind is taken to mean a restricted set of capabilities, first manifest at about the age of 4, the proposal of Frith is consistent with mine, and with Garety and Freeman. These capabilities presumably reflect a stage in the maturation of prefrontal and related circuitry that allows the emergence of introspection, and with it, an enhanced conception of the inner–outer distinction, empathy, and increased efficiency of evaluative and monitoring systems.

SUMMARY

As far as I am aware, there is no extended consideration of delusion formation in borderline personality disorder available in the literature. Perhaps unsurprisingly, the proposal put forward here has much in common with those derived from investigations of schizophrenia.

In this chapter, a distinction is made between paranoid ideas and delusion formation. Paranoid ideas are conceived as the manifestation of a reactivation of the traumatic memory system, which involves "malignant internalization" (Meares, 1999b). Certain figures in the social environment are experienced as the original traumatizer. Paranoid ideation is accompanied by a paranoid stance that is determined by the expectation of the damaged individual that he or she will be harmed once again. The stance is part of strategy designed to protect against intrusion into, and possible damage to, areas of psychic life that are highly valued and sensed as intensely personal.

Delusion formation involves somewhat different mechanisms. It is most likely to arise in states of enfeeblement of the self system due to relative inactivity of those prefrontal systems that are also necessary to sensory input regulation. The individual is now vulnerable to states of high arousal in which the inner–outer distinction is impaired or lost. The privacy of self is breached or, in another language, the theory of mind is lost, when this term is understood in terms of the inner–outer distinction.

The high arousal is likely to be associated with a feeling of estrangement analogous to dissociation. The feeling may be frightening. The delusion is organized around the subject's immediate experience in relation to the meaning given to it. For example, the delusion may arise from a disturbance of the inner–outer distinction so that the subject may conclude that his or her thoughts are being read. The meaning attributed to the feeling of estrangement and its accompaniments is likely to lower arousal through its effect in creating coherence. This meaning is unchallenged by an effective monitoring system because the prefrontal mechanisms involved in this process are hypoactive. In essence, the mechanisms underlying paranoid delusions in BPD may have much in common with those associated with dissociation, as implied by the linkage of the two phenomena of dissociation and paranoid ideation in DSM-IV's ninth criterion for the diagnosis of BPD (American Psychiatric Association, 1994).

Chapter 15

IS BPD A PARTICULARLY RIGHT-HEMISPHERIC DISORDER?

IT IS SOMETHING OF an abstraction to speak of the functions of the cerebral hemispheres in dichotomized terms, since, in usual circumstances, they are always coordinated, working together, with one hemisphere often dominant. For example, although speech is commonly held to be a left-hemisphere function, both hemispheres are involved. Jackson suggested "the left to the leading side, and the right the involuntary or automatic" (Jackson, 1958, II p. 221). He also noted that patients rendered speechless by a left-sided stroke may sing (Jackson, 1958, I p. 73). The observations of Roger Sperry (1966) on "split-brain" patients made clear that different functions were subserved by the isolated hemispheres. Even in this setting, absolute distinctions cannot be made. For example, it is usually found that the language function of the left hemisphere includes not only speaking but also reading and writing. But this is not always so. Kathleen Baynes and her colleagues (1998), for example, reported the case of a woman with left-hemisphere dominance for spoken language who, after resection of the corpus callosum, demonstrated a dissociation between spoken and written language, in which her capacity to write depended on the right hemisphere.

With these reservations in mind, a consideration is given, in this chapter, to the possibility that BPD is a particularly right hemispheric disorder and that this deficiency is the origin of the essential disconnectedness of brain–mind function in BPD.

SYNTHETIC FUNCTION OF THE RIGHT HEMISPHERE

Despite such unusual findings as those found by Baynes et al. (1998), generalization can be made, at least in the case of right-handed people. The left hemisphere is believed to be concerned with succession, the way in which one thing follows another. It is related to the unfolding of patterns over time, as in the structure of syntax. Such patterns may have their evolutionary origins in the complex sequences of muscle activity necessary to learned movements (Calvin, 2004). Whereas the left hemisphere is designated "sequential," the right hemisphere is designated "simultaneous," involved in the processing of patterns of immediate perception that appear all at once. The right hemisphere, then, is seen as having visuospatial capacities.

Elkhonon Goldberg (2005) considers that a principal difference between the two hemispheres is the capacity to find a solution to a previously unencountered problem or situation. The right hemisphere underpins creativity. He explains the functional characteristics of each hemisphere in terms of subtle differences in their wiring that have major consequences.

The first difference is in the way the cortical regions are connected in the two hemispheres. In the left hemisphere the connections tend to be local whereas the right-hemisphere connections involve distant regions. Such distant connections by means of white tracts that link widely dispersed and different brain domains are associated with creativity (Takeuchi et al., 2010). Another way in which connectivity is achieved in the right hemisphere, Goldberg points out (p. 187), is through spindle cells that are far more prevalent in the right hemisphere than the left. Spindle cells relay information between distant brain regions.

Goldberg goes on to describe the second main difference in the wiring of the hemispheres. This difference

> . . . relates to the way in which the overall hemispheric surface is allocated to different types of cortex. In the right hemisphere it seems to favor the *heteromodal association cortex;* but in the left hemisphere it seems to favor the *modality-specific association cortex.* Both types of cortex are engaged in complex information processing, but in different ways. The modality-specific cortex is restricted to processing information arriving via a particular sensory system, visual, auditory, or tactile, and separate areas exist in the cortex for each of these sensory systems. Modality-specific cortex dismantles the world around us into separate representations. By way of analogy, think of an object in a three-dimensional space projected onto the *x, y,* and *z* coordinates, which generate three partial representations: This is what the modality-specific association cortex does with the incoming information. By contrast, the heteromodal association cortex is in charge of integrating the information arriving via different sensory channels, for putting the synthetic picture of the multimedia world around us back together. (Goldberg, 2005, p. 196, italics in original)

This formulation sees the left hemisphere as analytic, focused on the details, whereas the right hemisphere has a synthetic function enabling us to create coherence out of the mass of sensory data impinging upon us at any moment. Since the main hypothesis concerning the core deficit in BPD proposed in this book is that the manifestations of the disorder reflect a failure of "personal synthesis," it might be supposed that the basic neural fault in BPD is a deficit in right-hemisphere function. A test of this hypothesis is reported in the next section and the implications of such a deficit are discussed.

Lateralization of Enhanced P3a Amplitudes

The hypothesis of a right-hemisphere dysfunction or deficit in BPD was tested using the notion that enlarged P3a, as suggested in Chapters 4 and 5, is a marker of the central disturbance of BPD. This hypothesis predicts that P3a will be more greatly enlarged on the right side of the brain than the left. Seventeen patients with BPD were compared with 17 age- and sex-matched controls. They were the same as those who participated in the investigation described in Chapter 5. The full report of the study appears in Meares, Schore, & Melkonian (2011).

The data from the previous study were reanalyzed in order to consider the issue of lateralization. We measured lateralization of brain potentials by comparing the potentials at homologous electrodes (e.g., locations F3 and F4) over both hemispheres. The interhemispheric relationships were estimated using the pairs of quantities (AL, AR), where AL and AR denote P3a peak amplitudes at the right- and left-homologous electrodes, respectively. The difference between the peak amplitudes, $\Delta A = AR - AL$, was taken as a measure of lateralization.

A comparison of P3a over homologous electrode sites in the patients with BPD showed that the amplitudes of P3a are significantly greater on the right side. The differences are displayed in Figure 15.1.

A similar comparison was made in the control patients. The amplitudes of P3a at homologous recording sites showed no significant differences. A third comparison, between patients with BPD and control subjects, was made at homologous frontal and middle recording sites. Table 15.1 shows the differences. There is no significant difference between amplitudes of P3a for the left-hemispheric comparisons. However, the differences between the groups were highly significant for the right-hemispheric comparisons.

These findings are consistent with the possibility that the neu-

TABLE 15.1

Recording Site	BPD patients (N = 17)			Normal subjects (N = 17)			Analysis[a]	
	N_S	Mean (μV)	SD	N_S	Mean (μV)	SD	Z	p
Left hemisphere, F7	463	7.0	5.1	443	7.5	3.7	1.89	ns[b]
Left hemisphere, F3	446	13.4	8.0	363	12.1	6.0	1.88	ns[b]
Middle site, Fz	427	14.8	9.3	328	12.6	6.4	3.88	0.001
Right hemisphere, F4	457	14.2	8.4	377	11.9	5.4	4.85	0.001
Right hemisphere, F8	440	8.4	5.8	429	7.3	3.3	3.28	0.002

rophysiological disorder underlying the manifestations of BPD is particularly right-hemispheric. The findings are also suggestive of a dissociative core in BPD because they have been replicated in patients with PTSD who dissociate (Meares, Melkonian, Felmingham et al., 2011). They are not replicated in another disorder characterized by a particular kind of disintegration of mental life, namely, schizophrenia. (Data in preparation for publication concerning comparison between borderline states and first-episode psychosis.)

Deficient Inhibitory Control and the Right Hemisphere

The enlarged P3a is considered to reflect a failure of inhibitory activity associated with prefrontally connected neurocircuitry. A certain amount of evidence indicates that the right hemisphere is particularly implicated in inhibitory control (Garavan et al., 1999). Failure of inhibition in a social context is significantly related to brain lesions leading to "dysfunction of orbitofrontal and basotemporal cortices of the right hemisphere" (Starkstein &

Robinson, 1997, p. 108). In a group of 28 patients with BPD, 10 of whom also met criteria for antisocial personality disorder, those with a history of aggression had significantly more right-sided neurological soft signs than those without a history of aggression (Stein et al., 1993). Tranel et al. (2002) found profound disturbance in the modulation of social and interpersonal behavior of four people who had right ventromedial cortical lesions, whereas another three who had similar left-sided lesions had normal social and interpersonal behaviour. The right-sided subjects also had profound abnormalities of emotional processing and decision making. Several authorities have seen disturbance of OFC function as a principal deficit underlying the manifestations of BPD (e.g., Blair, 2004; Berlin et al., 2005). The possibility that this is part of a right-hemispheric basis to BPD is consistent with the findings of Ruocco (2005), who concludes a meta-analysis of neuropsychological observations in BPD with: "The findings suggest a fronto-temporal dysfunction lateralized to the right hemisphere" (p. 197). He also remarks that the findings "provide support for the Jacksonian bio-psychosocial model of BPD (Meares et al., 1999)" (p. 197).

Disturbances of interpersonal behavior, however, cannot be conceived simply in terms of inhibitory control. They must be seen as the outcome of a number of factors acting in concert. These factors include empathy, a main aspect of a theory of mind. Stuss et al. (2001) found that this capacity appears to depend particularly upon right-sided neurocircuitry. Beyond the capacity for empathy, however, is a vast array of right-hemisphere-dependent skills that are necessary to relating satisfactorily with others. These skills and their cortical underpinnnings are reviewed by Schutz (2005), who focuses on the inability of people with a particular form of right-hemispheric damage to create a new pattern of behavioral response such that old patterns are repeated.

Inhibitory Control and "Painful Incoherence"

It has been suggested by a number of authorities that the dysphoria that is a main feature of BPD is a reflection of the person's inability to use the ordinary mechanism of controlling, or modifying, the intensity of unpleasant or distressing affect (see Chapter 11). It might be expected, then, that the experience of negative affect would be particularly associated with right-hemispheric dysfunction.

One observation suggesting that this might be so is the phenomenon of an *asomatognosia*, in which an individual who has had damage (e.g., a stroke) to the right hemisphere fails to recognize, and seems to deny the existence of, the left side of the body, including paralysis of the left arm. The patient is undistressed by this profound disability, even claiming that the arm is functional or that it belongs to someone else (Feinberg, 2001). On the other hand, people with similar damage in the left hemisphere do not deny their paralysis and show an appropriate emotional response to it. The odd behavior of the right-hemispheric patient has been explained in terms of the spatial functions of the right hemisphere. De Renzi (1982), for example, has suggested that the phenomenon is a reflection of the right hemisphere's involvement in the construction of central representations of space.

The apparently cheerful demeanor of the asomatognosic patient cannot be directly explained in this way. Some observers have suggested that the patient's absence of distress might indicate that the right hemisphere is, in some way, the basis of negative affect. Richard Davidson and his colleagues (2004) have demonstrated that negative affect, "particularly those forms of negative affect that involve heightened vigilance toward threat related cues in the environment, are preferentially represented in specific right-sided lateral prefrontal territories" (p. 390). The right-frontal hyperactivity related to negative mood state identified in Davidson's work (2003) appears to be replicated in our finding for P3a. The large amplitude indicative of diminished inhibitory activity reflects, as a consequence, overexcitation. Since P3a is a main component of the orienting system, it also reflects hypervigilance, a feature of trauma-associated disorders.

Our findings do not allow us to infer the precise physiology of the failure of inhibitory control that may be related to the dysphoria of BPD, but findings such as those of Tranel et al. (2002) suggest that deficient function of the right OFC may be implicated. A report from van Reekum et al. (2007) also implicates the ventral anterior cingulate cortex (BA24). These researchers found that higher psychological well-being was highly associated with increased activation in this area. It would be predicted, then, that low activation would be associated dysphoria. Diminished activation in BA24 has also been linked to treatment-resistant depression (Mayberg, 2007). In contrast, control of pain by placebo is associated with increased activity in BA 24 (Petrovic, 2005).

A search for the origins of well-being and its opposite state of dysphoria is complicated by the fact that neither well-being nor dysphoria is a single state but exist as a variety of emotional states that have subtle differences. The complexity of the subject is illustrated by Davidson's work on well-being, which focuses on the approach–withdrawal dimension. Approach-related positive affect that involves the implementation of appetitive goals is preferentially represented in specific left-sided dorsolateral prefrontal territories (Davidson, 2004; Pizzagalli et al., 2005). It is not known, as far as I am aware, whether a different physiology is found in the performance of autotelic behaviors, such as play in which there is no appetitive or other apparent purpose, the behavior seemingly having its own purpose. The hypothesis is suggested that the well-being associated with such behaviors might depend upon the right-side of the brain. Panksepp and

Trevarthen (2009) point out that well-being is associated with two forms of regulation, one of which is externally directed and subserved by the left brain, whereas the other, which can be conceived as more inner-directed, is a right-brain activity. Music appreciation is an example.

Activation of inhibitory mechanisms, however, cannot be considered the only factor involved in well-being. For example, Barbara Fredrickson's (Fredrickson & Branigan, 2005) experiments show that those in a state of well-being tend to perceive the environment holistically, whereas those in a negative mood state see the environment in a more fragmented way, according to its details. These experiments suggest a reciprocal relationship between coherence and well-being, in which one creates the other.

Inhibitory control is also related to coherence. The observations noted earlier in this book (Chapter 5) indicate that coherence, or coordination among brain areas, is related to enhanced inhibitory activity. This relationship is paralleled in the clinical situation by an association between a reduction in the sense of personal fragmentation and improved emotional and behavioral control.

Finally, the notion that the experience of coherence might influence the quality of inhibitory control has therapeutic implications. For example, it implies that inhibitory control in individuals who have not suffered actual brain damage, such as those suffering from BPD, is an aspect of a dynamic system in which the degree of inhibitory activation is not immutable but a variable condition. That this condition can be influenced by interpersonal factors is suggested by an interesting study from Richard Davidson's lab. Neural responses to threat (an electric shock) were found to be attenuated in women when they were holding their husband's hand. This effect was greater than hand-holding with a stranger and when the quality of the marital relationship was good (Coan et al., 2006).

SELF AND THE RIGHT BRAIN

The main theme of this book is woven around the idea that the symptoms of BPD are manifestations of a failure in the development of self. The data put forward in this chapter suggest, by inference, that the fundamental experience of self is a right-hemispheric affair and that, when right-hemispheric function is diminished, so also are those features associated with the over-arching concept of self, including inhibitory control and a background state of well-being. Both are impaired in BPD and both, on the basis of the evidence currently available, appear to be associated with deficient right-hemispheric function.

The possibility that a normally functioning right hemisphere is the basis of selfhood and that its loss is associated with a severe disturbance of self is supported by two case reports. The first of these is particularly remarkable. It came from the great neuropsychologist, Alexander Luria. He described, in lucid and moving terms, the case of a young soldier who suffered a severe brain injury in World War II, when a bullet penetrated his left parietal–occipital area. The frontal areas were spared. As a consequence of the injury he lost the normal use of speech; syntactical patterns were unfathomable to him. Although he could barely speak, he could write as part of automatic right-hemisphere function. However, he had a profound amnesia and could neither read nor remember what he had written. Despite his terrible disabilities, he strove, almost superhumanly, day after day, to overcome them, particularly by writing. It was an immense struggle to write one page a day, yet he wrote thousands and was "able to present a vivid account of his past." Above all, he retained his self. "He still had a powerful imagination, a marked capacity for fantasy and empathy" (Luria, 1972, p. 155).

This story is consistent with the view that what we call *self* is particularly dependent upon right-hemisphere function. Another account of a situation in which the experience and function of self was retained when the right hemisphere was intact but the left hemisphere was removed is described by Fournier et al. (2008). They compared two people who had received hemispherectomies for the treatment of severe epilepsy. One ablation was on the right, the other on the left. The person whose right hemisphere had been removed was severely disabled in social and interpersonal terms, showing disturbances in emotional recognition and the formation of social inferences. He showed a deficiency in mentalizing, as demonstrated by theory-of-mind tests. On the other hand, the man whose right hemisphere remained was highly skilled interpersonally, despite his problems with language.

The possibility that the generation of self is particularly right-sided is also supported by studies of autobiographical memory, which is a principal marker of the appearance of self. Retrieval of this kind of memory depends upon right prefrontal cortical regions. The left prefrontal cortical regions are more involved in retrieval of information from semantic memory (Tulving et al., 1994). This distinction between a memory for personal events, as they were experienced, and for facts, which contribute to communal knowledge, mirrors the distinction between the two zones of human experience: the private, personal world and the public domain. The right side of the brain seems to be more involved than the left in the creation of "inner," emotionally laden experience.

Predictably, right-sided lesions of the brain impair autobiographical memory more than lesions on the left (Kopelman et al., 1999). The default mode network, which overlaps the network for autobiographical memory (Spreng et al., 2009), shows more disturbances by trauma on the right side than on the left. Bluhm, Williamson, Osuch and their colleagues (2009) studied patients with chronic PTSD related to early life trauma. Their brains showed less connectivity than controls between the posterior cingulate gyrus and right amygdala, right hippocampus, and right insula. These disconnections were understood as reflections of altered connectivity in the default mode network, that system of cortical midline structures believed to underpin "introspective" mental activity (Fair et al., 2008)—that is, the self. Bluhm and her colleagues remark that their findings are resonant with Schore's proposal that early life trauma interferes with the development of the right brain (Schore, 2002).

TRAUMA AND THE RIGHT BRAIN

A main hypothesis developed in this book is that relational traumata, probably allied with certain genetic vulnerabilities, cause a disruption in the development of the neural network underpinning the experience of self, thus leading to the emergence of the symptom profile of BPD. Observations in the previous sections suggest that the disruption is likely to involve the right hemisphere and to result in negative affect and impaired inhibitory control. Findings from Justine Gatt and colleagues (2010), working with Lea Williams's group, suggest the main elements of this hypothesis. Their subjects included 363 volunteers who completed the 19-item Life Stress Questionnaire (ELS) and a self-report measure of "negativity bias." They also measured emotion-elicited heart rate and recorded the EEG. Trauma, as indicated by ELS scores, predicted negativity bias, which is related to negative mood states. Trauma, in combination with genetic factors, predicted right-sided frontal hyperactivation and right parietal hypoactivation.

This profile is in accord with observations from Richard Davidson's group (Davidson et al., 1999) that not only found right frontal hyperactivation in people scoring high on depression scales but also right parietal hypoactivation (Henriques & Davidson, 1997). This latter state was associated with selective impairment in a spatial, compared with a verbal, task, suggesting a deficiency of right-hemispheric function. Gatt and her colleagues (2010) also demonstrated an effect of trauma on heart rate that could be interpreted as indicative of diminished inhibitory control. High ELS scores predicted high emotion-elicited heart rate. The right frontal hyperactivation in these studies is in accord with our findings of large right-sided P3a in individuals with BPD, which reflects excitation consequent upon inhibitory failure.

Davidson and his colleagues have recently provided further evidence of the effect of early traumata on the development of the right brain. They studied 31 children who had suffered confirmed physical abuse. The data concerned structural changes shown by MRI. One of the largest differences between abused and control children was in the right OFC: The abused children showed reduced volumes in this region. Large reductions were also found in the dorsolateral prefrontal cortices, with smaller changes in the right temporal, right frontal, and bilateral parietal lobes (Hanson et al., 2010).

Finally, since the proposal that drives this book is that the core of BPD is dissociative, it might be expected that those who dissociate will exhibit right-hemisphere dysfunction. This appears to be the case. Spitzer et al. (2004), for example, found that subjects with a Dissociative Experience Scale (DES) score of over 30 showed right-hemispheric dysfunction in response to transcranial magnetic stimulation, relative to left-hemipheric function, that was greater than those scoring below 30. Their results suggested "a lack of integration in the right hemisphere" in those who dissociate.

Enriquez and Bernabeu (2008) presented high and low dissociators from an undergraduate population with target words and target emotional tones. The target words produced no differences in responding between the two groups, with words being processed left hemispherically. However, the participants performed differently in response to the emotional tones that involve right-hemisphere function. The low dissociators were superior to the high dissociators. The processing of tone is a right-hemispheric function.

Helton et al. (2011) produced further data supportive of the proposal that dissociation is a reflection of right-hemispheric dysfunction. Their subjects performed a vigilance task under two conditions, one emotional and the other neutral. Dissociative subjects were less vigilant than nondissociators only in the emotional condition. Since emotion processing is particularly right-hemispheric, it was inferred that the experience of dissociation is related to right-hemispheric dysfunction.

Chapter 16

TOWARD COHESION
Analogical Relatedness

THE AIM OF THIS BOOK has been to develop an understanding of BPD based on evidence currently available to us, which gives us a logical basis for treatment. The pieces of evidence brought together in the foregoing chapters suggest that the central disturbance of BPD is disconnectedness among the elements of neural function necessary to higher-order consciousness, or self. The outcome is a state of mind in which there is a failure in the integration of consciousness, a disconnectedness that fluctuates in degree from mild and barely perceptible to severe and florid, manifest in sharp and shifting changes in mood, relatedness, and behavior. These vicissitudes are usually the result of different forms of encounters that occur in the individual's daily life. The condition, then, cannot be understood simply in terms of a single individual, as an isolated entity, but as an aspect of the function of a larger organism that includes the social world. It is in the sphere of interpersonal relations that much of the DSM syndrome of BPD is defined.

The disconnectedness among the neural systems underpinning self is reflected not only in psychic life but in the totality of self, including the body. Those who suffer from BPD have, for example, unusual experiences of pain and show disturbances of autonomic function.

A particularly important aspect of the general disconnectedness of the body–self–other dynamism of BPD is the effect of unconscious traumatic memories, which operate as systems largely split off from everyday consciousness, as forms of psychic life sensed as alien and having a quality Charcot likened to the parasitic. These intrusions into the fragile zone of self distort, break up, or even overthrow this peculiarly human form of experience, which has appeared only very recently in evolutionary history. It is easily lost, and not inevitably gained, during a human lifetime.

A major aspect of the therapy of individuals with BPD is the recognition of the intrusion of these systems into the therapeutic conversation and into the conduct of the patient's everyday life, followed by work toward their transformation, of a kind that will allow their integration into the larger consciousness of self. Most of the better known therapies for BPD have a main focus on these systems that are the basis of negative self and other attributes, and of maladaptive forms of relating and behaving. Each therapy has its own theory and language, in which the words *trauma* and *dissociation* may or may not be prominent. Nevertheless, in different ways, the focus and therapeutic objective are shared. It is particularly well developed in Linehan's dialectical behavior therapy (DBT) model (Linehan, 1993). This is not the place to make comparisons between these various approaches, nor is it appropriate to detail our own approach, since that description is the purpose of a parallel volume (Meares et al., 2012). It is, however, important to remark that although the therapy must aim to change the maladaptive "script" of the traumatic memory system, the principal objective must be integration. This integration will depend, in my view, on a transformation of the thought processes implicit in traumatic consciousness, which is asymbolic. Assimilation into the different consciousness of self, which involves a coordination of two thought forms, literal (logical) and symbolic (analogical), depends upon a transformation of traumatic material in which the symbolic mode emerges. This assimilation, however, can take place only if self is established. Attempting to work on traumatic memory in a relational context in which higher-order consciousness is not operative is likely to be ineffective or worse.

THE BASIS OF THE CONVERSATIONAL MODEL

The paramount objective in working with BPD, according to the thesis developed in this book, must be to establish the self system, which, following the neo-Jacksonian theory outlined in earlier chapters, arises through cohesion. This cohesion has its basis in a brain state. The brain, however, is an abstraction when considered as an isolated entity. There is no such thing as a "brain" in functional terms. A brain is always in interplay with the environment of which, in the case of BPD, the social environment is the most important part. It is this interplay that produces particular forms of brain activity from which spring different kinds of mental life. The kind of mental life, which, following Jackson and James, I am calling *self*, arises in the context of a specific way of relating. This relationship, like every other, is conducted by means of conversation. The evolution of self, then, depends upon the co-creation of a specific form of conversation designed to foster a sense of cohesion, or coherence, in the ongoing experience of those living with BPD, whose central disorder, it is argued, is "painful incoherence." The notion that the relationship itself is therapeutic is given support by a recent study led by Brin Grenyer. He and his colleagues show, for the first time, that a specific form of conversation, involving a particular linguistic interplay, effects structural personality change (McCarthy, Mergenthaler, Schneider, & Grenyer, 2011). This idea is the basis of the Conversational Model (CM), which the parallel volume (i.e., Meares et al., in press) introduces. The therapy of BPD, seen in this way, is primarily relational in nature.

How Does Reflective Awareness Arise?

Self is identified, both Jackson and James agree, by the capacity for introspection. How is this capacity related to cohesion?

The emergence of reflective awareness of inner events at about 4 years of age is sometimes spoken of as if a mental searchlight has somehow been turned on, lighting up previously inaccessible areas of mental life. This conception implies that a capacity has appeared in primate evolution as a new mental system, apparently unrelated to previous developments. Nothing new, however, has been added to the human's basic primate brain. Instead, the elaboration of previously existing structures, notably the prefrontal cortex, allows greater coordination to occur between areas of brain activity, which results in a larger access of conscious mental life to areas not previously open to consciousness. Coordination of a neural kind has the consequence of coordination, or connectedness, between the elements of psychic life. This amplification of consciousness, in which, as it were, the individual can travel around to places in the past and in imagination via the "mind's eye," is the basis of the reflective capacity. Understood in this way, the introspective capacity arises out of mental cohesion and is lost or gained, depending on a relative sense of personal unity.

Another question might now be asked. If lack of cohesion is the fundamental disturbance of BPD, how is it manifest in someone like Adele, whose personal story was touched upon in Chapter 1? Although she struggled to find words, what she said made sense and was not, in the ordinary sense, incoherent. In order to answer this question we return to the hierarchical neo-Jacksonian concept of self. When coordination between systems of neural activity is diminished, there is then a reduced "spatiality" of consciousness. Consciousness is constricted rather than amplified. Adele lives in a psychic zone that is restricted relative to those who do not suffer from BPD. The past tends to be very recent, and the future is also limited. Janet, when talking about those states in which "personal synthesis" is impaired, often spoke of "constriction" or "restriction." In the case of Adele, diminished cohesion of psychic life was most evident, at least in our first meeting, in its aspect of constriction.

The constricted consciousness of those with BPD might be compared with the characteristics of child thought in which, as Piaget has pointed out, cohesion of psychic life is ill developed relative to the adult. Successive elements of thought, as manifest in language, do not properly connect and might involve unrecognized contradictions. Caregivers, however, do not notice the diminished cohesion relative to adult thought. They are more likely to be aware that past and future are barely developed and that to ask what will happen next week is a stupid question.

A MATURATIONAL THERAPEUTIC APPROACH

Grinker and his colleagues (1968) considered that the disturbances of BPD are a consequence of stunted or arrested development of a particular kind. A hypothesis concerning maturational failure of self as the basis of BPD is supported by the findings concerning P3a in BPD reported in Chapter 5. A significant component, however, of BPD symptomatology can be understood in terms of the effect of the continuing influence, both conscious and unconscious, of traumatic impacts on the individual's prevailing personal experience. There are, then, two main etiological factors to consider in constructing a suitable therapeutic approach to BPD. They are clearly related, since the repetitive impacts of traumatic memory impede maturation. Nevertheless, the primary therapeutic concern, as intimated earlier in this chapter, must be to foster the emergence of the self system.

The principles that guide such a therapeutic approach are derived from developmental observations. Despite the complexities added to the mental state of people with BPD by a pathogenic environment, the way in which the emergence of self is fostered remains the same.

The progress of maturation depends upon integration. Multiple studies of infant development show that the child's perceptual world is as if made of pieces. These pieces are integrated into progressively larger wholes. This process involves both biogenesis— the unfolding of phylogenetically given patterns—and "sociogenesis"—the provision of the requisite social environment (Vygotsky & Luria, 1994). For the higher psychological functions (i.e., self) the sociogenetic component is crucial. What, then, is the nature of the interplay between child and caregivers that is necessary to foster integration and that would serve as a model for the therapeutic situation? An answer is suggested by Vygotsky.

Vygotsky borrowed an idea from Janet and James Mark Baldwin that he stated in the following way: "The child's higher psychological functions, his higher attributes which are specific to humans, originally manifest themselves as forms of the child's collective behaviour, as a form of co-operation with other people, and it is only afterwards that they become the individual functions of the child himself" (Vygotsky, 1935, p. 353). This principle implies that the sense of personal coherence, of connectedness among the elements of psychic life, was first experienced as a feeling of connection between the child and the caregivers. It implies, furthermore, that the form of relatedness mirrors, and is part of, a state of mind. A remarkable study from Kasia Kozlowska and her colleagues (2011) illustrates this idea. In a study of conversion disorders in children, in which these disorders were categorized in a way that was broadly consistent with the concept of "somatoform dissociation" (Nijenhuis et al., 1999), the researchers measured each child's characteristic way of relating and processing emotion. Four patterns were identified: inhibitory, normative/balanced, coercive-preoccupied, and mixed inhibitory and coercive-preoccupied. The children in the inhibitory cluster used "extreme inhibition to minimize subjective awareness of distressing self-relevant feelings and memories. Instead, these children emphasize[d] positive feelings and memories, positive aspects of their attachment relationships, and the feelings, perspectives, and needs of others, but not their own" (p. 778) Such psychological inhibition was associated with negative conversion symptoms, that is, symptoms such as paresis/paralysis presumed to arise on the bases of an activation of inhibitory mechanisms.

These findings give some evidential support to the principle derived from Vygotsky, which proposes that a form of consciousness, or a kind of brain–mind function, arises in a state of relatedness which resembles it in an essential way. In the Kozlowska example, the inhibition was both "inner" and "outer," i.e., relational. This principle suggests that the sense of personal unity arises in the context of a form of relatedness in which there is a feeling of unity between the partners in this conversation. What, then, is the nature of this style of relating? I am suggesting that it involves a reciprocal shaping, or picturing, of the immediate central and emotional experience of the other, which might be called an *analogical relatedness*.

DEVELOPMENTAL MODELS
OF ANALOGICAL RELATEDNESS

The human being has two main forms of thought, dependent on different hemispheres, which usually operate together. One has the quality of synthesis, the other of analysis, of splitting things into their parts. The right hemisphere processes configurative information whereas the analytic functions of the left hemisphere subserve the processing of details, of feature-based information

(Bourne et al., 2009). Following the Vygotskian principle, each mode of thinking reflects, and is a part of, a form of relatedness between a person and his or her world.

These thought modes are manifest linguistically. Their different characteristics are discerned most easily in the earliest phases of life, in the language of the child, which was studied by Vygotsky (1962). The child speaks as if in two different tongues, reflecting different states of mind. The first language is that of ordinary day-to-day living, in which the child is engaged with others, responding to them, asking questions, expressing wishes, and so forth. This language is communicative and social; its purpose is evident and its function is clearly adaptive. This ordinary language, involving syntax and having within it the notion of succession, of a reality in which one thing follows another, is left-hemispheric. The second form of language, which in its purest form is almost without syntax, is a reflection of right-hemispheric function. This kind of language, "inner speech," is spoken much less frequently, during that activity that Piaget called *symbolic play*, when the child is absorbed in a game using objects as part of telling a little story, told as if to him- or herself, apparently oblivious toward other people. The characteristics of inner versus social speech are shown in the Table 16.1.

I am calling the language and the thought process of the child at symbolic play *analogical*, whereas social speech is more or less *logical*. An analogue, in the original meaning of the word, is a thing having a similar proportion, or shape, as another thing. This meaning has been extended to include a shared quality or attribute, common to the two things, which are thus analogically related. The child uses analogical thinking to represent elements of the story being told—a stick is a man, a large leaf is a boat, and so forth. This process is dependent upon right-hemispheric function. The right hemisphere might be considered an analogue detector, involved in finding shapes among sensory data, and at a

TABLE 16.1

Inner Speech	Social Speech
1. Nonlinear	1. Linear
2. Nongrammatical	2. Grammatical
3. Analogical, associative	3. Logical
4. Positive affect	4. Variable affect
5. Noncommunicative	5. Communicative
6. Inner-directed	6. Outer directed
7. Intimate	7. Nonintimate
8. Self-related	8. Identity-related
9. Synchronic time (Saussuer)	9. Diachronic time

high level, in the detection and understanding of the figurative aspects of language, such as metaphor use (Bottini et al., 1994).

Before the age of about 4, the two thought forms are relatively separable. However, with the integration that comes with maturation, they are soon coordinated. Ordinary conversation by about the age of 5 is composed of the two language forms combined, the linear language being the vehicle for the second, nonlinear and emotional language (Meares, 1993a, 2005).

The game of symbolic play is preceded by another game, played between mother and child in early life, which Trevarthen has called a *proto-conversation*. This activity predicts, and is likely to be a necessary precursor to, the emergence of symbolic play in the second year of life. Bornstein and Tamis Le Monda (1997) showed that maternal responsiveness during periods when the baby was in no distress predicted the later appearance of symbolic play, whereas responses to distress did not.

The proto-conversation is established by 2–3 months (Trevarthen, 1974). The to-and-fro reciprocity of this game has a structure that resembles that of mature conversation. The responses of each partner are closely coupled to the other's expression. The mother's responses have a particular character, and they differ from those she makes when the child is in distress. Not only are they sensitively linked to the child's experience at that moment, they represent, in her face and in her voice, an amplified version of that experience. It is a re-representation but not a copy. She shows to her baby, in another form, the shape and contours of the baby's experience, and most importantly, its emotional core. She behaves, in other words, as an analogue of her baby's experience. *The mother is the baby's first analogue.* The principles underlying the proto-conversation provide a model for an analogical relatedness of adult life.

THE RIGHT HEMISPHERE AND THE PROTO-CONVERSATION

The right hemisphere seems to be peculiarly set up for the proto-conversation. Recognition of faces (Kim et al., 1999), and especially the emotions they represent (Buchanan et al., 2000; Harciarek & Heilman, 2009; Iidaka et al., 2003; Tamietto et al., 2006), is largely right-hemispheric, as is the processing of prosody (Riecker et al., 2002) and rhythm (Jongsma, Desain, & Honing, 2004). P3a that is evoked by auditory stimuli is sensitive to changes in rhythm (Jongsma et al., 2004).

Women are more biologically adapted for proto-conversation than men. They are also superior in processing face-specific information (McBain et al., 2009), an ability that is correlated with right-hemispheric activation (Rueckert & Naybar, 2007).

Maturation of the right hemisphere may be particularly vulnerable during the first years of life. The right hemisphere is in a growth spurt during the first 2 years of life, a period of right-brain dominance, and so right-hemispheric resources are the first to develop (Chiron et al., 1997; Decety & Chaminade, 2003). This growth is not totally encoded in the genome, but is indelibly shaped by experiences with the environment. The neurobiological maturation of the emotion-processing right hemisphere in the early critical period of the first 2 years of life is thus "experience-dependent." It is specifically the affect-communicating and analogically representing interplay between mother and child—involving prosody, facial expressions, and rhythm—that impacts the experience-dependent maturation of prefrontal cortical–limbic circuits of the early developing right cortical hemisphere (Schore, 2005). The baby's right brain seems to be particularly set up to respond to the mother's face. For example, babies of 4–9 months move their eyes more quickly to the mother's face than to a stranger's face when the stimuli are presented in the left visual field. In contrast, simple geometric shapes are discriminated equally well in either field (Rapp & Bachevalier, 2008, p. 1046). Lyons and colleagues demonstrate that varying maternal behaviors in infancy produce "significant differences in right, not left, adult prefrontal volumes, with experience-dependent asymmetric variation most clearly expressed in ventral medial cortex measured *in vivo* by magnetic resonance imaging" (Lyons et al., 2002, p. 51).

A deficit in appropriate responding may produce the structural changes reported by Chanen et al. (2008) in a group of patients with first-presentation BPD, in whom secondary effects of the disorder over time were likely to be minimized. They showed right-sided OFC loss of gray matter, relative to controls, but no hippocampal or amygdaloid difference.

The findings of Chanen and his colleagues mirror our findings of functional disturbance of the P3a, believed to be dependent upon prefrontal OFC function. It leads to a two-stage proposal for the genesis of BPD. The first stage involves an external disconnection in which the child is deprived of analogical relatedness. The second stage is one of inner disconnection, in which failure of maturation of specific neurocircuitry involving the prefrontal OFC results in the failure of connection between brain systems that are connected and coordinated under normal circumstances.

It seems important that the interplay of the proto-conversation involves neurophysiological activation of a similar kind in both partners. For example, affective prosody is not only processed right hemispherically but is also delivered as a consequence of right-brain activation (Ross & Monnot, 2008). It might be said, then, in a partially figurative way, that the proto-conversation represents an interplay between two right brains. In the case of the mother, at least, OFC activation is prominent. It occurs when mothers view pictures of their babies (Nitschke et al., 2004). The OFC, periaqueductal grey matter, anterior insula, and dorsal and ventrolateral putamen become active when a mother views her baby smiling at her while she plays with him or her (Noriuchi, Kikuchi, & Senoo, 2008). Viewing her infant's distress evokes a different neural response in the mother. The smile is likely to enhance activation in the medial OFC beyond that evoked by the image of the baby alone (O'Doherty et al., 2003). Such observations lead to the speculation that the analogical matching behavior of the mother during the proto-conversation might evoke a mirrored neurophysiology in her baby and tend to stimulate activation and maturation of circuitry involving the OFC. The findings reported by Minagawa-Kawai et al. (2009) support the possibility of such reciprocity. These researchers showed OFC activation in the brains of mothers and babies when each was shown a video of the other. In the mother's case, the activation was right-sided. In another study, the mother's joy in observing and mirroring her baby's facial expressions was also found to be right-sided, in this case, mainly in right limbic and paralimbic areas (Lenzi et al., 2009).

The notion that early forms of "analogical relatedness" might be conceived as if an interplay between two right brains provides a structure for the therapeutic engagement. Translating principles derived from the proto-conversation into the more complex one of the therapeutic situation involves the use of right-hemispheric language. It is abbreviated, with the utterances often incomplete and lacking formal syntactical structure. In particular, the subject of a sentence tends to be left out, including pronouns. It is a language of predicates (Vygotsky, 1962). Furthermore, the language is emotionally expressive. As a consequence, the phonology is salient, the toning and inflections of the voice having a powerful communicative effect that is combined with facial expressions and the movements of the body. This kind of language creates the feeling of "being with" in a way that is greater than a logical, completely syntactical, left-hemisphere utterance, which sets up a different kind of relatedness.

ANALOGICAL RELATEDNESS, "FIT," AND HEDONIC TONE

The outcome of the proto-conversation is its partial internalization manifest in the scene of symbolic play. The connectedness between mother and child has become the child's own connectedness. The scene of symbolic play is now as if an external, and embryonic, form of the later reflective awareness of inner events. The child watches his or her own story evolving in the living room floor, or wherever it is being created. The early cohesion of analogical relating has now become a sort of inner conversation, an experience beautifully described by Piaget:

> What he says does not seem to him to be addressed to himself but is enveloped with the feeling of a presence, so that to speak of himself or to speak to his mother appear to him to be the same thing. His activity is thus bathed in an atmosphere of communion or syntonization, one might almost speak of "the life of union" to use the terms of mysticism, and this atmosphere excludes all consciousness of egocentrism. But, on the other hand, one cannot but be struck by the soliloquistic character of these same remarks. The child does not ask questions and expects no answer, neither does he attempt to give any definite information to his mother who is present. He does not

ask himself whether she is listening or not. He speaks for himself just as an adult does when he speaks within himself. (Piaget, 1959, p. 243)

This scene suggests that the child has internalized, at least in part, the feelings of "being with" mother as part of his own experience. The child acts as if alone but in the presence of someone else. The curious feeling is denied those who have not been given the generative form of responsiveness from caregivers.

In addition to this feeling, and part of it, is pleasure. It is not unreasonable to suppose that the early experience of cohesion is, in itself, a production of the positive affective state that is at the heart of healthy selfhood. This experience is not given to those with BPD, who live in a state of "painful incoherence." The remainder of this section is devoted to the idea that a particular form of interpersonal coordination creates a feeling of well-being.

It is evident that both proto-conversation and symbolic play are enjoyable. The participants do it because they like doing it, not because they are told to. The interplay of the proto-conversation creates a kind of pleasure that would not have been gained by either partner alone. It may be that the sense of "fit" that arises in the game of proto-conversation produces the sense of warmth and value that is at the heart of healthy selfhood (Meares, 1999a).

The hedonic tone that arises from "fit" (Meares, 1993, 2005b) presumably derives from our evolutionary heritage. We are phylogenetically endowed with systems of social signaling that are designed to connect in a particular way with receptive systems in the other. The neurotransmission involved in the proto-conversation is likely to involve the hormone oxytocin, which is known to enhance hedonic tone and to be released during maternal behaviors such as breast-feeding and skin-to-skin contact between mothers and their newborn babies (Carter, 1998; Light et al., 2000). It plays a part in attachment formation and in the development of social and afflictive behavior (Carter, 1998; Don-aldson & Young, 2008; Insel, 1997; Insel & Fernald, 2004; Insel & Young, 2001). An interesting recent study from Gordon et al. (2010) suggests that oxytocin release is not confined to the maternal figure or to birth and lactation. It occurs in father as well. Fathers had levels of oxytocin similar to the mothers both at the postpartum period and 6 months later. The maternal and paternal levels were interrelated and interdependent. The amount of oxytocin released is related to the amount of affectionate parenting behavior each displayed.

These observations suggest the possibility that the experience of a maturational relationship, in which a feeling of connectedness arises, is necessary not only to the cohesion of self but also to the positive feeling, the "warmth and intimacy," which William James (1890) found to be at the core of healthy existing. As a corollary, it is proposed that a lack of this relationship results not only in subtle and continuing states of diminished cohesion but also a lack of positive feeling, reaching, at times, profound dysphoria. Put another way, the early relational deficit has the outcome of "painful incoherence."

NARRATIVE COHESION: FROM THE SIMULTANEOUS TO SUCCESSIVE

The conclusion to the inquiry reflected in this book is that a "painful incoherence" lies at the heart of BPD and that, as a consequence, the principal therapeutic approach should have the effects of enhancing both cohesion and hedonic tone. It is suggested that an important component of this approach is a form of therapeutic conversation that can be conceived, only partly figuratively, as a dynamic interplay between two right hemispheres. This kind of language has a picturing and shaping function in which a representation of an immediate reality includes its emotional basis. Robert Hobson (1985) called these representations "forms of feeling." The form of the language is typically condensed, affectively toned, often incomplete and asyntactical, with subjects of sentences, particularly pronouns, omitted. This is the form of what Vygotsky (1962) called "inner speech."

Although a conversation having the structure of "analogical relatedness" is seen as a main component in the treatment of BPD, it is not the only kind of conversation involved. Analogical relatedness, as shown in the normal interplay of mother and child, is conducted in a state of positive affect. The game begins with the mother picking up some latent positivity in her child, an interest in some object, for example. She couples her response to this, at times, merely potential positivity. Her response amplifies and represents what she infers from her baby's face and bodily movements. Coupling, amplification, and representation are the main elements of a self-organizing system. The emergence of self can be conceived in this way, as a self-organizing system (Meares, 2000). Many of the conversations of those with BPD cannot have this effect, since they are negatively affectively toned.

Negatively toned styles of conversation characteristic of BPD include "chronicles" and "scripts" (Meares, 1998). The former reflects a depleted self, bereft of right-hemispheric language. The latter manifests a traumatic relatedness. The therapist must enter these and other similar "forms of life" (Wittgenstein, 1953) in order to transform them into a different and generative form of relatedness.

The capacity for analogical relatedness is part of our biological makeup. It comes to us naturally as does the proto-conversation to a mother. It seems likely that natural propensity, harnessed and enhanced by a particular interest in helping those who suffer from the borderline condition, may contribute substantially to the beneficial effects reported for all the main approaches to the treatment of BPD. Such nonspecific factors are powerful but often unacknowledged (Wampold et al., 1997). An innate propensity, like any inborn aptitude, needs training to develop into a skill. Therapists using the Conversational Model are trained intensively by means of audio- and videotaping, which allow focus on the "minute particulars" of the conversation.

Analogical representations range from nonverbal vocalizations to larger pictures of a personal reality, which may depend upon the co-creation of metaphor. If things go well, some of these depictions become scenes, and scenes are the units of narrative. In turn, narrative creates coherence in a dimension different from the analogical, which represents, and resonates with, a personal reality at a particular moment. Narrative contributes to coherence over time, to the sense of continuity. There is coordination, then, of the simultaneous and successive elements of human experiencing.

The narrative that emerges is not perceived, at first, by either partner in the conversation, since it does not move in the manner of a chronicle, one thing after another. Like the story being told in symbolic play, it seems to have no purpose, making its own wandering way. Like the child, the patient has little awareness of the proto-symbolic or symbolic mode in which the evolving story is told. The elements of the story are not merely spoken about, but visualized in words, and sometimes pictorially (Meares, A., 1958).

Narrative of a particular kind, usually having an analogical or mythic structure, is an important component not only of personal cohesion but in the creation of unified and coordinated groups of people, such as the tribe. "Narration," wrote Pierre Janet, "created humanity" (1928, p. 261).

Credits

I acknowledge with "thanks" permission to reproduce aspects of other publications in this book. The permissions are as follows.

Wolters Kluwer for Meares, R., Melkonian, D., Gordon, E., & Williams, L. (2005). Distinct pattern of P3a event-related potential in borderline personality disorder. *Neuroreport, 16*(3), 289–293. Diagrams and a table are taken from that paper.

Proceeding of the National Academy of Sciences for images used in Fair, D. A., Cohen, A. L., Dosenbach, N. U., Church, J. A., Miezin, F. M., Barch, D. M., et al. (2008). The maturing architecture of the brain's default network. *Proceedings of the National Academy of Sciences of the United States of America, 105*(10), 4028–4032.

Hogrefe Publishing for use of images appearing in Williams, L., Senior, C., David, A., Loughland, C. M., & Gordon, E. (2001). In search of the "Duchene" smile: evidence from eye movements. *Journal of Psychophysiology, 15*, 122–127.

Australian and New Zealand Journal of Psychiatry for aspects of the text of the following articles:

Meares, R., Gerull, F., Stevenson, J., & Korner, A. (2011b). Is Self Disturbance the core of borderline personality disorder? An outcome study of borderline personality factors. *Australian and New Zealand Journal of Psychiatry, 45*(3), 214.

Meares, R., Schore, A., & Melkonian, D. (2011a). Is borderline personality a particularly right hemispheric disorder? A study of P3a using single trial analysis. *Australian and New Zealand Journal of Psychiatry, 45*(2), 131–139.

Guildford Press for reproduction of large parts of the following article:

Meares, R., Gerull, F., Korner, A., Melkonian, D., Stevenson, J., & Samir, H. (2008). Somatization and stimulus entrapment. *The Journal of the American Academy of Psychoanalysis and Dynamic Psychiatry, 36*(1), 165–180.

Test library of the department of Linguistic and Psychology, Macquarie University, Sydney, for permitting Friederike Gerull, a PhD student of the department, to use for research purposes, the SCL 90-R of Derogatis, L. R. (1994). Manual for the Symptom Checklist 90-Revised. Minneapolis: NCS, for which the test library had secured right of usage.

References

Addis, D. R., Wong, A. T., & Schacter, D. L. (2007). Remembering the past and imagining the future: Common and distinct neural substrates during event construction and elaboration. *Neuropsychologia, 45*(7), 1363–1377.

Adler, G. (1985). *Borderline psychopathology and its treatment.* New York, NY: Jason Aronson.

Adler, G., & Buie, D. H., Jr. (1979). Aloneness and borderline psychopathology: The possible relevance of child development issues. *International Journal of Psycho-Analysis, 60*(1), 83–96.

Aggen, S. H., Neale, M. C., Roysamb, E., Reichborn-Kjennerud, T., & Kendler, K. S. (2009). A psychometric evaluation of the DSM-IV borderline personality disorder criteria: Age and sex moderation of criterion functioning. *Psychological Medicine, 39,* 1–12.

Ainsworth, M. D. S., Blehar, M., Waters, E., & Wall, S. (1978). *Patterns of attachment: A psychological study of the Strange Situation.* Hillsdale, NJ: Erlbaum.

Allen, B. (2008). An analysis of the impact of diverse forms of childhood psychological maltreatment on emotional adjustment in early adulthood. *Child Maltreatment, 13*(3), 307–312.

Als, H., Tronick, E., Lester, B. M., & Brazelton, T. B. (1977). The Brazelton Neonatal Behavioral Assessment Scale (BNBAS). *Journal of Abnormal Child Psychology, 5*(3), 215–231.

Altshuler, L. L., Bartzokis, G., Grieder, T., Curran, J., & Mintz, J. (1998). Amygdala enlargement in bipolar disorder and hippocampal reduction in schizophrenia: An MRI study demonstrating neuroanatomic specificity. *Archives General Psychiatry, 55*(7), 663–664.

Amaral, D. G., & Price, J. L. (1984). Amygdalo-cortical projections in the monkey (*Macaca fascicularis*). *Journal of Comparative Neurology, 230*(4), 465–496.

American Psychiatric Association. (1994). *Diagnostic and statistical manual of mental disorders* (4th ed.). Washington, DC: Author.

Amsterdam, B. (1972). Mirror self image reactions before age two. *Developmental Psychology, 5,* 297–305.

Armstrong, D. M. (1981). *The nature of mind.* New York, NY: Cornell University Press.

Armstrong, D. M. (1999). *The mind–body problem.* Boulder, CO: Westview.

Arnold, M. (1864/1964). The function of criticism at the present time." In J.M. Dent, *Essays in Criticism* (pp. 9–34). London: Everyman's Library.

Arntz, A., Bernstein, D., Oorschot, M., & Schobre, P. (2009). Theory of mind in borderline and Cluster-C personality disorder. *Journal Nervous Mental Disease, 197*(11), 801–807.

Arzy, S., Idel, M., Landis, T., & Blanke, O. (2005). Why revelations have occurred on mountains? Linking mystical experiences and cognitive neuroscience. *Medical Hypotheses, 65*(5), 841–845.

Atance, C. M., & O'Neill, D. K. (2001). Episodic future thinking. *Trends in Cognitive Sciences, 5*(12), 533–539.

Austin, M. A., Riniolo, T. C., & Porges, S. W. (2007). Borderline personality disorder and emotion regulation: Insights from the polyvagal theory. *Brain and Cognition, 65*(1), 69–76.

Axelrod, S. R., Morgan, C. A., 3rd, & Southwick, S. M. (2005). Symptoms of posttraumatic stress disorder and borderline personality disorder in veterans of Operation Desert Storm. *American Journal of Psychiatry, 162*(2), 270–275.

Baguley, I. J. (2008). The excitatory:inhibitory ratio model (EIR model): An integrative explanation of acute autonomic overactivity syndromes. *Medical Hypotheses, 70*(1), 26–35.

Baguley, I. J., Nott, M. T., Slewa-Younan, S., Heriseanu, R. E., & Perkes, I. E. (2009). Diagnosing dysautonomia after acute traumatic brain injury: Evidence for overresponsiveness to afferent stimuli. *Archives of Physical Medicine and Rehabilitation, 90*(4), 580–586.

Bakkevig, J. F., & Karterud, S. (2010). Is the *Diagnostic and Statistical Manual of Mental Disorders,* fourth edition, histrionic personality disorder category a valid construct? *Comprehensive Psychiatry, 51*(5), 462–470.

Bantick, S. J., Wise, R. G., Ploghaus, A., Clare, S., Smith, S. M., & Tracey, I. (2002). Imaging how attention modulates pain in humans using functional MRI. *Brain, 125*(Pt. 2), 310–319.

Barcelo, F., Perianez, J. A., & Knight, R. T. (2002). Think differently: A brain orienting response to task novelty. *NeuroReport, 13*(15), 1887–1892.

Barnett, D., Ganiban, J., & Cicchetti, D. (1999). Maltreatment, negative expressivity, and the development of type D attachments from 12 to 24 months of age. *Monographs of the Society for Research in Child Development, 64*, 97–118.

Baron-Cohen, S. (2001). Theory of mind in normal development and autism. *Prisme, 34*, 174–183.

Baron-Cohen, S., Wheelwright, S., Hill, J., Raste, Y., & Plumb, I. (2001). The "Reading the Mind in the Eyes" Test revised version: A study with normal adults, and adults with Asperger syndrome or high-functioning autism. *Journal of Child Psychology and Psychiatry, 42*(2), 241–251.

Barsky, A. J., & Klerman, G. L. (1983). Overview: Hypochondriasis, bodily complaints, and somatic styles. *American Journal of Psychiatry, 140*(3), 273–283.

Bartlett, F. (1932). *Remembering.* Cambridge, UK: Cambridge University Press.

Bateman, A., & Fonagy, P. (1999). Effectiveness of partial hospitalization in the treatment of borderline personality disorder: A randomized controlled trial. *American Journal of Psychiatry, 156*(10), 1563–1569.

Bateman, A., & Fonagy, P. (2004). *Psychotherapy for borderline personality disorder: Mentalization based treatment.* Oxford, UK: Oxford University Press.

Baudena, P., Halgren, E., Heit, G., & Clarke, J. M. (1995). Intracerebral potentials to rare target and distractor auditory and visual stimuli: III. Frontal cortex. *Electroencephalography and Clinical Neurophysiology, 94*(4), 251–264.

Bayer, T. L., Baer, P. E., & Early, C. (1991). Situational and psychophysiological factors in psychologically induced pain. *Pain, 44*(1), 45–50.

Baynes, K., Eliassen, J. C., Lutsep, H. L., & Gazzaniga, M. S. (1998). Modular organization of cognitive systems masked by interhemispheric integration. *Science, 280*(5365), 902–905.

Bechara, A., Damasio, A. R., Damasio, H., & Anderson, S. W. (1994). Insensitivity to future consequences following damage to human prefrontal cortex. *Cognition, 50*(1–3), 7–15.

Bechara, A., Damasio, H., Tranel, D., & Damasio, A. R. (2005). The Iowa Gambling Task and the somatic marker hypothesis: Some questions and answers. *Trends in Cognitive Science, 9*(4), 159–162; discussion, 162–164.

Bender, D. S., Dolan, R. T., Skodol, A. E., Sanislow, C. A., Dyck, I. R., McGlashan, T. H., et al. (2001). Treatment utilization by patients with personality disorders. *American Journal of Psychiatry, 158*(2), 295–302.

Berlin, H. A., Rolls, E. T., & Iversen, S. D. (2005). Borderline personality disorder, impulsivity, and the orbitofrontal cortex. *American Journal of Psychiatry, 162*(12), 2360–2373.

Bernstein, E. M., & Putnam, F. W. (1986). Development, reliability, and validity of a dissociation scale. *Journal of Nervous Mental Disease, 174*(12), 727–735.

Biggs, J. T., Wylie, L. T., & Ziegler, V. E. (1978). Validity of the Zung Self-Rating Depression Scale. *British Journal of Psychiatry, 132*, 381–385.

Blair, R. J. (2004). The roles of orbital frontal cortex in the modulation of antisocial behavior. *Brain Cognition, 55*(1), 198–208.

Blais, M. A., Hilsenroth, M. J., & Castlebury, F. D. (1997). Content validity of the DSM-IV borderline and narcissistic personality disorder criteria sets. *Comprehensive Psychiatry, 38*(1), 31–37.

Bland, A. R., Williams, C. A., Scharer, K., & Manning, S. (2004). Emotion processing in borderline personality disorders. *Issues in Mental Health Nursing, 25*(7), 655–672.

Blanke, O., Landis, T., Spinelli, L., & Seeck, M. (2004). Out-of-body experience and autoscopy of neurological origin. *Brain, 127*(Pt. 2), 243–258.

Blatt, S. J., & Auerbach, J. S. (1988). Differential cognitive disturbances in three types of borderline patients. *Journal of Personality Disorders, 2*, 198–211.

Blatt, S. J., D'Afflitti, J. P., & Quinlan, D. M. (1976). Experiences of depression in normal young adults. *Journal Abnormal Psychology, 85*(4), 383–389.

Blatt, S. J., Zohar, A. H., Quinlan, D. M., Zuroff, D. C., & Mongrain, M. (1995). Subscales within the dependency factor of the Depressive Experiences Questionnaire. *Journal of Personality Assessment, 64*(2), 319–339.

Bluhm, R. L., Williamson, P. C., Lanius, R., Theberge, J., Densmore, M., Bartha, R., et al. (2009). Resting state default-mode network connectivity in early depression using a seed region-of-interest analysis: Decreased connectivity with caudate nucleus. *Psychiatry and Clinical Neurosciences, 63*(6), 754–761.

Bluhm, R. L., Williamson, P. C., Osuch, E. A., Frewen, P. A., Stevens, T. K., Boksman, K., et al. (2009). Alterations in default network connectivity in posttraumatic stress disorder related to early-life trauma. *Journal of Psychiatry and Neuroscience, 34*(3), 187–194.

Bohus, M., Limberger, M., Ebner, U., Glocker, F. X., Schwarz, B., Wernz, M., et al. (2000). Pain perception during self-reported distress and calmness in patients with borderline personality disorder and self-mutilating behavior. *Psychiatry Research, 95*(3), 251–260.

Boon, S., & Draijer, N. (1993). Multiple personality disorder in The Netherlands: A clinical investigation of 71 patients. *American Journal of Psychiatry, 150*(3), 489–494.

Bornstein, M., & Tamis Le Monda, C. (1997). Maternal responsiveness and infant mental abilities: Specific predictive relations. *Infant Behavior and Development, 20*(3), 283–296.

Bornstein, R. F., Becker-Matero, N., Winarick, D. J., & Reichman, A. L. (2010). Interpersonal dependency in borderline personality disorder: Clinical context and empirical evidence. *Journal of Personality Disorders, 24*(1), 109–127.

Bottini, G., Corcoran, R., Sterzi, R., Paulesu, E., Schenone, P., Scarpa, P., et al. (1994). The role of the right hemisphere in the interpretation of figurative aspects of language: A positron emission tomography activation study. *Brain, 117*(Pt. 6), 1241–1253.

Bourne, V. J., Vladeanu, M., & Hole, G. J. (2009). Lateralised repetition priming for featurally and configurally manipulated familiar faces: Evidence for differentially lateralised processing mechanisms. *Laterality, 14*(3), 287–299.

Bower, T. (1971). The object in the world of the infant. *Scientific American, 225*, 30–38.

Bowlby, J. (1969). *Attachment*. London: Hogarth.

Bowlby, J. (1973). *Attachment and loss*. Vol. 2. *Separation: Anxiety and anger*. London, UK: Hogarth Press.

Brambilla, P., Soloff, P. H., Sala, M., Nicoletti, M. A., Keshavan, M. S., & Soares, J. C. (2004). Anatomical MRI study of borderline personality disorder patients. *Psychiatry Research, 131*(2), 125–133.

Brandchaft, B., Doctors, S., & Sorter, D. (2010). *Toward an emancipatory psychoanalysis: Brandchaft's intersubjective vision*. London, UK: Routledge.

Brazelton, T. B. (1975). *Early mother–infant reciprocity*. Paper presented at the Parent–Infant Interaction, Ciba Foundation Symposium, New York.

Brazelton, T. B. (1979). Behavioral competence of the newborn infant. *Seminars in Perinatology, 3*, 35–44.

Bremner, J. D., Licinio, J., Darnell, A., Krystal, J. H., Owens, M. J., Southwick, S. M., et al. (1997). Elevated CSF corticotropin-releasing factor concentrations in posttraumatic stress disorder. *American Journal of Psychiatry, 154*(5), 624–629.

Bremner, J. D., Narayan, M., Anderson, E. R., Staib, L. H., Miller, H. L., & Charney, D. S. (2000). Hippocampal volume reduction in major depression. *American Journal of Psychiatry, 157*(1), 115–118.

Bremner, J. D., Randall, P., Scott, T. M., Capelli, S., Delaney, R., McCarthy, G., et al. (1995). Deficits in short-term memory in adult survivors of childhood abuse. *Psychiatry Res, 59*(1–2), 97–107.

Breuer, J., & Freud, S. (1895). *Studies in hysteria* (A. A. Brill, Trans.). New York, NY: *Nervous and Mental Disorders Monograph*, No. 61.

Briquet, P. (1859). *Traité clinique et thérapeutique de l'hystérie*. Paris: J.B. Bailliere.

Broussard, E. R., & Hartner, M. S. S. (1971). Further considerations regarding maternal perception of the first born. In J. Helmuth (Ed.), *The exceptional infant* (Vol. II). New York, NY: Brunner/Mazel.

Brown, G. W., Harris, T. O., & Hepworth, C. (1995). Loss, humiliation and entrapment among women developing depression: A patient and nonpatient comparison. *Psychoogical Medicine, 25*(1), 7–21.

Brown, M. Z., Linehan, M. M., Comtois, K. A., Murray, A., & Chapman, A. L. (2009). Shame as a prospective predictor of self-inflicted injury in borderline personality disorder: A multi-modal analysis. *Behaviour Research and Therapy, 47*(10), 815–822.

Broyd, S. J., Demanuele, C., Debener, S., Helps, S. K., James, C. J., & Sonuga-Barke, E. J. (2009). Default-mode brain dysfunction in mental disorders: A systematic review. *Neuroscience and Biobehavioral Reviews, 33*(3), 279–296.

Brunner, R., Henze, R., Parzer, P., Kramer, J., Feigl, N., Lutz, K., et al. (2010). Reduced prefrontal and orbitofrontal gray matter in female adolescents with borderline personality disorder: Is it disorder specific? *NeuroImage, 49*(1), 114–120.

Bryant, R. A., & Panasetis, P. (2001). Panic symptoms during trauma and acute stress disorder. *Behaviour Research and Therapy, 39*(8), 961–966.

Buchanan, T. W., Lutz, K., Mirzazade, S., Specht, K., Shah, N. J., Zilles, K., et al. (2000). Recognition of emotional prosody and verbal components of spoken language: An fMRI study. *Cognitive Brain Research, 9*(3), 227–238.

Buchel, C., Bornhovd, K., Quante, M., Glauche, V., Bromm, B., & Weiller, C. (2002). Dissociable neural responses related to pain intensity, stimulus intensity, and stimulus awareness within the anterior cingulate cortex: A parametric single-trial laser functional magnetic resonance imaging study. *Journal of Neuroscience, 22*(3), 970–976.

Buchsbaum, M., & Pfefferbaum, A. (1971). Individual differences in stimulus intensity response. *Psychophysiology, 8*(5), 600–611.

Buchsbaum, M. (1974). Average evoked response and stimulus intensity in identical and fraternal twins. *Physiological Psychology, 2*, 365–370.

Buchsbaum, M., Goodwin, F., Murphy, D., & Borge, G. (1971). AER in affective disorders. *American Journal of Psychiatry, 128*(1), 19–25.

Buchsbaum, M., Landau, S., Murphy, D., & Goodwin, F. (1973). Average evoked response in bipolar and unipolar affective disorders: Relationship to sex, age of onset, and monoamine oxidase. *Biological Psychiatry, 7*(3), 199–212.

Buchsbaum, M., & Silverman, J. (1968). Stimulus intensity control and the cortical evoked response. *Psychosomatic Medicine, 30*(1), 12–22.

Buckner, R. L., & Carroll, D. C. (2007). Self-projection and the brain. *Trends in Cognitive Sciences, 11*(2), 49–57.

Bush, G., Luu, P., & Posner, M. I. (2000). Cognitive and emotional influences in anterior cingulate cortex. *Trends in Cognitive Sciences, 4*(6), 215–222.

Butt, D. G., Moore, A. R., Henderson-Brooks, C., Meares, R., & Haliburn, J. (2010). Dissociation, relatedness, and "cohesive harmony": A linguistic measure of degrees of "fragmentation"? *Linguistics and Human Sciences, 3.3*(2007), 263–293.

Calvin, W. (2004). *A brief history of the mind.* Oxford, UK: Oxford University Press.

Cantello, R., Boccagni, C., Comi, C., Civardi, C., & Monaco, F. (2001). Diagnosis of psychogenic paralysis: The role of motor evoked potentials. *Journal of Neurology, 248*(10), 889–897.

Carlson, E. A. (1998). A prospective longitudinal study of attachment disorganization/ disorientation. *Child Development, 69*, 1107–1128.

Caron, C., & Rutter, M. (1991). Comorbidity in child psychopathology: Concepts, issues and research strategies. *Journal of Child Psychology and Psychiatry, 32*, 1063–1080.

Carrion, V. G., Weems, C. F., Watson, C., Eliez, S., Menon, V., & Reiss, A. L. (2009). Converging evidence for abnormalities of the prefrontal cortex and evaluation of midsagittal structures in pediatric posttraumatic stress disorder: An MRI study. *Psychiatry Research, 172*(3), 226–234.

Carter, C. S. (1998). Neuroendocrine perspectives on social attachment and love. *Psychoneuroendocrinology, 23*(8), 779–818.

Champoux, M., Bennett, A., Shannon, C., Higley, J. D., Lesch, K. P., & Suomi, S. J. (2002). Serotonin transporter gene polymorphism, differential early rearing, and behavior in rhesus monkey neonates. *Molecular Psychiatry, 7*(10), 1058–1063.

Chanen, A. M., Jovev, M., & Jackson, H. J. (2007). Adaptive functioning and psychiatric symptoms in adolescents with borderline personality disorder. *Journal of Clinical Psychiatry, 68*(2), 297–306.

Chanen, A. M., Velakoulis, D., Carison, K., Gaunson, K., Wood, S. J., Yuen, H. P., et al. (2008). Orbitofrontal, amygdala and hippocampal volumes in teenagers with first-presentation borderline personality disorder. *Psychiatry Research: Neuroimaging, 163*(2), 116–125.

Chiron, C., Jambaque, I., Nabbout, R., Lounes, R., Syrota, A., & Dulac, O. (1997). The right brain hemisphere is dominant in human infants. *Brain, 120*(Pt. 6), 1057–1065.

Choi-Kain, L. W., Fitzmaurice, G. M., Zanarini, M. C., Laverdiere, O., &

Gunderson, J. G. (2009). The relationship between self-reported attachment styles, interpersonal dysfunction, and borderline personality disorder. *Journal of Nervous and Mental Disease, 197*(11), 816–821.

Chopra, H. D., & Beatson, J. A. (1986). Psychotic symptoms in borderline personality disorder. *American Journal of Psychiatry 143*(12), 1605–1607.

Claparéde, E. (1911/1951). Recognition and "me-ness." In D. Rapaport (Ed.), *Organization and pathology of thought: Selected sources* (pp. 58–75). New York, NY: Columbia University Press.

Clarkin, J. F., Hull, J. W., & Hurt, S. W. (1993). Factor structure of borderline personality disorder criteria. *Journal of Personality Disorders, 7*(2), 137–143.

Clarkin, J. F., & Posner, M. (2005). Defining the mechanisms of borderline personality disorder. *Psychopathology, 38*(2), 56–63.

Clarkin, J. F., Levy, K. N., Lenzenweger, M. F., & Kernberg, O. F. (2007). Evaluating three treatments for borderline personality disorder: A multiwave study. *American Journal of Psychiatry, 164*(6), 922–928.

Coan, J. A., Schaefer, H. S., & Davidson, R. J. (2006). Lending a hand: Social regulation of the neural response to threat. *Psychological Science, 17*(12), 1032–1039.

Coccaro, E. F., McCloskey, M. S., Fitzgerald, D. A., & Phan, K. L. (2007). Amygdala and orbitofrontal reactivity to social threat in individuals with impulsive aggression. *Biological Psychiatry, 62*(2), 168–178.

Coid, J., Yang, M., Bebbington, P., Moran, P., Brugha, T., Jenkins, R., et al. (2009). Borderline personality disorder: Health service use and social functioning among a national household population. *Psychological Medicine, 39*(10), 1721–1731.

Conte, H. R., Plutchik, R., Karasu, T. B., & Jerrett, I. (1980). A self-report borderline scale: Discriminative validity and preliminary norms. *Journal of Nervous and Mental Disease, 168*(7), 428–435.

Copolov, D. L., Seal, M. L., Maruff, P., Ulusoy, R., Wong, M. T., Tochon-Danguy, H. J., et al. (2003). Cortical activation associated with the experience of auditory hallucinations and perception of human speech in schizophrenia: A PET correlation study. *Psychiatry Research, 122*(3), 139–152.

Corbetta, M., Patel, G., & Shulman, G. L. (2008). The reorienting system of the human brain: From environment to theory of mind. *Neuron, 58*(3), 306–324.

Corcoran, R., Cahill, C., & Frith, C. D. (1997). The appreciation of visual jokes in people with schizophrenia: A study of "mentalizing" ability. *Schizophrenia Research, 24*(3), 319–327.

Corcoran, R., Mercer, G., & Frith, C. D. (1995). Schizophrenia, symptomatology and social inference: Investigating "theory of mind" in people with schizophrenia. *Schizophrenia Research, 17*(1), 5–13.

Corrigan, F. M., Davidson, A., & Heard, H. (2000). The role of dysregulated amygdalic emotion in borderline personality disorder. *Medical Hypotheses, 54*(4), 574–579.

Courchesne, E., Hillyard, S. A., & Galambos, R. (1975). Stimulus novelty, task relevance and the visual evoked potential in man. *Electroencephalography and Clinical Neurophysiology, 39*(2), 131–143.

Crandell, L. E., Patrick, M. P., & Hobson, R. P. (2003). "Still-face" interactions between mothers with borderline personality disorder and their 2-month-old infants. *British Journal of Psychiatry, 183*, 239–247.

Critchley, H. D., Tang, J., Glaser, D., Butterworth, B., & Dolan, R. J. (2005). Anterior cingulate activity during error and autonomic response. *NeuroImage, 27*(4), 885–895.

Crockenberg, S. B. (1981). Infant irritability, mother responsiveness, and social support influences on the security of infant–mother attachment. *Child Development, 52*(3), 857–865.

Crombez, G., Eccleston, C., Van den Broeck, A., Goubert, L., & Van Houdenhove, B. (2004). Hypervigilance to pain in fibromyalgia: The mediating role of pain intensity and catastrophic thinking about pain. *Clinical Journal of Pain, 20*(2), 98–102.

Crocq, L., & De Verbizier, J. (1989). Le traumatisme psychologique dans l'oeuvre de Pierre Janet [The psychology of trauma in the work of Pierre Janet]. *Annales Medico-Psychologiques, 147*, 983–987.

Damasio, A. R. (1996). *Descartes' error*. London, UK: Papermac/Macmillan. (Original U.S. edition published 1994)

Damasio, A. R. (1998). The somatic marker hypothesis and the possible functions of the prefrontal cortex. In A. C. Roberts, T. W. Robbins, & L. Weiskrantz (Eds.), *The prefrontal cortex: Executive and cognitive function* (pp. 103–116). Oxford, UK: Oxford University Press.

Damasio, A. R. (1999). *The feeling of what happens: Body, emotion, and the making of consciousness*. New York, NY: Harcourt-Brace.

Damasio, H., Grabowski, T., Frank, R., Galaburda, A. M., & Damasio, A. R. (1994). The return of Phineas Gage: Clues about the brain from the skull of a famous patient. *Science, 264*(5162), 1102–1105.

Darwin, C. (1859). *On the origin of species by natural selection*. London: J. Murray.

Darwin, C. (1872/1934). *The expression of emotions in man and animals* (abridged ed.). London, UK: Watts.

David, A. S. (2004). The cognitive neuropsychiatry of auditory verbal hallucinations: An overview. *Cognitive Neuropsychiatry, 9*(1–2), 107–123.

Davidson, M. C., Amso, D., Anderson, L. C., & Diamond, A. (2006). Development of cognitive control and executive functions from 4 to 13 years:

Evidence from manipulations of memory, inhibition, and task switching. *Neuropsychologia, 44*(11), 2037–2078.

Davidson, R. J. (2003). Affective neuroscience and psychophysiology: Toward a synthesis. *Psychophysiology, 40*(5), 655–665.

Davidson, R. J. (2004). Well-being and affective style: Neural substrates and biobehavioural correlates. *Philosophical Transactions of the Royal Society of London B Biological Sciences, 359*(1449), 1395–1411.

Davidson, R. J., Abercrombie, H., Nitschke, J. B., & Putnam, K. (1999). Regional brain function, emotion and disorders of emotion. *Current Opinion in Neurobiology, 9*(2), 228–234.

Davidson, R. J., Putnam, K. M., & Larson, C. L. (2000). Dysfunction in the neural circuitry of emotion regulation: A possible prelude to violence. *Science, 289*(5479), 591–594.

Davidson, R. J., Shackman, A. J., & Maxwell, J. S. (2004). Asymmetries in face and brain related to emotion. *Trends in Cognitive Sciences, 8*(9), 389–391.

De Bellis, M. D., Keshavan, M. S., Clark, D. B., Casey, B. J., Giedd, J. N., Boring, A. M., et al. (1999). A. E. Bennett Research Award. Developmental traumatology: Part II. Brain development. *Biological Psychiatry, 45*(10), 1271–1284.

De Bellis, M. D., Keshavan, M. S., Shifflett, H., Iyengar, S., Beers, S. R., Hall, J., et al. (2002). Brain structures in pediatric maltreatment-related posttraumatic stress disorder: A sociodemographically matched study. *Biological Psychiatry, 52*(11), 1066–1078.

De Bellis, M. D., & Kuchibhatla, M. (2006). Cerebellar volumes in pediatric maltreatment-related posttraumatic stress disorder. *Biological Psychiatry, 60*(7), 697–703.

de Certeau, M. (1988). *The practice of everyday life* (S. Rendall, Trans.). Berkeley, CA: University of California Press.

Decety, J., & Chaminade, T. (2003). When the self represents the other: A new cognitive neuroscience view on psychological identification. *Consciousness and Cognition, 12*(4), 577–596.

De La Fuente, J. M., Goldman, S., Stanus, E., Vizuete, C., Morlan, I., Bobes, J., et al. (1997). Brain glucose metabolism in borderline personality disorder. *Journal of Psychiatric Research, 31*(5), 531–541.

Dell, P. F. (1998). Axis II pathology in outpatients with dissociative identity disorder. *Journal of Nervous and Mental Disease, 186*(6), 352–356.

Dell, P. (2009). The phenomena of pathological dissociaton. In P. Dell & J. O'Neil (Eds.), *Dissociation and the dissociative disorders: DSM-V and beyond* (pp. 225–237). New York and London: Routledge.

Dell, P. F., & O'Neil, J. A. (2009). Chronic dissociation. In P. F. Dell & J. A.

O'Neil (Eds.), *Dissociation and the dissociative disorders* (pp. 225–328). London, UK: Routledge.

Depue, R. A., & Lenzenwger, M. F. (2001). A neurobehavioral dimensional model of personality disturbance. In W. J. Livesley (Ed.), *Handbook of personality disorders: Theory, research, and treatment* (pp. 136–176). New York, NY: Guildford Press.

Depue, R. A., & Lenzenwger, M. F. (2005). A neurobehavioral dimensional model of personality disturbance. In M. F. Lenzenwger & J. F. Clarkin (Eds.), *Major theories of personality disorder* (2nd ed., pp. 391–453). New York, NY: Guildford Press.

De Renzi, E. (1982). *Disorders of space exploration and cognition.* New York, NY: Wiley.

Derogatis, L. R. (1994). *Manual for the Symptom Checklist 90-Revised.* Minneapolis, MN: NCS.

Derogatis, L. R., & Cleary, P. A. (1977). Factorial invariance across gender for the primary symptom dimensions of the SCL-90. *British Journal of Social and Clinical Psychology, 16*(4), 347–356.

Deutsch, H. (1942). Some forms of emotional disturbance and the relationship to schizophrenia. *Psychoanalytic Quarterly, 11,* 301–321.

Di Lollo, V., Enns, J. T., & Rensink, R. A. (2000). Competition for consciousness among visual events: The psychophysics of reentrant visual processes. *Journal of Experimental Psychology, General, 129*(4), 481–507.

Distel, M. A., Hottenga, J. J., Trull, T. J., & Boomsma, D. I. (2008). Chromosome 9: Linkage for borderline personality disorder features. *Psychiatric Genetics, 18*(6), 302–307.

Distel, M. A., Rebollo-Mesa, I., Willemsen, G., Derom, C. A., Trull, T. J., Martin, N. G., et al. (2009). Familial resemblance of borderline personality disorder features: Genetic or cultural transmission? *PLoS One, 4*(4), e5334, 1–8.

Domes, G., Czieschnek, D., Weidler, F., Berger, C., Fast, K., & Herpertz, S. C. (2008). Recognition of facial affect in borderline personality disorder. *Journal of Personality Disorders, 22*(2), 135–147.

Domes, G., Schulze, L., & Herpertz, S. C. (2009). Emotion recognition in borderline personality disorder: A review of the literature. *Journal of Personality Disorders, 23*(1), 6–19.

Domes, G., Winter, B., Schnell, K., Vohs, K., Fast, K., & Herpertz, S. C. (2006). The influence of emotions on inhibitory functioning in borderline personality disorder. *Psychological Medicine, 36*(8), 1163–1172.

Donaldson, Z. R., & Young, L. J. (2008). Oxytocin, vasopressin, and the neurogenetics of sociality. *Science, 322*(5903), 900–904.

Donchin, E., & Coles, M. G. H. (1988). Is the P300 component a manifestation of context updating? *Behavioral and Brain Sciences, 11*, 357–374.

Donegan, N. H., Sanislow, C. A., Blumberg, H. P., Fulbright, R. K., Lacadie, C., Skudlarski, P., et al. (2003). Amygdala hyperreactivity in borderline personality disorder: Implications for emotional dysregulation. *Biological Psychiatry, 54*(11), 1284–1293.

Drevets, W. C., & Raichle, M. E. (1998). Reciprocal suppression of regional cerebral blood during emotional versus higher cognitive implications for interactions between emotion and cognition. *Cognition and Emotion, 12*(3), 353–385.

Driessen, M., Herrmann, J., Stahl, K., Zwaan, M., Meier, S., Hill, A., et al. (2000). Magnetic resonance imaging volumes of the hippocampus and the amygdala in women with borderline personality disorder and early traumatization. *Archives of General Psychiatry, 57*(12), 1115–1122.

Dutra, L., & Lyons-Ruth, K. (2005). *Maltreatment, maternal and child psychopathology, and quality of early care as predictors of adolescent dissociation.* Paper presented at the Biennial Meeting of the Society for Research in Child Development, Atlanta, GA.

Eames, P. (1992). Hysteria following brain injury. *Journal of Neurosurgery and Psychiatry, 55*(11), 1046–1053.

Ebner-Priemer, U. W., Badeck, S., Beckmann, C., Wagner, A., Feige, B., Weiss, I., et al. (2005). Affective dysregulation and dissociative experience in female patients with borderline personality disorder: A startle response study. *Journal of Psychiatry Research, 39*(1), 85–92.

Ebner-Priemer, U. W., Welch, S. S., Grossman, P., Reisch, T., Linehan, M. M., & Bohus, M. (2007). Psychophysiological ambulatory assessment of affective dysregulation in borderline personality disorder. *Psychiatry Research, 150*(3), 265–275.

Edelman, G. (1992). *Bright air, brilliant fire.* New York, NY: Basic Books.

Edelman, G. (2004). *Wider than the sky.* London, UK: Penguin, Allen Lane.

Edelman, G., & Tononi, G. (2000). *A universe of consciousness.* New York, NY: Basic Books.

Eichele, T., Debener, S., Calhoun, V. D., Specht, K., Engel, A. K., Hugdahl, K., et al. (2008). Prediction of human errors by maladaptive changes in event-related brain networks. *Proceedings of the National Academy of Sciences of the United States of America, 105*(16), 6173–6178.

Eisenberger, N. I., Lieberman, M. D., & Williams, K. D. (2003). Does rejection hurt?: An fMRI study of social exclusion. *Science, 302*(5643), 290–292.

Ellenberger, H. F. (1970). *The discovery of the unconscious.* London, UK: Allen Lane.

Elliott, R., Dolan, R. J., & Frith, C. D. (2000). Dissociable functions in the medial and lateral orbitofrontal cortex: Evidence from human neuroimaging studies. *Cerebral Cortex, 10*(3), 308–317.

Enriquez, P., & Bernabeu, E. (2008). Hemispheric laterality and dissociative tendencies: Differences in emotional processing in a dichotic listening task. *Consciousness and Cognition, 17*(1), 267–275.

Erikson, E. (1956). *Identity: Youth and crisis.* New York, NY: Norton.

Erikson, E. (1963). *Childhood and society* (2nd ed.). New York, NY: Norton.

Erikson, E. (1968). *Identity: Youth and crisis.* New York, NY: Norton.

Eysenck, H. J. (1967). *The biological basis of personality.* Springfield, IL: Charles C. Thomas.

Fair, D. A., Cohen, A. L., Dosenbach, N. U., Church, J. A., Miezin, F. M., Barch, D. M., et al. (2008). The maturing architecture of the brain's default network. *Proceedings of the National Academy of Sciences of the United States of America, 105*(10), 4028–4032.

Fair, D. A., Dosenbach, N. U., Church, J. A., Cohen, A. L., Brahmbhatt, S., Miezin, F. M., et al. (2007). Development of distinct control networks through segregation and integration. *Proceedings of the National Academy of Sciences of the United States of America, 104*(33), 13507–13512.

Farmer, A. E., & McGuffin, P. (2003). Humiliation, loss, and other types of life events and difficulties: A comparison of depressed subjects, healthy controls and their siblings. *Psychological Medicine, 33*(7), 1169–1175.

Feinberg, T. (2001). *Altered egos: How the brain creates the self.* New York, NY: Oxford University Press.

Felmingham, K., Kemp, A. H., Williams, L., Falconer, E., Olivieri, G., Peduto, A., et al. (2008). Dissociative responses to conscious and non-conscious fear impact underlying brain function in post-traumatic stress disorder. *Psychological Medicine, 38*(12), 1771–1780.

Fertuck, E. A., Jekal, A., Song, I., Wyman, B., Morris, M. C., Wilson, S. T., et al. (2009). Enhanced "reading the mind in the eyes" in borderline personality disorder compared to healthy controls. *Psychological Medicine, 39*(12), 1979–1988.

Feske, U., Kirisci, L., Tarter, R. E., & Pilkonis, P. A. (2007). An application of item response theory to the DSM-III-R criteria for borderline personality disorder. *Journal of Personality Disorders, 21*(4), 418–433.

Field, T. M. (1981). Infant gaze aversion and heart rate during face-to-face interactions. *Infant Behavior and Development, 4,* 307–315.

Flanagan, O. (1992). *Consciousness reconsidered.* Cambridge: MIT.

Flavell, J. (1968). *The development of role-taking and communication skills in children.* New York, NY: Wiley.

Fletcher, P. C., Frith, C. D., Baker, S. C., Shallice, T., Frackowiak, R. S., &

Dolan, R. J. (1995). The mind's eye: Precuneus activation in memory-related imagery. *NeuroImage, 2*(3), 195–200.

Flournoy, T. (1899/1994). *From India to Planet Mars*. Princeton, NJ: Princeton University Press.

Fonagy, P., & Bateman, A. (2008). The development of borderline personality disorder: A mentalizing model. *Journal of Personality Disorders, 22*(1), 4–21.

Fonagy, P., Leigh, T., Steele, M., Steele, H., Kennedy, R., Mattoon, G., et al. (1996). The relation of attachment status, psychiatric classification, and response to psychotherapy. *Journal of Consulting and Clinical Psychology, 64*(1), 22–31.

Fonagy, P., Target, M., Gergely, G., Allen, J. G., & Bateman, A. W. (2003). The developmental roots of borderline personality disorder in early attachment relationships: A theory and some evidence. *Psychoanalytic Inquiry, 23*, 412–459.

Ford, J. M., Sullivan, E. V., Marsh, L., White, P. M., Lim, K. O., & Pfefferbaum, A. (1994f). The relationship between P300 amplitude and regional gray matter volumes depends upon the attentional system engaged. *Electroencephalography and Clinical Neurophysiology, 90*(3), 214–228.

Fossati, A., Beauchaine, T. P., Grazioli, F., Borroni, S., Carretta, I., De Vecchi, C., et al. (2006). Confirmatory factor analyses of DSM-IV Cluster C personality disorder criteria. *Journal of Personality Disorders, 20*(2), 186–203.

Fossati, A., Maffei, C., Bagnato, M., Battaglia, M., Donati, D., Donini, M., et al. (2000). Patterns of covariation of DSM-IV personality disorders in a mixed psychiatric sample. *Comprehensive Psychiatry, 41*(3), 206–215.

Fournier, N. M., Calverley, K. L., Wagner, J. P., Poock, J. L., & Crossley, M. (2008). Impaired social cognition 30 years after hemispherectomy for intractable epilepsy: The importance of the right hemisphere in complex social functioning. *Epilepsy and Behavior, 12*(3), 460–471.

Fowler, D. (2000). Psychological formulation of early episodes of psychosis: A cognitive model. In M. Birchwood, D. Fowler, & C. Jackson (Eds.), *Early intervention in psychosis: A guide to concepts, evidence and interventions* (pp. 101–127). Chichester, UK: Wiley.

Fox, M. D., Corbetta, M., Snyder, A. Z., Vincent, J. L., & Raichle, M. E. (2006). Spontaneous neuronal activity distinguishes human dorsal and ventral attention systems. *Proceedings of the National Academy of Sciences of the United States of America, 103*(26), 10046–10051.

Fransson, P. (2005). Spontaneous low-frequency BOLD signal fluctuations: An fMRI investigation of the resting-state default mode of brain function hypothesis. *Human Brain Mapping, 26*(1), 15–29.

Fransson, P., Skiold, B., Horsch, S., Nordell, A., Blennow, M., Lagercrantz, H., et al. (2007). Resting-state networks in the infant brain. *Proceedings of the National Academy of Sciences of the United States of America, 104*(39), 15531–15536.

Fredrickson, B. L., & Branigan, C. (2005). Positive emotions broaden the scope of attention and thought–action repertoires. *Cognition and Emotion, 19*(13), 313–332.

Freeman, D., Garety, P. A., Fowler, D., Kuipers, E., Dunn, G., Bebbington, P., et al. (1998). The London–East Anglia randomized controlled trial of cognitive-behaviour therapy for psychosis: IV. Self-esteem and persecutory delusions. *British Journal of Clinical Psychology, 37*(Pt. 4), 415–430.

Freeman, D., Garety, P. A., & Phillips, M. L. (2000). An examination of hypervigilance for external threat in individuals with generalized anxiety disorder and individuals with persecutory delusions using visual scan paths. *Quarterly Journal of Experimental Psychology, 53*(2), 549–567.

Freud, S. (1896). Further remarks on the defence neuro-psychoses. *Collected papers* (Vol. I, pp. 155–182). London, UK: Hogarth.

Freud, S. (1915a). *Mourning and melancholia* (Standard Ed.Vol. 14). London: Hogarth.

Freud, S. (1915b). A case of paranoia running counter to the psychoanalytic theory of the disease. *Standard Edition, 14*, 263–272. London, UK: Hogarth.

Freud, S. (1915c). *Instincts and their vicissitudes* (Standard Edition 14, 111–40 ed.).

Freud, S. (1924). *The economic problem of masochism* (Standard Edition 19,157–70 ed.). London: Hogarth.

Freud, S. (1925). An autobiographical study. *Standard Edition, 20*, 3–70. London, UK: Hogarth.

Freud, S. (1939). An outline of psychoanalysis. *Standard Edition, 23*, 145–146). London, UK: Hogarth.

Friedman, D., & Simpson, G. V. (1994). ERP amplitude and scalp distribution to target and novel events: Effects of temporal order in young, middle-aged, and older adults. *Cognitive Brain Research, 2*(1), 49–63.

Friedman, J., & Meares, R. (1979c). The effect of placebo and tricyclic antidepressants on cortical evoked potentials in depressed patients. *Biological Psychology, 8*(4), 291–302.

Friedman, J., & Meares, R. (1979b). Cortical evoked potentials and severity of depression. *American Journal of Psychiatry, 136*(9), 1218–1220.

Friedman, J., & Meares, R. (1979a). Cortical evoked potentials and extraversion. *Psychosomatic Medicine, 41*(4), 279–286.

Frith, C. D. (1992). *The cognitive neuropsychology of schizophrenia*. Hove, UK: Erlbaum.

Frith, C. D. (2004). The pathology of experience. *Brain, 127*(Pt. 2), 239–242.

Frith, C. D., & Frith, U. (1999). Interacting minds: A biological basis. *Science, 286*(5445), 1692–1695.

Frith, U., & Frith, C. D. (2003). Development and neurophysiology of mentalizing. *Philosophical Transactions of the Royal Society of London B Biological Sciences, 358*(1431), 459–473.

Frith, U., Morton, J., & Leslie, A. M. (1991). The cognitive basis of a biological disorder: Autism. *Trends in Neuroscience, 14*(10), 433–438.

Frodl, T., Meisenzahl, E. M., Zetzsche, T., Born, C., Groll, C., Jager, M., et al. (2002). Hippocampal changes in patients with a first episode of major depression. *American Journal of Psychiatry, 159*(7), 1112–1118.

Gallagher, H. L., & Frith, C. D. (2003). Functional imaging of "theory of mind." *Trends in Cognitive Sciences, 7*(2), 77–83.

Gallagher, H. L., Happé, F., Brunswick, N., Fletcher, P. C., Frith, U., & Frith, C. D. (2000). Reading the mind in cartoons and stories: An fMRI study of "theory of mind" in verbal and nonverbal tasks. *Neuropsychologia, 38*(1), 11–21.

Gallese, V., & Goldman, A. (1998). Mirror neurons and the simulation theory of mind-reading. *Trends in Cognitive Sciences, 2*, 493–501.

Gao, W., Zhu, H., Giovanello, K. S., Smith, J. K., Shen, D., Gilmore, J. H., et al. (2009). Evidence on the emergence of the brain's default network from 2-week-old to 2-year-old healthy pediatric subjects. *Proceedings of the National Academy of Sciences of the United States of America, 106*(16), 6790–6795.

Garavan, H., Ross, T. J., & Stein, E. A. (1999). Right hemispheric dominance of inhibitory control: An event-related functional MRI study. *Proceedings of the National Academy of Sciences of the United States of America, 96*(14), 8301–8306.

Garbutt, M. (1997). *Figure talk: Reported speech and thought in the discourse of psychotherapy.* Unpublished doctoral dissertation, Macquarie University, Sydney, AU.

Garety, P. A., Hemsley, D. R., & Wessely, S. (1991). Reasoning in deluded schizophrenic and paranoid patients. Biases in performance on a probabilistic inference task. *Journal of Nervous Mental Disease, 179*(4), 194–201.

Garety, P. A., & Freeman, D. (1999). Cognitive approaches to delusions: A critical review of theories and evidence. *British Journal of Clinical Psychology, 38*(Pt. 2), 113–154.

Gatt, J. M., Nemeroff, C. B., Schofield, P. R., Paul, R. H., Clark, C. R., Gordon, E., et al. (2010). Early life stress combined with serotonin 3A receptor and brain-derived neurotrophic factor valine 66 to methionine genotypes impacts emotional brain and arousal correlates of risk for depression. *Biological Psychiatry, 68*(9), 818–824.

Gavrilescu, M., Rossell, S., Stuart, G. W., Shea, T. L., Innes-Brown, H., Henshall, K., et al. (2010). Reduced connectivity of the auditory cortex in patients with auditory hallucinations: A resting state functional magnetic resonance imaging study. *Psychological Medicine, 40*(7), 1149–1158.

Gawler, I., & Bedson, P. (2010). *Meditation: An in-depth guide.* Sydney, AU: Allen & Unwin.

Gershon, E. S., & Buchsbaum, M. (1977). A genetic study of average evoked response augmentation/reduction in affective disorders. In C. Shagass, S. Gerson & A. H. Friedhoff (Eds.), *Psychopathology and brain dysfunction* (pp. 279–290). New York, NY: Raven Press.

Gerull, F., Meares, R., Stevenson, J., Korner, A., & Newman, L. (2008). The beneficial effect on family life in treating borderline personality. *Psychiatry, 71*(1), 59–70.

Ghaffar, O., Staines, W. R., & Feinstein, A. (2006). Unexplained neurologic symptoms: An fMRI study of sensory conversion disorder. *Neurology, 67*(11), 2036–2038.

Giesbrecht, T., Smeets, T., Merckelbach, H., & Jelicic, M. (2007). Depersonalization experiences in undergraduates are related to heightened stress cortisol responses. *Journal of Nervous and Mental Disease, 195*(4), 282–287.

Giesen-Bloo, J., van Dyck, R., Spinhoven, P., van Tilburg, W., Dirksen, C., van Asselt, T., et al. (2006). Outpatient psychotherapy for borderline personality disorder: randomized trial of schema-focused therapy vs. transference-focused psychotherapy. *Archives of General Psychiatry, 63*(6), 649–658.

Gladstone, G. L., Parker, G. B., Mitchell, P. B., Malhi, G. S., Wilhelm, K., & Austin, M. P. (2004). Implications of childhood trauma for depressed women: An analysis of pathways from childhood sexual abuse to deliberate self-harm and revictimization. *American Journal of Psychiatry, 161*(8), 1417–1425.

Glaser, J. P., Van Os, J., Mengelers, R., & Myin-Germeys, I. (2008). A momentary assessment study of the reputed emotional phenotype associated with borderline personality disorder. *Psychological Medicine, 38*(9), 1231–1239.

Goldberg, E. (2005). *The wisdom paradox.* New York, NY: Gotham Books.

Golier, J. A., Yehuda, R., Bierer, L. M., Mitropoulou, V., New, A. S., Schmeidler, J., et al. (2003). The relationship of borderline personality disorder to posttraumatic stress disorder and traumatic events. *American Journal of Psychiatry, 160*(11), 2018–2024.

Goodman, M., New, A. S., Triebwasser, J., Collins, K. A., & Siever, L. (2010). Phenotype, endophenotype, and genotype comparisons between borderline personality disorder and major depressive disorder. *Journal of Personality Disorders, 24*(1), 38–59.

Gordon, I., Zagoory-Sharon, O., Leckman, J. F., & Feldman, R. (2010). Oxytocin and the development of parenting in humans. *Biological Psychiatry,* *68*(4), 377–382.

Goyer, P. F., Andreason, P. J., Semple, W. E., Clayton, A. H., King, A. C., Compton-Toth, B. A., et al. (1994). Positron-emission tomography and personality disorders. *Neuropsychopharmacology, 10*(1), 21–28.

Graham, P., & van Biene, L. (2007). Hierarchy of engagement. In R. Meares & P. Nolan (Eds.), *The self in conversation* (Vol. VI, pp. 177–196). Sydney, AU: ANZAP Books.

Gratz, K. L., Rosenthal, M. Z., Tull, M. T., Lejuez, C. W., & Gunderson, J. G. (2010). An experimental investigation of emotional reactivity and delayed emotional recovery in borderline personality disorder: The role of shame. *Comprehensive Psychiatry, 51*(3), 275–285.

Gratz, K. L., Tull, M. T., & Gunderson, J. G. (2008). Preliminary data on the relationship between anxiety sensitivity and borderline personality disorder: The role of experiential avoidance. *Journal of Psychiatric Research, 42*(7), 550–559.

Greicius, M. D., Krasnow, B., Reiss, A. L., & Menon, V. (2003). Functional connectivity in the resting brain: A network analysis of the default mode hypothesis. *Proceedings of the National Academy of Sciences of the United States of America, 100*(1), 253–258.

Greicius, M. D., & Menon, V. (2004). Default-mode activity during a passive sensory task: Uncoupled from deactivation but impacting activation. *Journal of Cognitive Neuroscience, 16*(9), 1484–1492.

Grilo, C. M., & McGlashan, T. H. (2000). Convergent and discriminant validity of DSM-IV axis II personality disorder criteria in adult outpatients with binge eating disorder. *Comprehensive Psychiatry, 41*(3), 163–166.

Grinker, R. R., Werble, B., & Drye, R. (1968). *The borderline syndrome: A behavioral study of ego functions.* New York, NY: Basic Books.

Grossmann, K., Grossmann, K. E., Spangler, G., Suess, G., & Unzner, L. (1985). Maternal sensitivity and newborns' orientation responses as related to quality of attachment in northern Germany. *Monographs of the Society for Research in Child Development, 50*(1–2), 233–256.

Gunderson, J. G. (1977). Charcteristics of borderlines. In P. Hartocollis (Ed.), *Borderline personality disorders* (pp. 173–192). New York, NY: International Universities Press.

Gunderson, J. G. (1984). *Borderline personality disorder.* Washington, DC: American Psychiatric Association.

Gunderson, J. G. (1996). The borderline patient's intolerance of aloneness: Insecure attachments and therapist availability. *American Journal of Psychiatry, 153*(6), 752–758.

Gunderson, J. G., Carpenter, W. T., Jr., & Strauss, J. S. (1975). Borderline and schizophrenic patients: A comparative study. *American Journal of Psychiatry, 132*(12), 1257–1264.

Gunderson, J. G., & Elliott, G. R. (1985). The interface between borderline personality disorder and affective disorder. *American Journal of Psychiatry, 142*(3), 277–288.

Gunderson, J. G., & Kolb, J. E. (1978). Discriminating features of borderline patients. *American Journal of Psychiatry, 135*(7), 792–796.

Gunderson, J. G., Kolb, J. E., & Austin, V. (1981). The diagnostic interview for borderline patients. *American Journal of Psychiatry, 138*(7), 896–903.

Gunderson, J. G., & Lyons-Ruth, K. (2008). BPD's interpersonal hypersensitivity phenotype: A gene–environment–developmental model. *Journal of Personality Disorders, 22*(1), 22–41.

Gunderson, J. G., & Phillips, K. A. (1991). A current view of the interface between borderline personality disorder and depression. *American Journal of Psychiatry, 148,* 967–975.

Gunderson, J. G., & Sabo, A. N. (1993). The phenomenological and conceptual interface between borderline personality disorder and PTSD. *American Journal of Psychiatry, 150*(1), 19–27.

Gunderson, J. G., & Singer, M. T. (1975). Defining borderline patients: An overview. *American Journal of Psychiatry, 132,* 1–10.

Gupta, M. A., & Gupta, A. K. (2006). Medically unexplained cutaneous sensory symptoms may represent somatoform dissociation: An empirical study. *Journal of Psychosomatic Research, 60*(2), 131–136.

Gur, R. C., Erwin, R. J., Gur, R. E., Zwil, A. S., Heimberg, C., & Kraemer, H. C. (1992). Facial emotion discrimination: II. Behavioral findings in depression. *Psychiatry Research, 42*(3), 241–251.

Gusnard, D. A., Akbudak, E., Shulman, G. L., & Raichle, M. E. (2001). Medial prefrontal cortex and self-referential mental activity: Relation to a default mode of brain function. *Proceedings of the National Academy of Sciences of the United States of America, 98*(7), 4259–4264.

Gusnard, D. A., & Raichle, M. E. (2001). Searching for a baseline: Functional imaging and the resting human brain. *Nature Reviews Neuroscience, 2*(10), 685–694.

Haaland, V. O., & Landrø, N. I. (2007). Decision making as measured with the Iowa Gambling Task in patients with borderline personality disorder. *Journal of the International Neuropsychological Society, 13*(4), 699–703.

Hagoort, P., Brown, C. M., & Swaab, T. Y. (1996). Lexical-semantic event-related potential effects in patients with left hemisphere lesions and aphasia, and patients with right hemisphere lesions without aphasia. *Brain, 119*(Pt. 2), 627–649.

Halgren, E., & Marinkovic, K. (1993). Neurophysiological networks integrating human emotions. In M. S. Gazzaniga (Ed.), *The cognitive neurosciences* (pp. 1137–1151). Cambridge, MA: MIT Press.

Halgren, E., Baudena, P., Clarke, J. M., Heit, G., Liegeois, C., Chauvel, P., et al. (1995a). Intracerebral potentials to rare target and distractor auditory and visual stimuli: I. Superior temporal plane and parietal lobe. *Electroencephalography and Clinical Neurophysiology, 94*(3), 191–220.

Halgren, E., Baudena, P., Clarke, J. M., Heit, G., Marinkovic, K., Devaux, B., et al. (1995b). Intracerebral potentials to rare target and distractor auditory and visual stimuli: II. Medial, lateral and posterior temporal lobe. *Electroencephalography and Clinical Neurophysiology, 94*(4), 229–250.

Halliday, M. A. K. (1975–2007). *The collected works of M. A. K. Halliday: Language Society.* London & New York, NY: Continuum.

Hanson, J. L., Chung, M. K., Avants, B. B., Shirtcliff, E. A., Gee, J. C., Davidson, R. J., et al. (2010). Early stress is associated with alterations in the orbitofrontal cortex: A tensor-based morphometry investigation of brain structure and behavioral risk. *Journal of Neuroscience, 30*(22), 7466–7472.

Happaney, K., Zelazo, P. D., & Stuss, D. T. (2004). Development of orbitofrontal function: Current themes and future directions. *Brain Cognition, 55*(1), 1–10.

Happé, F. G. (1994). An advanced test of theory of mind: Understanding of story characters' thoughts and feelings by able autistic, mentally handicapped, and normal children and adults. *Journal of Autism Developmental Disorders, 24*(2), 129–154.

Harciarek, M., & Heilman, K. M. (2009). The contribution of anterior and posterior regions of the right hemisphere to the recognition of emotional faces. *Journal of Clinical and Experimental Neuropsychology, 31*(3), 322–330.

Harned, M. S., Rizvi, S. L., & Linehan, M. M. (2010). Impact of co-occurring posttraumatic stress disorder on suicidal women with borderline personality disorder. *American Journal of Psychiatry, 167*(10), 1210–1217.

Harter, S. (1983). Developmental perspectives on the self system. In P. Mussen (Ed.), *Handbook of child psychology* (Vol. 4, pp. 275–385). New York, NY: Wiley.

Hartvig, P., & Sterner, G. (1985). Childhood psychologic environmental exposure in women with diagnosed somatoform disorders. A case-control study. *Scandinavian Journal of Social Medicine, 13*(4), 153–157.

Hasan, R. (1984). Coherence and cohesive harmony. In J. Flood (Ed.), *Understanding reading comprehension: Cognition, language, and the structure of prose* (pp. 181–219). Newark, DE: International Reading Association.

Hasan, R. (1985). The texture of a text. In M. A. K. Halliday & R. Hasan (Eds.), *Language, context and text: Aspects of language in a social–semiotic perspective.* Geelong, Victoria, AU: Deakin University Press.

Hassabis, D., Kumaran, D., & Maguire, E. A. (2007). Using imagination to

Herpertz, S. C., Kunert, H. J., Schwenger, U. B., & Sass, H. (1999). Affective responsiveness in borderline personality disorder: A psychophysiological approach. *American Journal of Psychiatry, 156*(10), 1550–1556.

Herpertz, S. C., Schwenger, U. B., Kunert, H. J., Lukas, G., Gretzer, U., Nutzmann, J., et al. (2000). Emotional responses in patients with borderline as compared with avoidant personality disorder. *Journal of Personality Disorders, 14*(4), 339–351.

Hesse, E. (1996). Discourse, memory, and the Adult Attachment Interview: A note with emphasis on the emerging cannot classify category. *Infant Mental Health Journal, 17*(1), 4–11.

Hesse, E., Main, M., Abrams, K. Y., & Rifkin, A. (2003). Unresolved states regarding loss or abuse can have "second generation" effects: Disorganized, role-inversion and frightening ideation in the offspring of traumatized non-maltreating parents. In D. J. Siegel & M. F. Solomon (Eds.), *Healing trauma: Attachment, mind, body and brain* (pp. 57–106). New York, NY: Norton.

Hobson, R. F. (1985). *Forms of feeling: The heart of psychotherapy.* London, UK: Tavistock.

Hobson, R. P., Patrick, M. P., Crandell, L., Garcia-Perez, R., & Lee, A. (2005). Personal relatedness and attachment in infants of mothers with borderline personality disorder. *Development and Psychopathology, 17*(2), 329–347.

Hobson, R. P., Patrick, M. P., Hobson, J. A., Crandell, L., Bronfman, E., & Lyons-Ruth, K. (2009). How mothers with borderline personality disorder relate to their year-old infants. *British Journal of Psychiatry, 195*(4), 325–330.

Hobson, R. P., Patrick, M. P., & Valentine, J. D. (1998). Objectivity in psychoanalytic judgements. *British Journal of Psychiatry, 173,* 172–177.

Hoch, P., & Polatin, P. (1949). Pseudoneurotic forms of schizophrenia. *Psychiatric Quarterly, 23,* 248–276.

Hollander, E., Carrasco, J. L., Mullen, L. S., Trungold, S., DeCaria, C. M., & Towey, J. (1992). Left hemispheric activation in depersonalization disorder: A case report. *Biological Psychiatry, 31*(11), 1157–1162.

Holmes, E. A., Brown, R. J., Mansell, W., Fearon, R. P., Hunter, E. C., Frasquilho, F., et al. (2005). Are there two qualitatively distinct forms of dissociation?: A review and some clinical implications. *Clinical Psychological Review 25*(1), 1–23.

Honderich, T. (2005). *The Oxford companion to philosophy.* New York, NY: Oxford University Press.

Hornberger, M., Rugg, M. D., & Henson, R. N. (2006). fMRI correlates of retrieval orientation. *Neuropsychologia, 44*(8), 1425–1436.

Horowitz, J., & Telch, M. J. (2007). Dissociation and pain perception: An experimental investigation. *Journal of Traumatic Stress, 20*(4), 597–609.

Horvath, T., Friedman, J., & Meares, R. (1980). Attention in hysteria: A study of Janet's hypothesis by means of habituation and arousal measures. *American Journal of Psychiatry, 137*(2), 217–220.

Horvath, T., & Meares, R. (1979). The sensory filter in schizophrenia: A study of habituation, arousal, and the dopamine hypothesis. *British Journal of Psychiatry, 134*, 39–45.

Houston, R. J., Ceballos, N. A., Hesselbrock, V. M., & Bauer, L. O. (2005). Borderline personality disorder features in adolescent girls: P300 evidence of altered brain maturation. *Clinical Neurophysiology, 116*(6), 1424–1432.

Hozumi, A., Hirata, K., Tanaka, H., & Yamazaki, K. (2000). Perseveration for novel stimuli in Parkinson's disease: An evaluation based on event-related potentials topography. *Movement Disorder 15*(5), 835–842.

Hull, J. W., Clarkin, J. F., & Kakuma, T. (1993). Treatment response of borderline inpatients: A growth curve analysis. *Journal of Nervous and Mental Disease, 181*(8), 503–508.

Humboldt, W. (1988). *On language: The diveristy of human language—structure and its influence on the mental development of mankind* (P. Heath, Trans.). Cambridge, UK: Cambridge University Press.

Hunter, E. E., Penick, E. C., Powell, B. J., Othmer, E., Nickel, E. J., & Desouza, C. (2005). Development of scales to screen for eight common psychiatric disorders. *Journal of Nervous and Mental Disease, 193*(2), 131–135.

Hyler, S. E., & Spitzer, R. L. (1978). Hysteria split asunder. *American Journal of Psychiatry, 135*(12), 1500–1504.

Iidaka, T., Terashima, S., Yamashita, K., Okada, T., Sadato, N., & Yonekura, Y. (2003). Dissociable neural responses in the hippocampus to the retrieval of facial identity and emotion: An event-related fMRI study. *Hippocampus, 13*(4), 429–436.

Insel, T. R. (1997). A neurobiological basis of social attachment. *American Journal of Psychiatry, 154*(6), 726–735.

Insel, T. R., & Fernald, R. D. (2004). How the brain processes social information: Searching for the social brain. *Annual Review of Neuroscience, 27*, 697–722.

Insel, T. R., & Young, L. J. (2001). The neurobiology of attachment. *Nature Reviews Neuroscience, 2*(2), 129–136.

Irle, E., Lange, C., & Sachsse, U. (2005). Reduced size and abnormal asymmetry of parietal cortex in women with borderline personality disorder. *Biological Psychiatry, 57*(2), 173–182.

Jackowski, A. P., de Araujo, C. M., de Lacerda, A. L., Mari Jde, J., & Kaufman, J. (2009). Neurostructural imaging findings in children with post-traumatic stress disorder: Brief review. *Psychiatry and Clinical Neurosciences, 63*(1), 1–8.

Jackowski, A. P., Douglas-Palumberi, H., Jackowski, M., Win, L., Schultz, R. T., Staib, L. W., et al. (2008). Corpus callosum in maltreated children with posttraumatic stress disorder: A diffusion tensor imaging study. *Psychiatry Research, 162*(3), 256–261.

Jackson, J. H. (1958). *Selected writings of John Hughlings Hackson* (Vol.I & II). New York, NY: Basic Books.

Jacob, G. A., Hellstern, K., Ower, N., Pillmann, M., Scheel, C. N., Rusch, N., et al. (2009). Emotional reactions to standardized stimuli in women with borderline personality disorder: Stronger negative affect, but no differences in reactivity. *Journal of Nervous and Mental Disease, 197*(11), 808–815.

James, L., Gordon, E., Kraiuhin, C., Howson, A., & Meares, R. (1990). Augmentation of auditory evoked potentials in somatization disorder. *Journal of Psychiatric Research, 24*(2), 155–163.

James, L., Gordon, E., Kraiuhin, C., & Meares, R. (1989). Selective attention and auditory event-related potentials in somatization disorder. *Comprehensive Psychiatry, 30*(1), 84–89.

James, W. (1890). *Principles of psychology* (Vol. I & II). New York, NY: Holt.

James, W. (1892). *Psychology: Briefer course*. London, UK: Macmillan.

James, W. (1895/1968). The knowing of things together. In J. J. McDermott (Ed.), *The writings of William James* (pp. 152–168). Chicago: University of Chicago Press, 1968.

James, W. (1983). *Essays in psychology*. Cambridge, MA: Harvard University Press.

James, W. (1909/1996). *A pluralistic universe*. Lincoln, NE: University of Nebraska Press. (Original work published 1909 by Longmans Green, New York, NY)

Janet, P. (1889). *L'automatisme psychologique [Psychological automatism]*. Paris: Alcan.

Janet, P. (1901). *L'etat mental des hysteriques* [*The mental state of hystericals*] (C. R. Corson, Trans.). New York & London, UK: Putnam.

Janet, P. (1903). *Les obsessions and la psychasthénie*. Paris: Alcan.

Janet, P. (1907). *The major symptoms of hysteria*. New York & London: Macmillan.

Janet, P. (1911). *L'etat mental des hysteriques*. (2nd ed.,. Paris: Alcan.

Janet, P. (1924). *Principles of psychotherapy*. London, UK: Allen & Unwin.

Janet, P. (1925). *Psychological healing* (Vol. I, E. Paul & C. Paul, Trans.). London, UK: Allen & Unwin.

Janet, P. (1928). *L'évolution de la mémoire et la notion du temps*. Paris: Maloine.

Janet, P. (1929). *L' évolution psychologique de la personnalité*. Paris: A. Chahine.

Jaspers, K. (1997). *General psychopathology* (J. Hoenig & M. W. Hamilton, Trans.). Baltimore, MD: Johns Hopkins Press.

Jaynes, J. (1990). *The origin of consciousness in the break down of the bicameral mind.* New York, NY: Houghton Mifflin.

Johansen, M., Karterud, S., Pedersen, G., Gude, T., & Falkum, E. (2004). An investigation of the prototype validity of the borderline DSM-IV construct. *Acta Psychiatrica Scandinavica, 109*(4), 289–298.

Johnson, C., Dorahy, M. J., Courtney, D., Bayles, T., & O'Kane, M. (2009). Dysfunctional schema modes, childhood trauma and dissociation in borderline personality disorder. *Journal of Behavior Therapy and Experimental Psychiatry, 40,* 248–255.

Johnson, P. A., Hurley, R. A., Benkelfat, C., Herpertz, S. C., & Taber, K. H. (2003). Understanding emotion regulation in borderline personality disorder: Contributions of neuroimaging. *Journal of Neuropsychiatry and Clinical Neurosciences, 15*(4), 397–402.

Johnson, R., Jr. (1993). On the neural generators of the P300 component of the event-related potential. *Psychophysiology, 30*(1), 90–97.

Jones, B., Heard, H., Startup, M., Swales, M., Williams, J. M., & Jones, R. S. (1999). Autobiographical memory and dissociation in borderline personality disorder. *Psychological Medicine, 29*(6), 1397–1404.

Jones, E. (1953). *Sigmund Freud: Life and work.* London, UK: Hogarth.

Jongsma, M. L., Desain, P., & Honing, H. (2004). Rhythmic context influences the auditory evoked potentials of musicians and non-musicians. *Biological Psychology, 66*(2), 129–152.

Jung, C. G. (1957). *Psychiatric studies: C.G. Jung the collected works* (R. F. C. Hull, Trans. Vol. I). London: Routledge & Kegan Paul.

Kandel, E. R. (1976). *Cellular basis of behavior: An introduction to behavioral neurobiology.* San Francisco: Freeman.

Kaplan, M., & Klinetob, N. (2000). Childhood emotional trauma and chronic post traumatic stress disorder in adult patients with treatment resistant depression. *Journal of Nervous and Mental Disease, 188,* 596–600.

Karl, A., Schaefer, M., Malta, L. S., Dorfel, D., Rohleder, N., & Werner, A. (2006). A meta-analysis of structural brain abnormalities in PTSD. *Neuroscience and Biobehavioral Reviews, 30*(7), 1004–1031.

Kendler, K. S., Aggen, S. H., Czajkowski, N., Roysamb, E., Tambs, K., Torgersen, S., et al. (2008). The structure of genetic and environmental risk factors for DSM-IV personality disorders: A multivariate twin study. *Archives of General Psychiatry, 65*(12), 1438–1446.

Kendler, K. S., Hettema, J. M., Butera, F., Gardner, C. O., & Prescott, C. A. (2003). Life event dimensions of loss, humiliation, entrapment, and danger in the prediction of onsets of major depression and generalized anxiety. *Archives of General Psychiatry, 60*(8), 789–796.

Kendall, P. C., & Clarkin, J. F. (1992). Introduction to special section: Comorbidity and treatment implications. *Journal of Consulting and Clinical Psychology, 60*(6), 833–834.

Kernberg, O. F. (1967). Borderline personality organization. *Journal of the American Psychoanalytic Association, 15*(3), 641–685.

Kernberg, O. F. (1975). *Borderline conditions and pathological narcissism.* New York, NY: Jason Aronson.

Kernberg, O. F. (1984). *Severe personality disorders: Psychotherapeutic strategies.* New Haven, CT: Yale University Press.

Kim, J. J., Andreasen, N. C., O'Leary, D. S., Wiser, A. K., Ponto, L. L., Watkins, G. L., et al. (1999). Direct comparison of the neural substrates of recognition memory for words and faces. *Brain, 122*(Pt. 6), 1069–1083.

Klein, D. N., & Schwartz, J. E. (2002). The relation between depressive symptoms and borderline personality disorder features over time in dysthymic disorder. *Journal of Personality Disorders, 16*(6), 523–535.

Knight, R. P. (1953). Borderline states. *Bulletin of the Menninger Clinic, 17*(1), 1–12.

Knight, R. T., Scabini, D., Woods, D. L., & Clayworth, C. C. (1989). Contributions of temporal–parietal junction to the human auditory P3. *Brain Research, 502*(1), 109–116.

Knight, T., Grabowecky, M. F., & Scabini, D. (1995). Role of human prefrontal cortex in attention control. In H. H. Jasper, S. Riggio, & P. S. Goldman-Rakic (Eds.), *Epilepsy and the functional anatomy of the frontal lobe.* New York, NY: Raven Press.

Kochanska, G., Philibert, R. A., & Barry, R. A. (2009). Interplay of genes and early mother–child relationship in the development of self-regulation from toddler to preschool age. *Journal of Child Psychology and Psychiatry, 50*(11), 1331–1338.

Koenigsberg, H. W. (1982). A comparison of hospitalized and nonhospitalized borderline patients. *American Journal of Psychiatry, 139*(10), 1292–1297.

Koenigsberg, H. W. (2010). Affective instability: Toward an integration of neuroscience and psychological perspectives. *Journal of Personality Disorders, 24*(1), 60–82.

Koenigsberg, H. W., Harvey, P. D., Mitropoulou, V., New, A. S., Goodman, M., Silverman, J., et al. (2001). Are the interpersonal and identity disturbances in the borderline personality disorder criteria linked to the traits of affective instability and impulsivity? *Journal of Personality Disorders, 15*(4), 358–370.

Koenigsberg, H. W., Siever, L. J., Lee, H., Pizzarello, S., New, A. S., Goodman, M., et al. (2009). Neural correlates of emotion processing in borderline personality disorder. *Psychiatry Research, 172*(3), 192–199.

Kohut, H. (1971). *The analysis of the self.* New York, NY: International Universities Press.

Kohut, H. (1977). *The restoration of the self.* New York, NY: International Universities Press.

Kolb, B., & Whishaw, I. (1990). *Fundamentals of human neuropsychology* (3rd ed.). New York, NY: Freeman.

Kopelman, M. D. (1995). The assessment of psychogenic amnesia. In A. D. Baddeley, B. A. Wilson, & F. N. Watts (Eds.), *Handbook of memory disorders* (pp. 427–448). New York, NY: Wiley.

Kopelman, M. D., Stanhope, N., & Kingsley, D. (1999). Retrograde amnesia in patients with diencephalic, temporal lobe or frontal lesions. *Neuropsychologia, 37*(8), 939–958.

Korner, A., Gerull, F., Meares, R., & Stevenson, J. (2006). Borderline personality disorder treated with the conversational model: A replication study. *Comprehensive Psychiatry, 47*(5), 406–411.

Korner, A., Gerull, F., Stevenson, J., & Meares, R. (2007). Harm avoidance, self-harm, psychic pain, and the borderline personality: Life in a "haunted house." *Comprehensive Psychiatry, 48*(3), 303–308.

Korzekwa, M. I., Dell, P. F., Links, P. S., Thabane, L., & Fougere, P. (2009). Dissociation in borderline personality disorder: A detailed look. *Journal of Trauma and Dissociation, 10*(3), 346–367.

Korzekwa, M. I., Dell, P. F., & Pain, C. (2009). Dissociation and borderline personality disorder: An update for clinicians. *Current Psychiatry Reports, 11*(1), 82–88.

Kotze, B., & Meares, R. (1996). Erotic transference and a threatened sense of self. *British Journal of Medical Psychology, 69*(Pt. 1), 21–31.

Koyama, T., McHaffie, J. G., Laurienti, P. J., & Coghill, R. C. (2005). The subjective experience of pain: Where expectations become reality. *Proceedings of the National Academy of Sciences of the United States of America, 102*(36), 12950–12955.

Kozlowska, K., Scher, S., & Williams, L. M. (2011). Patterns of emotional-cognitive functioning in pediatric conversion patients: implications for the conceptualization of conversion disorders. *Psychosomatic Medicine, 73*(9), 775–788.

Kriechman, A. M. (1987). Siblings with somatoform disorders in childhood and adolescence. *Journal of the American Academy of Child Adolescent Psychiatry, 26*(2), 226–231.

Krystal, J. H., Woods, S. W., Hill, C. L., & Charney, D. S. (1991). Characteristics of panic attack subtypes: Assessment of spontaneous panic, situational panic, sleep panic, and limited symptom attacks. *Comprehensive Psychiatry, 32*(6), 474–480.

Kulkarni, B., Bentley, D. E., Elliott, R., Youell, P., Watson, A., Derbyshire, S. W., et al. (2005). Attention to pain localization and unpleasantness discriminates the functions of the medial and lateral pain systems. *European Journal of Neuroscience, 21*(11), 3133–3142.

Kullgren, G. (1988). Factors associated with completed suicide in borderline personality disorder. *Journal of Nervous and Mental Disease, 176*(1), 40–44.

Kumaran, D., & Maguire, E. A. (2007). Which computational mechanisms operate in the hippocampus during novelty detection? *Hippocampus, 17*(9), 735–748.

Kuo, J. R., & Linehan, M. M. (2009). Disentangling emotion processes in borderline personality disorder: Physiological and self-reported assessment of biological vulnerability, baseline intensity, and reactivity to emotionally evocative stimuli. *Journal of Abnormal Psychology, 118*(3), 531–544.

Kuyken, W., & Brewin, C. R. (1995). Autobiographical memory functioning in depression and reports of early abuse. *Journal of Abnormal Psychology, 104*(4), 585–591.

Kuyken, W., Howell, R., & Dalgleish, T. (2006). Overgeneral autobiographical memory in depressed adolescents with, versus without, a reported history of trauma. *Journal of Abnormal Psychology, 115*(3), 387–396.

Lader, M. H. (1967). Palmar skin conductance measures in anxiety and phobic states. *Journal of Psychosomatic Research, 11*(3), 271–281.

Lader, M. H. (1969). Psychophysological aspects of anxiety. In M. H. Lader (Ed.), *Studies of anxiety* (pp. 53–61). Ashford, Kent, UK: Headley.

Lader, M. H., & Sartorius, N. (1968). Anxiety in patients with hysterical conversion symptoms. *Journal of Neurology, Neurosurgery, and Psychiatry, 31*(5), 490–495.

Lagopoulos, J., Gordon, E., Barhamali, H., Lim, C. L., Li, W. M., Clouston, P., et al. (1998). Dysfunctions of automatic (P300a) and controlled (P300b) processing in Parkinson's disease. *Neurological Research, 20*(1), 5–10.

Lancet, Editors of.. (1952). *Disabilities and how to live with them*. London: Lancet.

Lane, R. D., Reiman, E. M., Axelrod, B., Yun, L. S., Holmes, A., & Schwartz, G. E. (1998). Neural correlates of levels of emotional awareness: Evidence of an interaction between emotion and attention in the anterior cingulate cortex. *Journal of Cognitive Neuroscience, 10*(4), 525–535.

Langdon, R., Michie, P. T., Ward, P. B., McConaghy, N., Catts, S. V., & Coltheart, M. (1997). Defective self and/or other mentalising in shizophrenia: A cognitive neuropsychological approach. *Cognitive Neuropsychiatry,* 2, 167–193.

Lange, C., & Irle, E. (2004). Enlarged amygdala volume and reduced hippocampal volume in young women with major depression. *Psychological Medicine, 34*(6), 1059–1064.

Lanius, R. A., Bluhm, R., Lanius, U., & Pain, C. (2006). A review of neuroimaging studies in PTSD: Heterogeneity of response to symptom provocation. *Journal of Psychiatric Research, 40*(8), 709–729.

Lanius, R. A., Williamson, P. C., Boksman, K., Densmore, M., Gupta, M., Neufeld, R. W., et al. (2002). Brain activation during script-driven imagery induced dissociative responses in PTSD: A functional magnetic resonance imaging investigation. *Biological Psychiatry, 52*(4), 305–311.

Laplanche, J., & Pontalis, J. B. (1973). *The language of psycho-analysis* (D. Nicholson-Smith, Trans.). London, UK: Hogarth.

LeDoux, J. (2003). *Synaptic self.* London, UK: Penguin.

Lee, S. H., Lee, K. J., Lee, H. J., Ham, B. J., Ryu, S. H., & Lee, M. S. (2005). Association between the 5-HT6 receptor C267T polymorphism and response to antidepressant treatment in major depressive disorder. *Psychiatry of Clinical Neuroscience, 59*(2), 140–145.

Leichsenring, F., Leibing, E., Kruse, J., New, A. S., & Leweke, F. (2011). Borderline personality disorder. *Lancet, 377*(9759), 74–84.

Lenzenweger, M. F., Lane, M. C., Loranger, A. W., & Kessler, R. C. (2007). DSM-IV personality disorders in the National Comorbidity Survey replication. *Biological Psychiatry, 62*(6), 553–564.

Lenzi, D., Trentini, C., Pantano, P., Macaluso, E., Iacoboni, M., Lenzi, G. L., et al. (2009). Neural basis of maternal communication and emotional expression processing during infant preverbal stage. *Cerebral Cortex, 19*(5), 1124–1133.

Levine, D., Marziali, E., & Hood, J. (1997). Emotion processing in borderline personality disorders. *Journal of Nervous and Mental Disease, 185*(4), 240–246.

Levitan, R. D., Parikh, S. V., Lesage, A. D., Hegadoren, K. M., Adams, M., Kennedy, S. H., et al. (1998). Major depression in individuals with a history of childhood physical or sexual abuse: Relationship to neurovegetative features, mania, and gender. *American Journal of Psychiatry, 155*(12), 1746–1752.

Levitin, D. J. (2007). *This is your brain on music.* New York, NY: Plume, Penguin.

Levy, K. N., Edell, W. S., & McGlashan, T. H. (2007). Depressive experiences in inpatients with borderline personality disorder. *Psychiatric Quarterly, 78*(2), 129–143.

Lewin, R. (1993). *Complexity: Life on the edge of chaos*. London, UK: Phoenix.

Lewis, K. L., & Grenyer, B. F. (2009). Borderline personality or complex posttraumatic stress disorder?: An update on the controversy. *Harvard Review of Psychiatry, 17*(5), 322–328.

Lewis, M. (1992). *Shame: The exposed self*. New York, NY: Free Press.

Lewis, M., & Brooks-Gunn, J. (1979). *Social cognition and the acquisition of self*. New York, NY: Plenum.

Lewis, M., & Carmody, D. P. (2008). Self-representation and brain development. *Developmental Psychology, 44*(5), 1329–1334.

Libet, B., Gleason, C. A., Wright, E. W., & Pearl, D. K. (1983). Time of conscious intention to act in relation to onset of cerebral activity (readiness-potential): The unconscious initiation of a freely voluntary act. *Brain, 106*(Pt. 3), 623–642.

Libet, B., Pearl, D. K., Morledge, D. E., Gleason, C. A., Hosobuchi, Y., & Barbaro, N. M. (1991). Control of the transition from sensory detection to sensory awareness in man by the duration of a thalamic stimulus: The cerebral "time-on" factor. *Brain, 114*(Pt. 4), 1731–1757.

Liddell, B. J., Brown, K. J., Kemp, A. H., Barton, M. J., Das, P., Peduto, A., et al. (2005). A direct brainstem–amygdala–cortical "alarm" system for subliminal signals of fear. *NeuroImage, 24*(1), 235–243.

Liddell, B. J., Williams, L. M., Rathjen, J., Shevrin, H., & Gordon, E. (2004). A temporal dissociation of subliminal versus supraliminal fear perception: An event-related potential study. *Journal of Cognitive Neuroscience, 16*(3), 479–486.

Lieb, K., Zanarini, M. C., Schmahl, C., Linehan, M. M., & Bohus, M. (2004). Borderline personality disorder. *Lancet, 364*(9432), 453–461.

Light, K. C., Smith, T. E., Johns, J. M., Brownley, K. A., Hofheimer, J. A., & Amico, J. A. (2000). Oxytocin responsivity in mothers of infants: A preliminary study of relationships with blood pressure during laboratory stress and normal ambulatory activity. *Health Psychology, 19*(6), 560–567.

Linehan, M. (1993). *Cognitive–behavioral treatment of borderline personality disorder*. New York, NY: Guilford Press.

Linehan, M., Armstrong, H., Suarez, A., Allman, D., & Heard, H. (1991). Cognitive behavioral treatment of chronically parasuicidal borderline patients. *Archives of General Psychiatry, 48*, 1060–1064.

Linehan, M. M., Heard, H. L., & Armstrong, H. E. (1993). Naturalistic follow-up of a behavioral treatment for chronically parasuicidal borderline patients. *Archives of General Psychiatry, 50*(12), 971–974.

Links, P. S., Heslegrave, R., & van Reekum, R. (1999). Impulsivity: Core aspect of borderline personality disorder. *Journal of Personality Disorders, 13*(1), 1–9.

Links, P. S., Steiner, M., & Mitton, J. (1989). Characteristics of psychosis in borderline personality disorder. *Psychopathology, 22*(4), 188–193.

Liotti, G. (1992). Disorganized/disoriented attachment in the etiology of the dissociative disorders. *Dissociation, 5*, 196–204.

Liotti, G. (1994). *La dimensione interpersonale dell coscienza [The interpersonal dimension of consciousness]*. Rome, IT: NIS.

Liotti, G. (1995). Disorganized/disoriented attachment in the psychotherapy of the dissociative disorders. In S. Goldberg, R. Muir, & J. Kerr (Eds.), *Attachment theory: Social, developmenta,l and clinical perspectives* (pp. 343–363). Hillsdale, NJ: Analytic Press.

Liotti, G. (1999). Disorganized attachment as a model for the understanding of dissociative psychopathology. In J. Solomon & C. George (Eds.), *Disorganized attachment as a model for the understanding of dissociative psychopathology* (pp. 291–317). New York, NY: Guilford Press.

Liotti, G. (2000). Disorganized attachment, models of borderline states, and evolutionary psychotherapy. In P. Gilbert & K. Bailey (Eds.), *Genes on the couch: Essays in evolutionary psychotherapy* (pp. 232–256). Hove, UK: Psychology Press.

Liotti, G. (2004). Trauma, dissociation, and disorganized attachment: Three strands of a single braid. *Psychotherapy: Theory, Research, Practice, and Training, 41*, 472–486.

Liotti, G. (2006). A model of dissociation based on attachment theory and research. *Journal of Trauma and Dissociation, 7*(4), 55–73.

Liotti, G. (2009). Attachment and dissociation. In P. Dell & D. K. O'Neill (Eds.), *Dissociation and the dissociative disorders* (pp. 53–65). New York & London: Routledge.

Liotti, G., & Pasquini, P. (2000). Predictive factors for borderline personality disorder: Patients' early traumatic experiences and losses suffered by the attachment figure. The Italian Group for the Study of Dissociation. *Acta Psychiatrica Scandinavica, 102*(4), 282–289.

Lipowski, Z. J. (1988). Somatization: The concept and its clinical application. *American Journal of Psychiatry, 145*(11), 1358–1368.

Livesley, J. (2008). Toward a genetically-informed model of borderline personality disorder. *Journal of Personality Disorders, 22*(1), 42–71.

Lucki, I. (1998). The spectrum of behaviors influenced by serotonin. *Biological Psychiatry, 44*(3), 151–162.

Ludascher, P., Bohus, M., Lieb, K., Philipsen, A., Jochims, A., & Schmahl, C. (2007). Elevated pain thresholds correlate with dissociation and aversive arousal in patients with borderline personality disorder. *Psychiatry Research, 149*(1–3), 291–296.

Ludolph, P., Westen, D., Misle, B., & Jackson, A. (1990). The borderline diagnosis in adolescents: Symptoms and developmental history. *American Journal of Psychiatry, 147,* 470–476.

Lupien, S. J., McEwen, B. S., Gunnar, M. R., & Heim, C. (2009). Effects of stress throughout the lifespan on the brain, behavior, and cognition. *Nature Reviews Neuroscience, 10*(6), 434–445.

Luria, A. R. (1972). *The man with a shattered world.* Cambridge, MA: Harvard University Press.

Lynch, T. R., Rosenthal, M. Z., Kosson, D. S., Cheavens, J. S., Lejuez, C. W., & Blair, R. J. (2006). Heightened sensitivity to facial expressions of emotion in borderline personality disorder. *Emotion, 6*(4), 647–655.

Lyons, D. M., Afarian, H., Schatzberg, A. F., Sawyer-Glover, A., & Moseley, M. E. (2002). Experience-dependent asymmetric variation in primate prefrontal morphology. *Behavioural Brain Research, 136*(1), 51–59.

Lyons-Ruth, K., Bronfman, E., & Parsons, E. (1999). Maternal frightened, frightening, or atypical behaviour and disorganized infant attachment patterns. *Monographs of the Society for Research in Child Development, 64,* 67–96.

Lyons-Ruth, K., Holmes, B., Sasvari-Szekely, M., Ronai, Z., Nemoda, Z., Pauls D. (2007). Serotonin transporter polymorphism and borderline or antisocial traits among low-income young adults. *Psychiatric Genetics, 17*(6), 339–343.

Lyons-Ruth, K., & Jacobvitz, D. (1999). Attachment disorganization: Unresolved loss, relational violence, and lapses in behavioral and attentional strategies. In J. Cassidy & P. Shaver (Eds.), *Handbook of attachment: Theory, research, and clinical implications* (pp. 520–554). New York, NY: Guilford Press.

Lyons-Ruth, K., Melnick, S., Patrick, M., & Hobson, R. P. (2007). A controlled study of hostile–helpless states of mind among borderline and dysthymic women. *Attachment and Human Development, 9*(1), 1–16.

Lyons-Ruth, K., Repacholi, B., McLeod, S., & Silva, E. (1991). Disorganized attachment behavior in infancy. Short-term stability, maternal and infant correlates, and risk-related subtypes. *Development and Psychopathology, 3,* 377–396.

Lyons-Ruth, K., Yellin, C., Melnick, S., & Atwood, G. (2005). Expanding the concept of unresolved mental states: Hostile/helpless states of mind on the Adult Attachment Interview are associated with disrupted mother–infant communication and infant disorganization. *Development and Psychopathology, 17*(1), 1–23.

Lyoo, I. K., Han, M. H., & Cho, D. Y. (1998). A brain MRI study in subjects with borderline personality disorder. *Journal of Affective Disorders, 50*(2–3), 235–243.

McBain, R., Norton, D., & Chen, Y. (2009). Females excel at basic face perception. *Acta Psychologica, 130*(2), 168–173.

McCarthy, K. L., Mergenthaler, E., Schneider, S., & Grenyer, B. F. (2011). Psychodynamic change in psychotherapy: cycles of patient-therapist linguistic interactions and interventions. *Psychotherapy Research, 21*(6), 722–731.

MacCarthy, F. (2003). *Byron: Life and legend.* London, UK: Faber & Faber.

MacLean, P. D. (1990). *The triune brain in evolution: Role in paleocerebral functions.* Toronto, ON: University of Toronto Press.

MacLeod, A. D. (1993). Putnam, Jackson, and post-traumatic stress disorder. *Journal of Nervous and Mental Disease, 181,* 709–710.

MacQueen, G. M., Campbell, S., McEwen, B. S., Macdonald, K., Amano, S., Joffe, R. T., et al. (2003). Course of illness, hippocampal function, and hippocampal volume in major depression. *Proceedings of the National Academy of Sciences of the United States of America, 100*(3), 1387–1392.

Madigan, S., Moran, G., & Pederson, D. R. (2006). Unresolved states of mind, disorganized attachment relationships, and disrupted interactions of adolescent mothers and their infants. *Developmental Psychology, 42*(2), 293–304.

Maguire, E. A., Frackowiak, R. S., & Frith, C. D. (1997). Recalling routes around London: Activation of the right hippocampus in taxi drivers. *Journal of Neuroscience, 17*(18), 7103–7110.

Maher, B. A. (1988). Anomalous experience and delusional thinking: The logic of explanations. In T. F. Oltmanns & B. A. Maher (Eds.), *Delusional beliefs* (pp. 15–33). New York, NY: Wiley.

Main, M. (1991). Metacognitive knowledge, metacognitive monitoring, and singular (coherent) vs. multiple (incoherent) model of attachment. In C. M. Parkes, J. Stevenson-Hinde, & P. Marris (Eds.), *Handbook of attachment* (pp. 127–159). London, UK: Routledge.

Main, M., & Hesse, E. (1990). Parents' unresolved traumatic experiences are related to infant disorganized attachment status: Is frightened and/or frightening parental behavior the linking mechanism? In M. T. Greenberg, D. Cicchetti, & E. M. Cummings (Eds.), *Attachment in the preschool years* (pp. 161–182). Chicago, IL: University of Chicago Press.

Main, M., & Solomon, J. (1990). *Attachment in the preschool years: Theory, research, and intervention.* Chicago, IL: University of Chicago Press.

Manian, N., & Bornstein, M. H. (2009). Dynamics of emotion regulation in infants of clinically depressed and nondepressed mothers. *Journal of Child Psychology and Psychiatry, 50*(11), 1410–1418.

Mar, R. A. (2004). The neuropsychology of narrative: Story comprehension, story production and their interrelation. *Neuropsychologia, 42*(10), 1414–1434.

Marchand, W. R. (1957). *Byron: A biography* (Vol. 1). New York, NY: Knopf.

Marcia, J. E. (1987). The identity status approach to the study of ego identity. In T. Honess & K. Yardely (Eds.), *Self and identity: Perspectives across the lifespan* (pp. 161–171). Boston, MA: Routledge & Kegan Paul.

Marcia, J. E. (1993). *Ego identity: A handbook for psychosocial research*. New York, NY: Springer-Verlag.

Marshall, J. C., Halligan, P. W., Fink, G. R., Wade, D. T., & Frackowiak, R. S. (1997). The functional anatomy of a hysterical paralysis. *Cognition, 64*(1), B1–8.

Mason, M. F., Norton, M. I., Van Horn, J. D., Wegner, D. M., Grafton, S. T., & Macrae, C. N. (2007). Wandering minds: The default network and stimulus-independent thought. *Science, 315*(5810), 393–395.

Masterson, J. (1972). *Treatment of borderline adolescents: A developmental approach*. New York, NY: Wiley.

Mauss, M. (1969). *The gift*. London: Routledge.

Mayberg, H. S. (2007). Defining the neural circuitry of depression: Toward a new nosology with therapeutic implications. *Biological Psychiatry, 61*(6), 729–730.

McCrory, E., De Brito, S. A., & Viding, E. (2010). Research review: The neurobiology and genetics of maltreatment and adversity. *Journal of Child Psychology and Psychiatry, 51*(10), 1079–1095.

McDermid, A. J., Rollman, G. B., & McCain, G. A. (1996). Generalized hypervigilance in fibromyalgia: Evidence of perceptual amplification. *Pain, 66*(2–3), 133–144.

McDougall, W. (1926). *An outline of abnormal psychology*. London, UK: Methuen.

McGlashan, T. H., Grilo, C. M., Skodol, A. E., Gunderson, J. G., Shea, M. T., Morey, L. C., et al. (2000). The Collaborative Longitudinal Personality Disorders Study: Baseline Axis I/II and II/II diagnostic co-occurrence. *Acta Psychiatrica Scandinavica, 102*(4), 256–264.

McGuire, P. K., Robertson, D., Thacker, A., David, A. S., Kitson, N., Frackowiak, R. S., et al. (1997). Neural correlates of thinking in sign language. *NeuroReport, 8*(3), 695–698.

McGuire, P. K., Silbersweig, D. A., Wright, I., Murray, R. M., David, A. S., Frackowiak, R. S., et al. (1995). Abnormal monitoring of inner speech: A physiological basis for auditory hallucinations. *Lancet, 346*(8975), 596–600.

McKiernan, K. A., D'Angelo, B. R., Kaufman, J. N., & Binder, J. R. (2006). Interrupting the "stream of consciousness": An fMRI investigation. *NeuroImage, 29*(4), 1185–1191.

Meares, A. (1958). *The door of serenity: A study in the therapeutic use of symbolic painting*. London: Faber & Faber.

Meares, R. (1976). The secret. *Psychiatry, 39*(3), 258–265.

Meares, R. (1977). *The pursuit of intimacy: An approach to psychotherapy.* Melbourne: Nelson.

Meares, R. (1980). Body feeling in human relations: The possible examples of Brancusi and Giacometti. *Psychiatry, 43*(2), 160–167.

Meares, R. (1983). Keats and the "impersonal" therapist: A note on empathy and the therapeutic screen. *Psychiatry, 46*(1), 73–82.

Meares, R. (1984). Inner space: Its constriction in anxiety states and narcissistic personality. *Psychiatry, 47*(2), 162–171.

Meares, R. (1988). The secret, lies and the paranoid process. *Contemporary Psychoanalysis, 24,* 650–666.

Meares, R. (1993a). *The metaphor of play: Disruption and restoration in the borderline experience.* Northvale, NJ: Jason Aronson.

Meares, R. (1993b). Reversals: on certain pathologies of identification. In E. Goldberg (Ed.), *Progress in Self Psychology* (Vol. 9, pp. 231–246). Hillsdale, New Jersey: Analytic Press.

Meares, R. (1997). Stimulus entrapment. *Psychoanalytic Inquiry, 17*(2), 223–234.

Meares, R. (1998). The self in conversation: On narratives, chronicles and scripts. *Psychoanalytic Dialogues, 8,* 875–891.

Meares, R. (1999a). The contribution of Hughlings Jackson to an understanding of dissociation. *American Journal of Psychiatry, 156*(12), 1850–1855.

Meares, R. (1999b). The "dualistic" representation of trauma: On malignant internalization. *American Journal of Psychotherapy, 53*(3), 392–402.

Meares, R. (1999c). Value, trauma, and personal reality. *Bulletin of the Menninger Clinic, 63*(4), 443–458.

Meares, R. (2000). *Intimacy and alienation: Memory, trauma and personal being.* London, UK: Routledge.

Meares, R. (2000b). Priming and projective identification. *Bulletin of the Menninger Clinic, 64*(1), 76–90.

Meares, R. (2001a). A specific developmental deficit in obsessive–compulsive disorder: The example of the wolf man. *Psychoanalytic Inquiry, 21,* 289–319.

Meares, R. (2001b). What happens next?: A developmental model of therapeutic spontaneity commentary on paper by Philip A. Ringstrom. *Psychoanalytic Dialogues, 11,* 755–769.

Meares, R. (2004a). Attacks upon value: A new approach to depression. In R. Meares & P. Nolan (Eds.), *Self in conversation* (pp. 10–22). Sydney, AU: ANZAP.

Meares, R. (2004b). The conversational model: An outline. *American Journal of Psychotherapy, 58*(1), 51–66.

Meares, R. (2005). *The metaphor of play: Origin and breakdown of personal being,* (Rev. & exp. ed.). London, UK: Routledge.

Meares, R., & Horvath, T. (1972). "Acute" and "chronic" hysteria. *British Journal of Psychiatry, 121*(565), 653–657.

Meares, R., & Horvath, T. (1974). A physiological approach to the study of attachment: The mother's attention and her infant's heart rate. *Australian and New Zealand Journal of Psychiatry, 8*(1), 3–7.

Meares, R. A., & Hobson, R. F. (1977). The persecutory therapist. *British Journal of Medical Psychology, 50*(4), 349–359.

Meares, R., Penman, R., Milgrom-Friedman, J., & Baker, K. (1982). Some origins of the 'difficult' child: the Brazelton scale and the mother's view of her new-born's character. *British Journal of Medical Psychology, 55*(Pt 1), 77–86.

Meares, R., & Orlay, W. (1988). On self-boundary: A study of the development of the concept of secrecy. *British Journal of Medical Psychology, 61*(Pt. 4), 305–316.

Meares, R., & Anderson, J. (1993). Intimate space: On the developmental significance of exchange. *Contemporary Psychoanalysis, 29*(4), 595–612.

Meares, R., Stevenson, J., & Comerford, A. (1999). Psychotherapy with borderline patients: I. A comparison between treated and untreated cohorts. *Australian and New Zealand Journal of Psychiatry, 33*(4), 467–472; discussion 478–481.

Meares, R., Stevenson, J., & Gordon, E. (1999a). A Jacksonian and biopsychosocial hypothesis concerning borderline and related phenomena. *Australian and New Zealand Journal of Psychiatry, 33*(6), 831–840.

Meares, R., & Sullivan, G. (2002). Two forms of human language. In G. Williams & A. Lukin (Eds.), *Language development: Functional perspective in evolution and autogenesis* (pp. 184–195). London, UK: Continuum.

Meares, R., Butt, D. G., Henderson-Brooks, C., & Samir, H. (2005). A poetics of change. *Psychoanalytic Dialogues, 15*(5), 661–680.

Meares, R., Melkonian, D., Gordon, E., & Williams, L. (2005). Distinct pattern of P3a event-related potential in borderline personality disorder. *NeuroReport, 16*(3), 289–293.

Meares, R., Gerull, F., Korner, A., Melkonian, D., Stevenson, J., & Samir, H. (2008). Somatization and stimulus entrapment. *Journal of the American Academy of Psychoanalysis and Dynamic Psychiatry, 36*(1), 165–180.

Meares, R., & Jones, S. (2009). Analogical relatedness in personal integration or coherence. *Contemporary Psychoanalysis, 45*(4), 504–519.

Meares, R., Schore, A., & Melkonian, D. (2011a). Is borderline personality a particularly right hemispheric disorder?: A study of P3a using single trial analysis. *Australian and New Zealand Journal of Psychiatry, 45*(2), 131–139.

Meares, R., Gerull, F., Stevenson, J., & Korner, A. (2011b). Is self disturbance the core of borderline personality disorder?: An outcome study of borderline personality factors. *Australian and New Zealand Journal of Psychiatry, 45*(3), 214.

Meares, R., Melkonian, D., Felmingham, K., Brown, K., Williams, L. M., & Bryant, R. (2011, March). *The impact of dissociation in posttraumatic stress disorder (PTSD) in electrical brain activity.* Paper presented at the 11th International Society for the Study of Personality Disorders Congress, Melbourne, Australia.

Meares, R., Bendit, N., Haliburn, J., Korner, A., Mears, D., & Butt, D. (2012). *Borderline Personality Disorder and the Conversational Model: A Clinician's Manual.* New York, NY: Norton.

Mechanic, D. (1980). The experience and reporting of common physical complaints. *Journal of Health and Social Behavior, 21*(2), 146–155.

Mehta, M. A., Golembo, N. I., Nosarti, C., Colvert, E., Mota, A., Williams, S. C., et al. (2009). Amygdala, hippocampal and corpus callosum size following severe early institutional deprivation: The English and Romanian adoptees study pilot. *Journal of Child Psychology and Psychiatry, 50*(8), 943–951.

Melkonian, D., Blumenthal, T. D., & Meares, R. (2003). High-resolution fragmentary decomposition: A model-based method of non-stationary electrophysiological signal analysis. *Journal of Neuroscience Methods, 131*(1–2), 149–159.

Melkonian, D., Gordon, E., & Bahramali, H. (2001). Single-event-related potential analysis by means of fragmentary decomposition. *Biological Cybernetics, 85*(3), 219–229.

Mervaala, E., Fohr, J., Kononen, M., Valkonen-Korhonen, M., Vainio, P., Partanen, K., et al. (2000). Quantitative MRI of the hippocampus and amygdala in severe depression. *Psychological Medicine, 30*(1), 117–125.

Milgrom-Friedman, J., Penman, R., & Meares, R. (1980). Some pilot studies of early attachment and detachment behaviour. In E. J. Anthony & C. Chiland (Eds.), *The child in his family: Preventive child psychiatry in an age of transition.* New York, NY: Wiley.

Miltner, W., Johnson, R., Jr., Braun, C., & Larbig, W. (1989). Somatosensory event-related potentials to painful and non-painful stimuli: Effects of attention. *Pain, 38*(3), 303–312.

Minagawa-Kawai, Y., Matsuoka, S., Dan, I., Naoi, N., Nakamura, K., & Kojima, S. (2009). Prefrontal activation associated with social attachment:

Facial-emotion recognition in mothers and infants. *Cerebral Cortex, 19*(2), 284–292.

Minzenberg, M. J., Fan, J., New, A. S., Tang, C. Y., & Siever, L. J. (2007). Fronto-limbic dysfunction in response to facial emotion in borderline personality disorder: An event-related fMRI study. *Psychiatry Research, 155*(3), 231–243.

Minzenberg, M. J., Fan, J., New, A. S., Tang, C. Y., & Siever, L. J. (2008). Frontolimbic structural changes in borderline personality disorder. *Journal of Psychiatric Research, 42*(9), 727–733.

Minzenberg, M. J., Poole, J. H., & Vinogradov, S. (2006). Social-emotion recognition in borderline personality disorder. *Comprehensive Psychiatry, 47*(6), 468–474.

Moldin, S. O., Rice, J. P., Erlenmeyer-Kimling, L., & Squires-Wheeler, E. (1994). Latent structure of DSM-III-R Axis II psychopathology in a normal sample. *Journal of Abnormal Psychology, 103*(2), 259–266.

Moody, R. L. (1946). Bodily changes during abreaction. *Lancet, 2*(6435), 934.

Moody, R. L. (1948). Bodily changes during abreaction. *Lancet, 1*(6512), 964.

Moreau de Tours, J. J. (1845/1973). *Du haschish et de l'Aliénation mentale: Études psychologiques* [Hashish and mental illness]. New York, NY: Raven Press.

Morris, J. S., DeGelder, B., Weiskrantz, L., & Dolan, R. J. (2001). Differential extrageniculostriate and amygdala responses to presentation of emotional faces in a cortically blind field. *Brain, 124*(Pt. 6), 1241–1252.

Moser, E. I., Kropff, E., & Moser, M. B. (2008). Place cells, grid cells, and the brain's spatial representation system. *Annual Review of Neuroscience, 31*, 69–89.

Munafo, M. R., Brown, S. M., & Hariri, A. R. (2008). Serotonin transporter (*5-HTTLPR*) genotype and amygdala activation: A meta-analysis. *Biological Psychiatry, 63*(9), 852–857.

Murphy, J. M., Nierenberg, A. A., Laird, N. M., Monson, R. R., Sobol, A. M., & Leighton, A. H. (2002). Incidence of major depression predictions from subthreshold categories in the Stirling County study. *Journal of Affective Disorders, 68*, 251–259.

Murray, H. A. (1938). *Explorations on personality*. New York, NY: Oxford University Press.

Myers, C. S. (1915). A contribution to the study of shell shock: Being an account of three cases of loss of memory, vision, smell and taste, admitted into the Duchess of Westminster's War Hospital, Le Touquet. *Lancet, 185*(4772), 316–320.

Myers, C. S. (1940). *Shell-shock in France 1914–18*. Cambridge, UK: Cambridge University Press.

Nelson, K. (1992). Emergence of autobiographical memory at four. *Human Development, 35,* 172–177.

Nemeroff, C. B., Heim, C. M., Thase, M. E., Klein, D. N., Rush, A. J., Schatzberg, A. F., et al. (2003). Differential responses to psychotherapy versus pharmacotherapy in patients with chronic forms of major depression and childhood trauma. *Proceedings of the National Academy of Sciences of the United States of America, 100*(24), 14293–14296.

New, A. S., & Siever, L. J. (2002). Neurobiology and genetics of borderline personality disorder. *Psychiatric Annals, 32*(6), 329–336.

Ni, X., Chan, D., McMain, S., & Kennedy, J. L. (2009). Serotonin genes and gene–gene *progress in neuro-psychopharmacology and biological psychiatry* interactions in borderline personality disorder in a matched case-control study., *33,* 128–133.

Nica, E. I., & Links, P. S. (2009). Affective instability in borderline personality disorder: Experience sampling findings. *Current Psychiatry Reports, 11*(1), 74–81.

Nijenhuis, E. R. (2000). Somatoform dissociation: Major symptoms of dissociative disorders. *Journal of Trauma and Dissociation, 1,* 7–32.

Nijenhuis, E. R., van Dyck, R., Spinhoven, P., van der Hart, O., Chatrou, M., Vanderlinden, J., et al. (1999). Somatoform dissociation discriminates among diagnostic categories over and above general psychopathology. *Australian and New Zealand Journal of Psychiatry, 33*(4), 511–520.

Nitschke, J. B., Nelson, E. E., Rusch, B. D., Fox, A. S., Oakes, T. R., & Davidson, R. J. (2004). Orbitofrontal cortex tracks positive mood in mothers viewing pictures of their newborn infants. *NeuroImage, 21*(2), 583–592.

Noriuchi, M., Kikuchi, Y., & Senoo, A. (2008). The functional neuroanatomy of maternal love: Mother's response to infant's attachment behaviors. *Biological Psychiatry, 63*(4), 415–423.

Nurnberg, H. G., Hurt, S. W., Feldman, A., & Suh, R. (1988). Evaluation of diagnostic criteria for borderline personality disorder. *American Journal of Psychiatry, 145*(10), 1280–1284.

O'Doherty, J., Winston, J., Critchley, H., Perrett, D., Burt, D. M., & Dolan, R. J. (2003). Beauty in a smile: The role of medial orbitofrontal cortex in facial attractiveness. *Neuropsychologia, 41*(2), 147–155.

Ogawa, J. R., Sroufe, L. A., Weinfield, N. S., Carlson, E. A., & Egeland, B. (1997). Development and the fragmented self: Longitudinal study of dissociative symptomatology in a nonclinical sample. *Development and Psychopathology, 9*(4), 855–879.

Ogden, T. (1982). *Projective identification and psychotherapeutic technique*. New York, NY: Aronson.

Ogden, T. (2002). A new reading of object relations theory. *International Journal of Psychoanalysis, 83*(76), 767–782.

O'Keefe, J., & Dostrovsky, J. (1971). The hippocampus as a spatial map: Preliminary evidence from unit activity in the freely-moving rat. *Brain Research, 34*(1), 171–175.

Olson, I. R., Chun, M. M., & Allison, T. (2001). Contextual guidance of attention: Human intracranial event-related potential evidence for feedback modulation in anatomically early temporally late stages of visual processing. *Brain, 124*(Pt. 7), 1417–1425.

Opitz, B., Mecklinger, A., Friederici, A. D., & von Cramon, D. Y. (1999). The functional neuroanatomy of novelty processing: Integrating ERP and fMRI results. *Cerebral Cortex, 9*(4), 379–391.

Oxford English Dictionary: Compact edition. (1971). Oxford: Clarendon Press, Oxford University.

Ozer, E. J., Best, S. R., Lipsey, T. L., & Weiss, D. S. (2003). Predictors of posttraumatic stress disorder and symptoms in adults: A meta-analysis. *Psychological Bulletin, 129*(1), 52–73.

Panksepp, J., & Trevarthen, C. (2009). The neuroscience of emotion in music. In S. Malloch & C. Trevarthen, *Communicative Musicality* (pp. 105–146). New York, NY: Oxford University Press.

Paris, J., Brown, R., & Nowlis, D. (1987). Long-term follow-up of borderline patients in a general hospital. *Comprehensive Psychiatry, 28*(6), 530–535.

Paris, J., Gunderson, J., & Weinberg, I. (2007). The interface between borderline personality disorder and bipolar spectrum disorders. *Comprehensive Psychiatry, 48*(2), 145–154.

Paris, J., & Zweig-Frank, H. (2001). A 27-year follow-up of patients with borderline personality disorder. *Comprehensive Psychiatry, 42*(6), 482–487.

Partridge, E. (1983). *Origins: A short etymological dictionary of modern English.* New York, NY: Greenwich House.

Pascual, J. C., Soler, J., Barrachina, J., Campins, M. J., Alvarez, E., Perez, V., et al. (2008). Failure to detect an association between the serotonin transporter gene and borderline personality disorder. *Journal of Psychiatric Research, 42*(1), 87–88.

Pasquini, P., Liotti, G., Mazzotti, E., Fassone, G., & Picardi, A. (2002). Risk factors in the early family life of patients suffering from dissociative disorders. *Acta Psychiatrica Scandinavica, 105*(2), 110–116.

Patrick, M. (1994). Personality disorder and the mental representation of early social experience. *Development and Psychopathology, 6*, 375–388.

Patterson, J. C., Ungerleider, L. G., & Bandettini, P. A. (2002). Task-independent functional brain activity correlation with skin conductance changes: An fMRI study. *NeuroImage, 17*(4), 1797–1806.

Pearlson, G. D., Barta, P. E., Powers, R. E., Menon, R. R., Richards, S. S., Aylward, E. H., et al. (1997). Medial and superior temporal gyral volumes and cerebral asymmetry in schizophrenia versus bipolar disorder. *Biological Psychiatry, 41,* 1–14.

Peirce, C. S. (1932). Elements of logic. In C. Hartshorne & P. Weiss (Eds.), *Collected papers of Charles Sanders Peirce* (Vol. 2). Cambridge, MA: Harvard University Press.

Penman, R., Meares, R., Baker, K., & Milgrom-Friedman, J. (1983). Synchrony in mother–infant interaction: A possible neurophysiological base. *British Journal of Medical Psychology, 56*(Pt. 1), 1–7.

Perez-Rodriguez, M. M., Weinstein, S., New, A. S., Bevilacqua, L., Yuan, Q., Zhou, Z., et al. (2010). Tryptophan-hydroxylase 2 haplotype association with borderline personality disorder and aggression in a sample of patients with personality disorders and healthy controls. *Journal of Psychiatric Research, 44*(15), 1075–1081.

Perley, M. J., & Guze, S. B. (1962). Hysteria—the stability and usefulness of clinical criteria: A quantitative study based on a follow-up period of six to eight years in 39 patients. *New England Journal of Medicine, 266,* 421–426.

Perner, J., & Ruffman, T. (1995). Episodic memory and autonoetic consciousness: Developmental evidence and a theory of childhood amnesia. *Journal of Experimental Child Psychology, 59*(3), 516–548.

Perner, J., & Wimmer, H. (1985). John thinks that Mary thinks that . . .": Attribution of second-order false beliefs by 5–10-year-old children. *Journal of Experimental Child Psychology, 39,* 437–471.

Perry, J. C., & Klerman, G. L. (1980). Clinical features of the borderline personality disorder. *American Journal of Psychiatry, 137*(2), 165–173.

Persad, S. M., & Polivy, J. (1993). Differences between depressed and non-depressed individuals in the recognition of and response to facial emotional cues. *Journal of Abnormal Psychology, 102*(3), 358–368.

Petrie, A. (1967). *Individuality in pain and suffering.* Chicago: University of Chicago Press.

Petrovic, P., Carlsson, K., Petersson, K. M., Hansson, P., & Ingvar, M. (2004). Context-dependent deactivation of the amygdala during pain. *Journal of Cognitive Neuroscience, 16*(7), 1289–1301.

Petrovic, P., Dietrich, T., Fransson, P., Andersson, J., Carlsson, K., & Ingvar, M. (2005). Placebo in emotional processing: Induced expectations of anxiety relief activate a generalized modulatory network. *Neuron, 46*(6), 957–969.

Phillips, M. L., Medford, N., Senior, C., Bullmore, E. T., Suckling, J., Brammer, M. J., et al. (2001). Depersonalization disorder: Thinking without feeling. *Psychiatry Research, 108*(3), 145–160.

Piaget, J. (1959). *The language and thought of the child* (M. R. Gabain, Trans., 3rd ed.). London, UK: Routledge & Kegan Paul.

Pine, F. (1986). On the development of the "borderline-child-to-be." *American Journal of Orthopsychiatry, 56,* 450–457.

Pizzagalli, D. A., Sherwood, R. J., Henriques, J. B., & Davidson, R. J. (2005). Frontal brain asymmetry and reward responsiveness: A source-localization study. *Psychological Science, 16*(10), 805–813.

Polich, J. (2004). Neuropsychology of P3a and P3b: A theoretical overview. In N. C. Moore &. K. Arikan (Eds.), *Brainwave and mind: Recent developments* (pp. 15–29). Wheaton, IL: Kjellberg.

Polich, J. (2007). Updating P300: An integrative theory of P3a and P3b. *Clinical Neurophysiology, 118*(10), 2128–2148.

Porges, S. W. (1992). Vagal tone: A physiologic marker of stress vulnerability. *Pediatrics, 90*(3 Pt. 2), 498–504.

Porges, S. W. (2007). The polyvagal perspective. *Biological Psychology, 74*(2), 116–143.

Porges, S. W. (2009). The polyvagal theory: New insights into adaptive reactions of the autonomic nervous system. *Cleveland Clinic Journal of Medicine, 76*(Suppl. 2), S86–90.

Posner, M. I., Rothbart, M. K., Vizueta, N., Levy, K. N., Evans, D. E., Thomas, K. M., et al. (2002). Attentional mechanisms of borderline personality disorder. *Proceedings of the National Academy of Sciences of the United States of America, 99*(25), 16366–16370.

Premack, D. G., & Woodruff, G. (1978). Does the chimpanzee have a theory of mind? *Behavioral and Brain Sciences, 4,* 515–526.

Putnam, J. J. (1898). On the aetiology and pathogenesis of the postraumatic psychoneuroses and neuroses. *Journal of Nervous and Mental Disease, 25,* 769–799.

Raichle, M. E., & Gusnard, D. A. (2002). Appraising the brain's energy budget. *Proceedings of the National Academy of Sciences of the United States of America, 99*(16), 10237–10239.

Raichle, M. E., MacLeod, A. M., Snyder, A. Z., Powers, W. J., Gusnard, D. A., & Shulman, G. L. (2001). A default mode of brain function. *Proceedings of the National Academy of Sciences of the United States of America, 98*(2), 676–682.

Raichle, M. E., & Mintun, M. A. (2006). Brain work and brain imaging. *Annual Review of Neuroscience, 29,* 449–476.

Rapp, P., & Bachevalier, J. (2008). Cognitive development and aging. In L. Squire et al. (Eds.), *Fundamental neuroscience* (pp. 1039–1066). Amsterdam, NL: Elsevier.

Reed, S. F., Ohel, G., David, R., & Porges, S. W. (1999). A neural explanation of fetal heart rate patterns: A test of the polyvagal theory. *Developmental Psychobiology, 35*(2), 108–118.

Reichborn-Kjennerud, T. (2008). Genetics of personality disorders. *Psychiatric Clinics of North America, 31*(3), 421–440.

Reisch, T., Ebner-Priemer, U. W., Tschacher, W., Bohus, M., & Linehan, M. M. (2008). Sequences of emotions in patients with borderline personality disorder. *Acta Psychiatrica Scandinavica, 118*(1), 42–48.

Resnick, H. S., Falsetti, S. A., Kilpatrick, D. G., & Foy, D. W. (1994). *Associations between panic attacks during rape assaults and follow-up PTSD or panic-attack outcomes.* Paper presented at the 10th annual meeting of the International Society of Traumatic Stress Studies.

Richardson, R. D. (2006). *William James: In the maelstrom of American modernism.* Boston, MA: Houghton Mifflin.

Riecker, A., Wildgruber, D., Dogil, G., Grodd, W., & Ackermann, H. (2002). Hemispheric lateralization effects of rhythm implementation during syllable repetitions: An fMRI study. *NeuroImage, 16*(1), 169–176.

Rivers, W. H. R. (1922). Dissociation. In *Instinct and the Unconscious: a contribution to a biological theory of psycho-neuroses* (2nd ed., Vol. viii, pp. 71–85). Cambridge, UK: Cambridge University Press.

Roberts, N. A., Beer, J. S., Werner, K. H., Scabini, D., Levens, S. M., Knight, R. T., et al. (2004). The impact of orbital prefrontal cortex damage on emotional activation to unanticipated and anticipated acoustic startle stimuli. *Cognitive Affective and Behavioral Neuroscience, 4*(3), 307–316.

Roberts, W. W. (1960). Normal and abnormal depersonalization. *Journal of Mental Science, 106,* 478–493.

Rodrigues, E., Wenzel, A., Ribeiro, M. P., Quarantini, L. C., Miranda-Scippa, A., de Sena, E. P., et al. (2010). Hippocampal volume in borderline personality disorder with and without comorbid posttraumatic stress disorder: A meta-analysis. *European Psychiatry, 26,* 452–456.

Rosenbaum, S., Stuss, D. T., Levine, B., & Tulving, E. (2007). Theory of mind is independent of episodic memory. *Science, 318,* 1257.

Ross, E. D., & Monnot, M. (2008). Neurology of affective prosody and its functional–anatomic organization in right hemisphere. *Brain and Language, 104*(1), 51–74.

Roth, M. (2004). Depersonalization. In R. L. Gregory (Ed.), *The companion to the mind* (pp. 247–248). Oxford, UK: Oxford University Press.

Rubinow, D. R., & Post, R. M. (1992). Impaired recognition of affect in facial expression in depressed patients. *Biological Psychiatry, 31*(9), 947–953.

Rueckert, L., & Naybar, N. (2008). Gender differences in empathy: The role of the right hemisphere. *Brain and Cognition, 67*(2), 162–167.

Rugg, M. D., Otten, L. J., & Henson, R. N. (2002). The neural basis of episodic memory: Evidence from functional neuroimaging. *Philosophical Transactions of the Royal Society of London B Biological Sciences, 357*(1424), 1097–1110.

Rule, R. R., Shimamura, A. P., & Knight, R. T. (2002). Orbitofrontal cortex and dynamic filtering of emotional stimuli. *Cognitive Affective Behavioural Neuroscience, 2*(3), 264–270.

Ruocco, A. C. (2005). The neuropsychology of borderline personality disorder: A meta-analysis and review. *Psychiatry Research, 137*(3), 191–202.

Rusch, N., van Elst, L. T., Ludaescher, P., Wilke, M., Huppertz, H. J., Thiel, T., et al. (2003). A voxel-based morphometric MRI study in female patients with borderline personality disorder. *NeuroImage, 20*(1), 385–392.

Russell, B. (1921). *The analysis of mind*. London, UK: Allen & Unwin; New York, NY: Macmillan.

Russell, B. (1971). *The autobiography of Bertrand Russell* (Vol. I). London, UK: George Allen Unwin.

Russell, J. J., Moskowitz, D. S., Zuroff, D. C., Sookman, D., & Paris, J. (2007). Stability and variability of affective experience and interpersonal behavior in borderline personality disorder. *Journal of Abnormal Psychology, 116*(3), 578–588.

Rycroft, C. (1972). *A critical dictionary of psychoanalysis*. Harmondsworth, UK: Penguin.

Ryle, G. (1949). *The concept of mind*. London: Hutchinson.

Sadikaj, G., Russell, J. J., Moskowitz, D. S., & Paris, J. (2010). Affect dysregulation in individuals with borderline personality disorder: Persistence and interpersonal triggers. *Journal of Personality Assessment, 92*(6), 490–500.

Sanislow, C. A., Grilo, C. M., & McGlashan, T. H. (2000). Factor analysis of the DSM-III-R borderline personality disorder criteria in psychiatric inpatients. *American Journal of Psychiatry, 157*(10), 1629–1633.

Sapolsky, R. M., Uno, H., Rebert, C. S., & Finch, C. E. (1990). Hippocampal damage associated with prolonged glucocorticoid exposure in primates. *Journal of Neuroscience, 10*(9), 2897–2902.

Sarfati, Y., Hardy-Bayle, M. C., Besche, C., & Widlocher, D. (1997). Attribution of intentions to others in people with schizophrenia: A non-verbal exploration with comic strips. *Schizophrenia Research, 25*(3), 199–209.

Sartre, J. P. (1966). *The psychology of imagination*. New York, NY: Citadel.

Schmahl, C. G., Elzinga, B. M., Ebner, U. W., Simms, T., Sanislow, C., Vermetten, E., et al. (2004). Psychophysiological reactivity to traumatic and abandonment scripts in borderline personality and posttraumatic stress disorders: A preliminary report. *Psychiatry Research, 126*(1), 33–42.

Schmahl, C. G., Vermetten, E., Elzinga, B. M., & Bremner, J. D. (2003). Magnetic resonance imaging of hippocampal and amygdala volume in women with childhood abuse and borderline personality disorder. *Psychiatry Research, 122*(3), 193–198.

Schmahl, C. G., Vermetten, E., Elzinga, B. M., & Bremner, J. D. (2004). A positron emission tomography study of memories of childhood abuse in borderline personality disorder. *Biological Psychiatry, 55*(7), 759–765.

Schneider, F., Bermpohl, F., Heinzel, A., Rotte, M., Walter, M., Tempelmann, C., et al. (2008). The resting brain and our self: Self-relatedness modulates resting state neural activity in cortical midline structures. *Neuroscience, 157*(1), 120–131.

Schore, A. N. (2000). Attachment and the regulation of the right brain. *Attachment and Human Development, 2*(1), 23–47.

Schore, A. N. (2001). The effects of relational trauma on right brain development, affect regulation, and infant mental health. *Infant Mental Health Journal, 22,* 201–269.

Schore, A. N. (2002). Dysregulation of the right brain: A fundamental mechanism of traumatic attachment and the psychopathogenesis of posttraumatic stress disorder. *Australian and New Zealand Journal of Psychiatry, 36*(1), 9–30.

Schore, A. N. (2003a). *Affect dysregulation and disorders of the self.* New York, NY: Norton.

Schore, A. N. (2003b). *Affect dysregulation and the repair of self.* New York, NY: Norton.

Schore, A. N. (2005). Back to basics: Attachment, affect regulation, and the developing right brain—linking developmental neuroscience to pediatrics. *Pediatrisc in Review, 26*(6), 204–217.

Schutz, L. E. (2005). Broad-perspective perceptual disorder of the right hemisphere. *Neuropsychological Review, 15*(1), 11–27.

Schwerdtfeger, A., & Friedrich-Mai, P. (2009). Social interaction moderates the relationship between depressive mood and heart rate variability: Evidence from an ambulatory monitoring study. *Health Psychology, 28*(4), 501–509.

Scott, J., Chant, D., Andrews, G., & McGrath, J. (2006). Psychotic-like experiences in the general community: The correlates of CIDI psychosis screen items in an Australian sample. *Psychological Medicine, 36*(2), 231–238.

Seal, M. L., Aleman, A., & McGuire, P. K. (2004). Compelling imagery, unanticipated speech and deceptive memory: neurocognitive models of auditory verbal hallucinations in schizophrenia. *Cognition and Neuropsychiatry, 9*(1–2), 43–72.

Segal, H. (1973). *Introduction to the Works of Melanie Klein.* New York, NY: Basic Books.

Seigel, J. (2005). *The idea of the self.* Cambridge, UK: Cambridge University Press.

Sestieri, C., Shulman, G. L., & Corbetta, M. (2010). Attention to memory and the environment: Functional specialization and dynamic competition in human posterior parietal cortex. *Journal of Neuroscience, 30*(25), 8445–8456.

Shah, P. J., Ebmeier, K. P., Glabus, M. F., & Goodwin, G. M. (1998). Cortical grey matter reductions associated with treatment-resistant chronic unipolar depression. Controlled magnetic resonance imaging study. *British Journal of Psychiatry, 172*, 527–532.

Shamay-Tsoory, S. G., & Aharon-Peretz, J. (2007). Dissociable prefrontal networks for cognitive and affective theory of mind: A lesion study. *Neuropsychologia, 45*(13), 3054–3067.

Shapiro, E., & Rosenfeld, A. (1986). *The somatizing child*. New York, NY: Springer.

Shearer, S. L. (1994). Dissociative phenomena in women with borderline personality disorder. *American Journal of Psychiatry, 151*(9), 1324–1328.

Shedler, J., & Westen, D. (1998). Refining the measurement of Axis II: A Q-sort procedure for assessing personality pathology. *Assessment, 5*(4), 333–353.

Sheehy, M., Goldsmith, L., & Charles, E. (1980). A comparative study of borderline patients in a psychiatric outpatient clinic. *American Journal of Psychiatry, 137*(11), 1374–1379.

Sheline, Y. I., Sanghavi, M., Mintun, M. A., & Gado, M. H. (1999). Depression duration but not age predicts hippocampal volume loss in medically healthy women with recurrent major depression. *Journal of Neuroscience, 19*(12), 5034–5043.

Sheline, Y. I., Wang, P. W., Gado, M. H., Csernansky, J. G., & Vannier, M. W. (1996). Hippocampal atrophy in recurrent major depression. *Proceedings of the National Academy of Sciences of the United States of America, 93*(9), 3908–3913.

Shergill, S. S., Brammer, M. J., Amaro, E., Williams, S. C., Murray, R. M., & McGuire, P. K. (2004). Temporal course of auditory hallucinations. *British Journal of Psychiatry, 185*, 516–517.

Shergill, S. S., Brammer, M. J., Fukuda, R., Williams, S. C., Murray, R. M., & McGuire, P. K. (2003). Engagement of brain areas implicated in processing inner speech in people with auditory hallucinations. *British Journal of Psychiatry, 182*, 525–531.

Shergill, S. S., Brammer, M. J., Williams, S. C., Murray, R. M., & McGuire, P. K. (2000). Mapping auditory hallucinations in schizophrenia using functional magnetic resonance imaging. *Archives of General Psychiatry, 57*(11), 1033–1038.

Shergill, S. S., Cameron, L. A., Brammer, M. J., Williams, S. C., Murray, R. M., & McGuire, P. K. (2001). Modality specific neural correlates of auditory and somatic hallucinations. *Journal of Neurology, Neurosurgery, and Psychiatry, 71*(5), 688–690.

Shulman, G. L., Fiez, J. A., Corbetta, M., Buckner, R. L., Miezin, F. M., Raichle, M. E., et al. (1997). Common blood flow changes across visual tasks: II. Decreases in cerebral cortex. *Cognitive Neuroscience, 9*, 648–663.

Sidgwick, H., Johnson, A., & Myers, F. W. H. (1894, ...). *Report on the census of hallucinations.* Paper presented at the Proceedings of the Society for Psychical Research.

Siever, L. J., Torgersen, S., Gunderson, J. G., Livesley, W. J., & Kendler, K. S. (2002). The borderline diagnosis: III. Identifying endophenotypes for genetic studies. *Biological Psychiatry, 51*(12), 964–968.

Silk, K. R. (2000). Overview of biological factors in borderline personality disorder. *Psychiatric Clinics of North America, 23*, 61–75.

Silk, K. R. (2011). Overview of the pharmacotherapy of Borderline Personality Disorder: Should we rethink the APA alogorithm? *Journal of Personality Disorders, 25 (Supplement),* 1–8.

Silk, K. R., Lohr, N. E., Western, D., & Goodrich, S. (1989). Psychosis in borderline patients with depression. *Journal of Personality Disorder, 3*, 92–100.

Simons, R. F., Graham, F. K., Miles, M. A., & Chen, X. (2001). On the relationship of P3a and the novelty–P3. *Biological Psychology, 56*(3), 207–218.

Singh, K. D., & Fawcett, I. P. (2008). Transient and linearly graded deactivation of the human default-mode network by a visual detection task. *NeuroImage, 41*(1), 100–112.

Skodol, A. E., Gunderson, J. G., Pfohl, B., Widiger, T. A., Livesley, W. J., & Siever, L. J. (2002). The borderline diagnosis: I. Psychopathology, comorbidity, and personality structure. *Biological Psychiatry, 51*(12), 936–950.

Slater, E. (1965). Diagnosis of "hysteria." *British Medical Journal, 1*(5447), 1395–1399.

Smith, C. S. (1978). Structural hierarchy in science, art and history. In J. Wechsler (Ed.), *On aesthetics in science* (pp. 9–54). Cambridge, MA: MIT Press.

Smith, M. E. (2005). Bilateral hippocampal volume reduction in adults with post-traumatic stress disorder: A meta-analysis of structural MRI studies. *Hippocampus, 15*(6), 798–807.

Sokolov, Y. N. (1960). Neuronal models and the orienting reflex. In M. Brazier (Ed.), *The central nervous system and behaviour* (pp. 187–276). New York, NY: J. Macey Foundation.

Soloff, P. H. (1981). A comparison of borderline with depressed and schizophrenic patients on a new diagnostic interview. *Comprehensive Psychiatry, 22*(3), 291–300.

Soloff, P. H., Meltzer, C. C., Becker, C., Greer, P. J., Kelly, T. M., & Constantine, D. (2003). Impulsivity and prefrontal hypometabolism in borderline personality disorder. *Psychiatry Research, 123*(3), 153–163.

Soltani, M., & Knight, R. T. (2000). Neural origins of the P300. *Critical Reviews in Neurobiology, 14*(3–4), 199–224.

Sommer, I. E., Diederen, K. M., Blom, J. D., Willems, A., Kushan, L., Slotema, K., et al. (2008). Auditory verbal hallucinations predominantly activate the right inferior frontal area. *Brain, 131*(Pt 12), 3169–3177.

Sonuga-Barke, E. J., & Castellanos, F. X. (2007). Spontaneous attentional fluctuations in impaired states and pathological conditions: A neurobiological hypothesis. *Neuroscience and Biobehavioral Reviews, 31*(7), 977–986.

Sorce, J., Emde, R., Campos, J., & Klinnet, M. (1985). Maternal emotional signaling: Its effect on the visual cliff behavior of 1-year-olds. *Developmental Psychology, 21*, 195–200.

Spangler, G., Fremmer-Bomik, E., & Grossmann, K. (1996). Social and individual determinants of attachment security and disorganization during the first year. *Infant Mental Health Journal, 17*, 127–139.

Spangler, G., Johann, M., Ronai, Z., & Zimmermann, P. (2009). Genetic and environmental influence on attachment disorganization. *Journal of Child Psychology and Psychiatry, 50*(8), 952–961.

Sperry, R. (1966). Brain bisection and mechanisms of consciousness. In J. C. Eccles (Ed.), *Brain and conscious experience* (pp. 298–313). New York, NY: Spinger Verlag.

Spinhoven, P., Bockting, C. L., Kremers, I. P., Schene, A. H., Mark, J., & Williams, G. (2007). The endorsement of dysfunctional attitudes is associated with an impaired retrieval of specific autobiographical memories in response to matching cues. *Memory, 15*(3), 324–338.

Spitzer, C., Willert, C., Grabe, H. J., Rizos, T., Moller, B., & Freyberger, H. J. (2004). Dissociation, hemispheric asymmetry, and dysfunction of hemispheric interaction: A transcranial magnetic stimulation approach. *Journal of Neuropsychiatry and Clinical Neuroscience, 16*(2), 163–169.

Spitzer, R. L., Endicott, J., & Gibbon, M. (1979). Crossing the border into borderline personality and borderline schizophrenia: The development of criteria. *Archives of General Psychiatry, 36*(1), 17–24.

Spreng, R. N., Mar, R. A., & Kim, A. S. (2009). The common neural basis of autobiographical memory, prospection, navigation, theory of mind, and the default mode: A quantitative meta-analysis. *Journal of Cognitive Neuroscience, 21*(3), 489–510.

Squires, N. K., Squires, K. C., & Hillyard, S. A. (1975). Two varieties of long-latency positive waves evoked by unpredictable auditory stimuli in man. *Electroencephalography and Clinical Neurophysiology, 38*(4), 387–401.

Starkstein, S. E., & Robinson, R. G. (1997). Mechanism of disinhibition after brain lesions. *Journal of Nervous Mental Disease, 185*(2), 108–114.

Steiger, H., Richardson, J., Joober, R., Gauvin, L., Israel, M., Bruce, K. R., et al. (2007). The *5HTTLPR* polymorphism, prior maltreatment, and dramatic-erratic personality manifestations in women with bulimic syndromes. *Journal of Psychiatry and Neuroscience, 32*(5), 354–362.

Stein, D. J., Hollander, E., Cohen, L., Frenkel, M., Saoud, J. B., DeCaria, C., et al. (1993). Neuropsychiatric impairment in impulsive personality disorders. *Psychiatry Research, 48*(3), 257–266.

Stengel, E. (1939). Studies on the psychopathology of compulsive wandering. *British Journal Medical of Psychology, 18,* 250–254.

Stengel, E. (1943). Further studies on pathological wandering (fugues with impulse to wander). *Journal of Mental Science, 89,* 224–241.

Stengel, E., & Vienna, M. D. (1941). On the aetiology of fugue states. *Journal of Mental Science, 87,* 572–599.

Stern, A. (1938). Psychoanalytic investigation of and therapy in the borderline group of neuroses. *Psychoanalytic Quarterly, 7,* 467–489.

Stern, D. (1977). *The first relationship.* Cambridge, MA: Harvard University Press.

Stevenson, J., Datyner, A., Boyce, P., & Brodaty, H. (2011). The effect of age on prevalence, type and diagnosis of personality disorder in psychiatric inpatients. *International Journal of Geriatric Psychiatry, 26*(9), 981–987.

Stevenson, J., & Meares, R. (1992). An outcome study of psychotherapy for patients with borderline personality disorder. *American Journal of Psychiatry, 149*(3), 358–362.

Stevenson, J., Meares, R., & Comerford, A. (2003). Diminished impulsivity in older patients with borderline personality disorder. *American Journal of Psychiatry, 160*(1), 165–166.

Stevenson, J., Meares, R., & D'Angelo, R. (2005). Five-year outcome of outpatient psychotherapy with borderline patients. *Psychological Medicine, 35*(1), 79–87.

Stiglmayr, C. E., Grathwol, T., Linehan, M. M., Ihorst, G., Fahrenberg, J., & Bohus, M. (2005). Aversive tension in patients with borderline personality disorder: A computer-based controlled field study. *Acta Psychiatrica Scandinavica, 111*(5), 372–379.

Stiglmayr, C. E., Shapiro, D. A., Stieglitz, R. D., Limberger, M. F., & Bohus, M. (2001). Experience of aversive tension and dissociation in female patients with borderline personality disorder: A controlled study. *Journal of Psychiatric Research, 35*(2), 111–118.

Stone, M. L. (1990). *The fate of borderline patients.* New York, NY: Guilford Press.

Strachey, J. (Ed.). (1961). *Editoral note: Complete psychological works of Sig-*

mund Freud standard edition, 19, 8. London, UK: Hogarth & Institute of Psycho-Analysis.

Strakowski, S. M., DelBello, M. P., Sax, K. W., Zimmerman, M. E., Shear, P. K., Hawkins, J. M., et al. (1999). Brain magnetic resonance imaging of structural abnormalities in bipolar disorder. *Archives of General Psychiatry, 56*(3), 254–260.

Strauss, E., & Wada, J. (1983). Lateral preferences and cerebral speech dominance. *Cortex, 19*(2), 165–177.

Streeter, C. C., Van Reekum, R., Shorr, R. I., & Bachman, D. L. (1995). Prior head injury in male veterans with borderline personality disorder. *Journal Nervous Mental Disease, 183*(9), 577–581.

Stuss, D. T., Gallup, G. G., Jr., & Alexander, M. P. (2001). The frontal lobes are necessary for "theory of mind." *Brain, 124*(Pt. 2), 279–286.

Sugiura, M., Sassa, Y., Watanabe, J., Akitsuki, Y., Maeda, Y., Matsue, Y., et al. (2009). Anatomical segregation of representations of personally familiar and famous people in the temporal and parietal cortices. *Journal of Cognitive Neuroscience, 21*(10), 1855–1868.

Sullivan, H. S. (1953). *The interpersonal theory of psychiatry.* New York, NY: Norton.

Suomi, S. J. (2006). Risk, resilience, and gene × environment interactions in rhesus monkeys. *Annals of the New York Academy of Sciences, 1094,* 52–62.

Supekar, K., Uddin, L. Q., Prater, K., Amin, H., Greicius, M. D., & Menon, V. (2010). Development of functional and structural connectivity within the default mode network in young children. *NeuroImage, 52*(1), 290–301.

Sutton, S., Braren, M., Zubin, J., & John, E. R. (1965). Evoked-potential correlates of stimulus uncertainty. *Science, 150*(700), 1187–1188.

Swirsky-Sacchetti, T., Gorton, G., Samuel, S., Sobel, R., Genetta-Wadley, A., & Burleigh, B. (1993). Neuropsychological function in borderline personality disorder. *Journal of Clinical Psychology, 49*(3), 385–396.

Szpunar, K. K., Watson, J. M., & McDermott, K. B. (2007). Neural substrates of envisioning the future. *Proceedings of the National Academy of Sciences of the United States of America, 104*(2), 642–647.

Tadic, A., Victor, A., Baskaya, O., von Cube, R., Hoch, J., Kouti, I., et al. (2009). Interaction between gene variants of the serotonin transporter promoter region (*5-HTTLPR*) and catechol O-methyltransferase (*COMT*) in borderline personality disorder. *American Journal of Medical Genetics, 150B*(4), 487–495.

Takahashi, T., Chanen, A. M., Wood, S. J., Walterfang, M., Harding, I. H., Yucel, M., et al. (2009). Midline brain structures in teenagers with first-presentation borderline personality disorder. *Progress in Neuropsychopharmacology and Biological Psychiatry, 33*(5), 842–846.

Takeuchi, H., Taki, Y., Sassa, Y., Hashizume, H., Sekiguchi, A., Fukushima, A., et al. (2010). White matter structures associated with creativity: Evidence from diffusion tensor imaging. *NeuroImage, 51*(1), 11–18.

Tamietto, M., Latini Corazzini, L., de Gelder, B., & Geminiani, G. (2006). Functional asymmetry and interhemispheric cooperation in the perception of emotions from facial expressions. *Experimental Brain Research, 171*(3), 389–404.

Tamm, L., Menon, V., & Reiss, A. L. (2002). Maturation of brain function associated with response inhibition. *Journal of the American Academy of Child and Adolescent Psychiatry, 41*(10), 1231–1238.

Tanskanen, A., Hintikka, J., Honkalampi, K., Haatainen, K., Koivumaa-Honkanen, H., & Viinamaki, H. (2004). Impact of multiple traumatic experiences on the persistence of depressive symptoms: A population-based study. *Nordic Journal of Psychiatry, 58*(6), 459–464.

Taylor, J. (Ed.). (1925). *Neurological fragments: With a biographical memoir of John Hughlings Jackson*. London, UK: Milford.

Taylor, J., & Reeves, M. (2007). Structure of borderline personality disorder symptoms in a nonclinical sample. *Journal of Clinical Psychology, 63*(9), 805–816.

Tebartz van Elst, L., Hesslinger, B., Thiel, T., Geiger, E., Haegele, K., Lemieux, L., et al. (2003). Frontolimbic brain abnormalities in patients with borderline personality disorder: A volumetric magnetic resonance imaging study. *Biological Psychiatry, 54*(2), 163–171.

Teicher, M. H., Dumont, N. L., Ito, Y., Vaituzis, C., Giedd, J. N., & Andersen, S. L. (2004). Childhood neglect is associated with reduced corpus callosum area. *Biological Psychiatry, 56*(2), 80–85.

Terr, L. (1988). What happens to early memories of trauma?: A study of twenty children under age five at the time of documented traumatic events. *Journal of the American Academy of Child and Adolescent Psychiatry, 27*(1), 96–104.

Thomas, A., Chess, S., & Birch, N. (1978). *Temperament and behavior disorder in children*. New York, NY: New York University Press.

Tolpin, L. H., Gunthert, K. C., Cohen, L. H., & O'Neill, S. C. (2004). Borderline personality features and instability of daily negative affect and self-esteem. *Journal of Personality, 72*(1), 111–137.

Tononi, G., Sporns, O., & Edelman, G. M. (1992). Reentry and the problem of integrating multiple cortical areas: Simulation of dynamic integration in the visual system. *Cerebral Cortex, 2*(4), 310–335.

Torgersen, S., Czajkowski, N., Jacobson, K., Reichborn-Kjennerud, T., Roysamb, E., Neale, M. C., et al. (2008). Dimensional representations of DSM-IV Cluster B personality disorders in a population-based sample of Norwegian twins: A multivariate study. *Psychological Medicine, 38*(11), 1617–1625.

Torgersen, S., Kringlen, E., & Cramer, V. (2001). The prevalence of personality disorders in a community sample. *Archives of General Psychiatry, 58*(6), 590–596.

Torgersen, S., Lygren, S., Oien, P. A., Skre, I., Onstad, S., Edvardsen, J., et al. (2000). A twin study of personality disorders. *Comprehensive Psychiatry, 41*(6), 416–425.

Toth, S. L., Cicchetti, D., Macfie, J., & Emde, R. N. (1997). Representations of self and other in the narratives of neglected, physically abused, and sexually abused preschoolers. *Developmental Psychopathology, 9*(4), 781–796.

Tranel, D., Bechara, A., & Denburg, N. L. (2002). Asymmetric functional roles of right and left ventromedial prefrontal cortices in social conduct, decision-making, and emotional processing. *Cortex, 38*(4), 589–612.

Tranel, D., Damasio, H., Denburg, N. L., & Bechara, A. (2005). Does gender play a role in functional asymmetry of ventromedial prefrontal cortex? *Brain, 128*(Pt. 12), 2872–2881.

Trevarthen, C. (1974). Conversations with a two-month-old. *New Scientist, 62*, 230–235.

Tronick, E. D., Als, H., & Brazelton, T. B. (1977). Mutuality in mother–infant interaction. *Journal of Communication, 27*(2), 74–79.

Tulving, E. (1972). Episodic and semantic memory. In E. Tulving & W. Donaldson (Eds.), *Organization of memory* (pp. 381–403). New York, NY: Academic Press.

Tulving, E. (1983). *Elements of episodic memory*. Oxford, UK: Clarendon Press (Oxford University Press).

Tulving, E. (2001). Episodic memory and common sense: How far apart? *Philosophical Transactions of the Royal Society of Lond B Biological Sciences, 356*(1413), 1505–1515.

Tulving, E. (2005). Episodic memory and autonoesis. In H. S. Terrace & J. Metcalfe (Eds.), *The missing link in cognition* (pp. 4–56). New York, NY: Oxford University Press.

Tulving, E., Kapur, S., Craik, F. I., Moscovitch, M., & Houle, S. (1994). Hemispheric encoding/retrieval asymmetry in episodic memory: Positron emission tomography findings. *Proceedings of the National Academy of Sciences of the United States of America, 91*(6), 2016–2020.

Tulving, E., & Schacter, D. L. (1990). Priming and human memory systems. *Science, 247*(4940), 301–306.

Tynjanov, J., & Jakobson, R. (19281981). Problems in the study of literature and Ian-gauge. In R. Jakobson (Ed.), *Selected Writings* (Vol. 3 3-6). The Hague: Mouton. (Original work published 1928)

Tyrer, P. (2009). Why borderline personality disorder is neither borderline nor a personality disorder. *Personality and Mental Health, 3,* 86–95.

Uddin, L. Q., Kelly, A. M., Biswal, B. B., Xavier Castellanos, F., & Milham, M. P. (2009). Functional connectivity of default mode network components: Correlation, anticorrelation, and causality. *Human Brain Mapping, 30*(2), 625–637.

Valentino, K., Toth, S. L., & Cicchetti, D. (2009). Autobiographical memory functioning among abused, neglected, and nonmaltreated children: The overgeneral memory effect. *Journal of Child Psychology and Psychiatry, 50*(8), 1029–1038.

Van Buuren, M., Gladwin, T. E., Zandbelt, B. B., Kahn, R. S., & Vink, M. (2010). Reduced functional coupling in the default-mode network during self-referential processing. *Human Brain Mapping, 31*(8), 1117–1127.

Van der Hart, O., van Dijke, A., van Son, M., & Steele, K. (2000). Somatoform dissociation in traumatized world war I combat soldiers: A neglected clinical heritage. *Journal of Trauma and Dissociation, 1*(4), 33–66.

Van der Hart, O., & Dorahy, M. (2006). Pierre Janet and the concept of dissociation. *American Journal of Psychiatry, 163*(9), 1646.

Van der Hart, O., Nijenhuis, E. R., & Steele, K. (2006). *The haunted self: Structural dissociation and the treatment of chronic traumatization.* New York/London: Norton.

Van der Kolk, B. A., & Van der Hart, O. (1989). Pierre Janet and the breakdown of adaptation in psychological trauma. *American Journal of Psychiatry, 146*(12), 1530–1540.

Van der Kolk, B., Van der Hart, O., & Marmar, C. (1996). Dissociation and information processing in post traumatic stress disorder. In B. van der Kolk, A. McFarlane, & L. Weisaeth (Eds.), *Traumatic stress* (pp. 303–330). New York, NY: Guilford Press.

Van der Veer, R., & Valsiner, J. (1988). Lev Vygotsky and Pierre Janet: On the origin of the concept of sociogenesis. *Developmental Review, 8,* 52–65.

Van IJzendoorn, M. H., & Schuengel, C. (1996). The measurement of dissociation in normal and clinical populations: Meta-analytic validation of the Dissociative Experience Scale (DES). *Clinical Psychology Review, 16,* 365–382.

Van IJzendoorn, M. H., Schuengel, C., & Bakermans-Kranenburg, M. J. (1999). Disorganized attachment in early childhood: Meta-analysis of precursors, concomitants, and sequelae. *Developmental Psychopathology, 11*(2), 225–249.

Van Lancker, D., & Cummings, J. L. (1999). Expletives: Neurolinguistic and neurobehavioral perspectives on swearing. *Brain Research Reviews, 31*(1), 83–104.

Van Reekum, C. M., Urry, H. L., Johnstone, T., Thurow, M. E., Frye, C. J., Jackson, C. A., et al. (2007). Individual differences in amygdala and ventromedial prefrontal cortex activity are associated with evaluation speed and psychological well-being. *Journal of Cognitive Neuroscience, 19*(2), 237–248.

Van Reekum, R., Conway, C. A., Gansler, D., White, R., & Bachman, D. L. (1993). Neurobehavioral study of borderline personality disorder. *Journal of Psychiatry Neuroscience, 18*(3), 121–129.

Veith, I. (1965). *The history of disease.* Chicago, IL: University of Chicago Press.

Verleger, R. (1988). Event-related potentials and cognition: A critique of the context updating hypothesis and an alternative interpretation of P3. *Behavioral and Brain Sciences, 11*, 343–356.

Verleger, R. (2002, September). *Fehlendes Bewusstsein fur Gesehenes bei maskierten Reizen und bei pathologischem Neglect: Auf dem Weg zu einem integrierten Modell [Lack of awareness for visual input with masked stimuli and with pathological neglect: Toward an integrated model].* Paper presented at the 43rd conference of German Society of Psychology.

Verleger, R., Gorgen, S., & Jaskowski, P. (2005). An ERP indicator of processing relevant gestalts in masked priming. *Psychophysiology, 42*(6), 677–690.

Verleger, R., Heide, W., Butt, C., & Kompf, D. (1994). Reduction of P3b in patients with temporo-parietal lesions. *Cognitive Brain Research, 2*(2), 103–116.

Vermetten, E., Schmahl, C., Lindner, S., Loewenstein, R. J., & Bremner, J. D. (2006). Hippocampal and amygdalar volumes in dissociative identity disorder. *American Journal of Psychiatry, 163*(4), 630–636.

Vincent, J. L., Snyder, A. Z., Fox, M. D., Shannon, B. J., Andrews, J. R., Raichle, M. E., et al. (2006). Coherent spontaneous activity identifies a hippocampal–parietal memory network. *Journal of Neurophysiology, 96*(6), 3517–3531.

Vinogradova, O. S. (2001). Hippocampus as comparator: role of the two input and two output systems of the hippocampus in selection and registration of information. *Hippocampus, 11*(5), 578–598.

Vogeley, K., Bussfeld, P., Newen, A., Herrmann, S., Happé, F., Falkai, P., et al. (2001). Mind reading: Neural mechanisms of theory of mind and self-perspective. *NeuroImage, 14*(Pt. 1), 170–181.

Vogt, B. A. (2005). Pain and emotion interactions in subregions of the cingulate gyrus. *Nature Reviews Neuroscience, 6*(7), 533–544.

Vogt, B. A., Finch, D. M., & Olson, C. R. (1992). Functional heterogeneity in cingulate cortex: The anterior executive and posterior evaluative regions. *Cerebral Cortex, 2*(6), 435–443.

Vogt, B. A., & Robert, W. C. (1993). Anterior cingulate cortex and the medial pain system. In B. A. Vogt & M. Gabriel (Eds.), *Neurobiology of cingulate cortex and limbic thalamus: A comprehensive handbook* (pp. 313–344). Boston, MA: Birkäuser.

Vollm, B. A., Zhao, L., Richardson, P., Clark, L., Deakin, J. F., Williams, S., et al. (2009). A voxel-based morphometric MRI study in men with borderline personality disorder: Preliminary findings. *Criminal Behaviour and Mental Health, 19*(1), 64–72.

Voon, V., Brezing, C., Gallea, C., Ameli, R., Roelofs, K., LaFrance, W. C., Jr., et al. (2010). Emotional stimuli and motor conversion disorder. *Brain, 133*(Pt. 5), 1526–1536.

Vygotsky, L. S. (1935). The problem of the environment. In R. Van der Veer & J. Valsiner (Eds.), *The Vygotsky reader* (pp. 338–354). Oxford, UK: Blackwell.

Vygotsky, L. S. (1962). *Thought and language* (E. Hanfmann & G. Vakar, Trans.; E. Hanfmann & G. Vakar, Eds.). Cambridge, MA: MIT Press.

Vygotsky, L. S., & Luria, A. (1994). Tool and symbol in child development. In R. Van der Veer & J. Valsiner (Eds.), *The Vygotsky reader* (pp. 99–174). Oxford, UK: Blackwell.

Vythilingam, M., Heim, C., Newport, J., Miller, A. H., Anderson, E., Bronen, R., et al. (2002). Childhood trauma associated with smaller hippocampal volume in women with major depression. *American Journal of Psychiatry, 159*(12), 2072–2080.

Wagner, A. D., Shannon, B. J., Kahn, I., & Buckner, R. L. (2005). Parietal lobe contributions to episodic memory retrieval. *Trends in Cognitive Sciences, 9*(9), 445–453.

Waller, N., Putnam, F. W., & Carlson, E. B. (1996). Types of dissociation and dissociative types: A taxometric analysis of dissociative experiences. *Psychological Methods, 1*(3), 300–321.

Wampold, B. E., Mondin, G. W., Moody, M., Stich, F., Benson, K., & Hyunnie, A. (1997). A meta-Analysis of outcome studies comparing bona fide psychotherapies: empircally, "All must have prizes". *Psychological Bulletin, 122*(3), 203–215.

Waters, E., Vaughn, B. E., & Egeland, B. R. (1980). Individual differences in infant–mother attachment relationships at age one: Antecedents in neonatal behavior in an urban, economically disadvantaged sample. *Child Development, 51*(1), 208–216.

Weiskrantz, L. (1986). *Blindsight: A case study and its implications*. Oxford, UK: Clarendon Press.

Weiskrantz, L., Warrington, E. K., Sanders, M. D., & Marshall, J. (1974). Visual capacity in the hemianopic field following a restricted occipital ablation. *Brain, 97*, 709–728.

West, R. (1971). The grey men. In R. Dalby (Ed.), *Modern ghost stories by noted women writers* (pp. 52–56). New York, NY: Barnes & Noble.

Westen, D. (1985). *Self and society: Narcissism, collectivism, and the development of morals*. New York, NY: Cambridge University Press.

Westen, D. (1992). The cognitive self and the psychoanalytic self: Can we put ourselves together? *Psychological Inquiry, 3*, 1–13.

Westen, D., Moses, M. J., & Silk, K. R., Lohr, N.E., Cohen, R., Segal, H. (1992). Quality of depressive experience in borderline personality disorder and major depression: When depression is not just depression. *Journal of Personality Disorders, 6*, 382–393.

Westen, D., & Shedler, J. (1999). Revising and assessing Axis II: Part II. Toward an empirically based and clinically useful classification of personality disorders. *American Journal of Psychiatry, 156*(2), 273–285.

Wheeler, M. A., Stuss, D. T., & Tulving, E. (1997). Toward a theory of episodic memory: The frontal lobes and autonoetic consciousness. *Psychological Bulletin, 121*(3), 331–354.

Whitehead, A. N., & Russell, B. (1910–1913). *Principia Mathematica* (Vol. 1–3). Cambridge: Cambridge University Press.

Whitfield-Gabrieli, S., Thermenos, H. W., Milanovic, S., Tsuang, M. T., Faraone, S. V., McCarley, R. W., et al. (2009). Hyperactivity and hyperconnectivity of the default network in schizophrenia and in first-degree relatives of persons with schizophrenia. *Proceedings of the National Academy of Sciences of the United States of America, 106*(4), 1279–1284.

Whitlock, F. A. (1967). The aetiology of hysteria. *Acta Psychiatrica Scandinavica, 43*(2), 144–162.

Whittle, S., Chanen, A. M., Fornito, A., McGorry, P. D., Pantelis, C., & Yucel, M. (2009). Anterior cingulate volume in adolescents with first-presentation borderline personality disorder. *Psychiatry Research, 172*(2), 155–160.

Widiger, T. A., & Frances, A. J. (1989). Epidemiology, diagnosis, and comorbidity of borderline personality disorder. In A. Tasman, R. E. Hales, & A. J. Frances (Eds.),American Psychiatry Press Review of Psychiatry *8*, (pp. 8–24). Washington, DC: American Psychiatric Press..

Widiger, T. A., Frances, A. J., Harris, M., Jacobsberg, L. B., Fyer, M., & Manning, D. (1991). Comorbidity among Axis II disorders. In J. M. Oldham (Ed.), *Personality disorders: New perspecitves on diagnostic validity*. Washington DC: American Psychiatric Association.

Wildgoose, A., Waller, G., Clarke, S., & Reid, A. (2000). Psychiatric symptomatology in borderline and other personality disorders: Dissociation and fragmentation as mediators. *Journal of Nervous and Mental Disease,* *188*(11), 757–763.

Wilkinson-Ryan, T., & Westen, D. (2000). Identity disturbance in borderline personality disorder: An empirical investigation. *American Journal of Psychiatry, 157*(4), 528–541.

Williams, J. M., & Scott, J. (1988). Autobiographical memory in depression. *Psychological Medicine, 18*(3), 689–695.

Williams, J. M., Barnhofer, T., Crane, C., Herman, D., Raes, F., Watkins, E., et al. (2007). Autobiographical memory specificity and emotional disorder. *Psychological Bulletin, 133*(1), 122–148.

Williams, J. M., & Broadbent, K. (1986). Autobiographical memory in suicide attempters. *Journal of Abnormal Psychology, 95*(2), 144–149.

Williams, L. M., Brammer, M. J., Skerrett, D., Lagopolous, J., Rennie, C., Kozek, K., et al. (2000). The neural correlates of orienting: An integration of fMRI and skin conductance orienting. *NeuroReport, 11*(13), 3011–3015.

Williams, L. M., Brown, K. J., Palmer, D., Liddell, B. J., Kemp, A. H., Olivieri, G., et al. (2006). The mellow years?: Neural basis of improving emotional stability over age. *Journal of Neuroscience, 26*(24), 6422–6430.

Williams, L. M., Gordon, E., Wright, J., & Bahramali, H. (2000). Late component ERPs are associated with three syndromes in schizophrenia. *International Journal of Neuroscience, 105*(1–4), 37–52.

Williams, L. M., Liddell, B. J., Kemp, A. H., Bryant, R. A., Meares, R. A., Peduto, A. S., et al. (2006). Amygdala–prefrontal dissociation of subliminal and supraliminal fear. *Human Brain Mapping, 27*(8), 652–661.

Williams, L. M., Phillips, M. L., Brammer, M. J., Skerrett, D., Lagopoulos, J., Rennie, C., et al. (2001). Arousal dissociates amygdala and hippocampal fear responses: Evidence from simultaneous fMRI and skin conductance recording. *NeuroImage, 14*(5), 1070–1079.

Williams, L. M., Senior, C., David, A., Loughland, C. M., & Gordon, E. (2001). In search of the "Duchenne" smile: Evidence from eye movements. *Journal of Psychophysiology, 15,* 122–127.

Wimmer, H., & Perner, J. (1983). Beliefs about beliefs: Representation and constraining function of wrong beliefs in young children's understanding of deception. *Cognition, 13*(1), 103–128.

Winhuisen, L., Thiel, A., Schumacher, B., Kessler, J., Rudolf, J., Haupt, W. F., et al. (2005). Role of the contralateral inferior frontal gyrus in recovery of language function in poststroke aphasia: A combined repetitive transcranial magnetic stimulation and positron emission tomography study. *Stroke, 36*(8), 1759–1763.

Winnicott, D. W. (1958). *Collected papers: Through paediatrics to psychoanalysis.* London, UK: Tavistock.

Winnicott, D. W. (1963). Communicating and not communicating leading to a study of certain opposites. In *The maturational processes and facilitating environment* (pp. 179–192). New York, NY: International Universities Press, 1965.

Winnicott, D. W. (1971). *Playing and reality*. London, UK: Tavistock–Harmondsworth–Penguin.

Wittgenstein, L. (1953). *Philosophical investigations*. Oxford, UK: Blackwell.

Woldorff, M. G., Liotti, M., Seabolt, M., Busse, L., Lancaster, J. L., & Fox, P. T. (2002). The temporal dynamics of the effects in occipital cortex of visual–spatial selective attention. *Cognitive Brain Research, 15*(1), 1–15.

Woodruff, P., Brammer, M., Mellers, J., Wright, I., Bullmore, E., & Williams, S. (1995). Auditory hallucinations and perception of external speech. *Lancet, 346*(8981), 1035.

Woon, F. L., & Hedges, D. W. (2008). Hippocampal and amygdala volumes in children and adults with childhood maltreatment-related posttraumatic stress disorder: A meta-analysis. *Hippocampus, 18*(8), 729–736.

Yamaguchi, S. (2004). Neural network for novelty processing. *Supplements to Clinical Neurophysiology, 57*, 635–641.

Yamaguchi, S., & Knight, R. T. (1991). Anterior and posterior association cortex contributions to the somatosensory P300. *Journal of Neuroscience, 11*(7), 2039–2054.

Yee, L., Korner, A. J., McSwiggan, S., Meares, R. A., & Stevenson, J. (2005). Persistent hallucinosis in borderline personality disorder. *Comprehensive Psychiatry, 46*(2), 147–154.

Young, J. E., Klosko, J. S., & Weishaar, M. E. (2003). *Schema therapy: A practitioner's guide*. London, UK: Guilford Press.

Zanarini, M. C. (2000). Childhood experiences associated with the development of borderline personality disorder. *Psychiatric Clinics of North America, 23*(1), 89–101.

Zanarini, M. C., & Frankenburg, F. R. (2007). The essential nature of borderline psychopathology. *Journal of Personality Disorders, 21*(5), 518–535.

Zanarini, M. C., Frankenburg, F. R., Chauncey, D. L., & Gunderson, J. G. (1987). The Diagnostic Interview for Personality Disorders: Interrater and test–retest reliability. *Comprehensive Psychiatry, 28*(6), 467–480.

Zanarini, M. C., Frankenburg, F. R., DeLuca, C. J., Hennen, J., Khera, G. S., & Gunderson, J. G. (1998). The pain of being borderline: Dysphoric states specific to borderline personality disorder. *Harvard Review of Psychiatry, 6*(4), 201–207.

Zanarini, M. C., Frankenburg, F. R., Dubo, E. D., Sickel, A. E., Trikha, A., Levin, A., et al. (1998). Axis I comorbidity of borderline personality disorder. *American Journal of Psychiatry, 155*(12), 1733–1739.

Zanarini, M. C., Frankenburg, F. R., Hennen, J., Reich, D. B., & Silk, K. R. (2004). Axis I comorbidity in patients with borderline personality disorder: 6-year follow-up and prediction of time to remission. *American Journal of Psychiatry, 161*(11), 2108–2114.

Zanarini, M. C., Frankenburg, F. R., Jager-Hyman, S., Reich, D. B., & Fitzmaurice, G. (2008). The course of dissociation for patients with borderline personality disorder and Axis II comparison subjects: A 10-year follow-up study. *Acta Psychiatrica Scandinavica, 118*(4), 291–296.

Zanarini, M. C., Frankenburg, F. R., Khera, G. S., & Bleichmar, J. (2001). Treatment histories of borderline inpatients. *Comprehensive Psychiatry, 42*(2), 144–150.

Zanarini, M. C., Frankenburg, F. R., Vujanovic, A. A., Hennen, J., Reich, D. B., & Silk, K. R. (2004). Axis II comorbidity of borderline personality disorder: Description of 6-year course and prediction to time-to-remission. *Acta Psychiatrica Scandinavica, 110*(6), 416–420.

Zanarini, M. C., Gunderson, J. G., & Frankenburg, F. R. (1990). Cognitive features of borderline personality disorder. *American Journal of Psychiatry, 147*(1), 57–63.

Zanarini, M. C., Gunderson, J. G., Marino, M. F., Schwartz, E. O., & Frankenburg, F. R. (1989). Childhood experiences of borderline patients. *Comprehensive Psychiatry, 30*(1), 18–25.

Zanarini, M. C., Ruser, T., Frankenburg, F. R., & Hennen, J. (2000). The dissociative experiences of borderline patients. *Comprehensive Psychiatry, 41*(3), 223–227.

Zanetti, M. V., Soloff, P. H., Nicoletti, M. A., Hatch, J. P., Brambilla, P., Keshavan, M. S., et al. (2007). MRI study of corpus callosum in patients with borderline personality disorder: A pilot study. *Progress in Neuro-Psychopharmacology and Biological Psychiatry, 31*(7), 1519–1525.

Zhou, Z., Roy, A., Lipsky, R., Kuchipudi, K., Zhu, G., Taubman, J., et al. (2005). Haplotype-based linkage of tryptophan hydroxylase 2 to suicide attempt, major depression, and cerebrospinal fluid 5-hydroxyindoleacetic acid in 4 populations. *Archives of General Psychiatry, 62*(10), 1109–1118.

Zimmerman, M., & Coryell, W. (1989). DSM-III personality disorder diagnoses in a nonpatient sample: Demographic correlates and comorbidity. *Archives of General Psychiatry, 46*(8), 682–689.

Zimmerman, M., & Coryell, W. H. (1990). DSM-III personality disorder dimensions. *Journal of Nervous and Mental disease, 178*(11), 686–692.

Zimmerman, M., Rothschild, L., & Chelminski, I. (2005). The prevalence of DSM-IV personality disorders in psychiatric outpatients. *American Journal of Psychiatry, 162*(10), 1911–1918.

Zimmermann, P., Mohr, C., & Spangler, G. (2009). Genetic and attachment influences on adolescents' regulation of autonomy and aggressiveness. *Journal of Child Psychology and Psychiatry, 50*(11), 1339–1347.

Zittel Conklin, C., & Westen, D. (2005). Borderline personality disorder in clinical practice. *American Journal of Psychiatry, 162*(5), 867–875.

Zlotnick, C., Johnson, D. M., Yen, S., Battle, C. L., Sanislow, C. A., Skodol, A. E., et al. (2003). Clinical features and impairment in women with borderline personality disorder (BPD) with posttraumatic stress disorder (PTSD), BPD without PTSD, and other personality disorders with PTSD. *Journal of Nervous Mental Disease, 191*(11), 706–713.

Zlotnick, C., Johnson, J., Kohn, R., Vicente, B., Rioseco, P., & Saldivia, S. (2008). Childhood trauma, trauma in adulthood, and psychiatric diagnoses: Results from a community sample. *Comprehensive Psychiatry, 49*(2), 163–169.

Zweig-Frank, H., Paris, J., & Guzder, J. (1994). Dissociation in male patients with borderilne and non-borderline personality disorders. *Journal of Personality Disorder, 8*, 210–218.

Index